SAUNDERS STRATEGIES FOR SUCCESS *for the* NCLEX-PN® EXAMINATION

SAUNDERS STRATEGIES FOR SUCCESS *for the* NCLEX-PN® EXAMINATION

LINDA ANNE SILVESTRI, MSN, RN

Instructor of Nursing
Salve Regina University
Newport, Rhode Island

President
Nursing Reviews, Inc.
and
Professional Nursing Seminars, Inc.
Charlestown, Rhode Island

SAUNDERS
ELSEVIER

SAUNDERS
ELSEVIER

11830 Westline Industrial Drive
St. Louis, Missouri 63146

SAUNDERS STRATEGIES FOR SUCCESS FOR THE NCLEX-PN® EXAMINATION

ISBN 13: 978-1-4160-0094-5
ISBN 10: 1-4160-0094-1

Notice

Pharmacology is an ever-changing field. Standard safety precautions must be followed, but as new research and clinical experience broaden our knowledge, changes in treatment and drug therapy may become necessary or appropriate. Readers are advised to check the most current product information provided by the manufacturer of each drug to be administered to verify the recommended dose, the method and duration of administration, and contraindications. It is the responsibility of the licensed prescriber, relying on experience and knowledge of the patient, to determine dosages and the best treatment for each individual patient. Neither the publisher nor the author assumes any liability for any injury and/or damage to persons or property arising from this publication.

Managing Editor: *Nancy O'Brien*
Associate Developmental Editor: *Charlene R.M. Ketchum*
Publishing Services Manager: *Jeff Patterson*
Project Manager: *Jeanne Genz*
Designer: *Jyotika Shroff*

ISBN 13: 978-1-4160-0094-5
ISBN 10: 1-4160-0094-1

Printed in the United States of America

Last digit is the print number: 9 8 7 6 5 4 3 2 1

To all nursing students,

Your commitment to becoming successful and your dedication to the profession of nursing will bring never-ending rewards!

About the Author

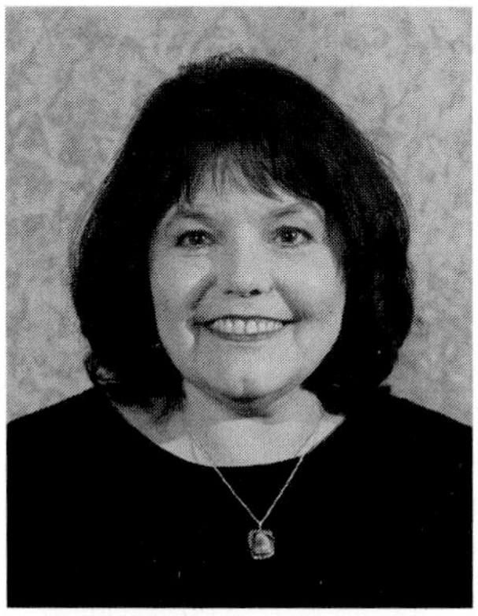

Photo by Laurent W. Valliere

Linda Anne Silvestri received her diploma in nursing at Cooley Dickinson Hospital School of Nursing in Northampton, Massachusetts. Afterward, she worked at Baystate Medical Center in Springfield, Massachusetts. At Baystate Medical Center, she worked in acute medical-surgical units, the intensive care unit, the emergency department, pediatric units, and other acute care units. She later received an associate degree from Holyoke Community College in Holyoke, Massachusetts, and then received her BSN from American International College in Springfield, Massachusetts.

A native of Springfield, Massachusetts, Linda began her teaching career as an instructor of medical-surgical nursing and leadership-management nursing at Baystate Medical Center School of Nursing in 1981. In 1985, she earned her MSN from Anna Maria College, Paxton, Massachusetts, with a dual major in nursing management and patient education. Linda is a member of Sigma Theta Tau.

Linda relocated to Rhode Island in 1989 and began teaching advanced medical-surgical nursing and psychiatric nursing to RN and LPN students at the Community College of Rhode Island. While teaching there, a group of students approached Linda, asking her to help them prepare for the NCLEX examination. Based on her experience as a nursing educator and as an NCLEX item writer, she developed a comprehensive review course to prepare nursing graduates for the NCLEX examination. In 1994, Linda began teaching medical-surgical nursing at Salve Regina University in Newport, Rhode Island. She also prepares nursing students at Salve Regina University for the NCLEX-RN® examination.

In 1991, Linda established Professional Nursing Seminars, Inc., and in 2000, she established Nursing Reviews, Inc. Both companies are dedicated to conducting NCLEX-RN and NCLEX-PN review courses and assisting nursing graduates to achieve their goals of becoming registered nurses and/or licensed practical/vocational nurses.

Today, Linda Silvestri's companies conduct NCLEX review courses throughout New England. She is the successful author of numerous NCLEX-RN and NCLEX-PN review products, including *Saunders Comprehensive Review for the NCLEX-RN® Examination*, *Saunders Q&A Review for the NCLEX-RN® Examination*, *Saunders Computerized Review for the NCLEX-RN® Examination*, *Saunders Instructor's Resource Package for the NCLEX-RN®*, *Saunders Strategies for Success for the NCLEX-RN® Examination*, *Saunders Comprehensive Review for the NCLEX-PN® Examination*, *Saunders Q&A Review for the NCLEX-PN® Examination*, *Saunders Review Cards for the NCLEX-PN® Examination*, and *Saunders Instructor's Resource*

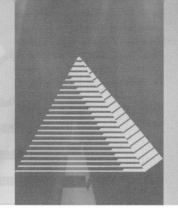

Package for NCLEX-PN®. Linda has also authored several online products including the online specialty tests titled *Adult Health, Mental Health, Maternal-Newborn, Pediatrics, and Pharmacology*, and the *Saunders Online Review Course for the NCLEX-RN® examination.*

Reviewers

Faculty Reviewers

Nancy Maebius, RN, PhD
Instructor, School of Nursing
Calen Health Institute
San Antonio, Texas

Lorene Payne, RN, MSN
Professor, School of Nursing
Tomball College

Sally Flesch, RN, BSN, MA, PhD
Professor, School of Nursing
Black Hawk College
Moline, Illinois

Margaret Gingrich, MSN, RN
Associate Professor
Harrisburg Area Community College
Harrisburg, PA

Student Reviewers

Therese Frederick
Minneapolis Community College
Minneapolis, Minnesota

Rhonda Singer
Lebanon County Career and Technology Center
Lebanon, Pennsylvania

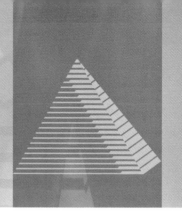

Preface

Welcome to Saunders Pyramid to Success!

The *Saunders Strategies for Success for the NCLEX-PN®* Examination is one of a series of products designed to assist you in achieving your goal of becoming a licensed practical/vocational nurse. This product provides you with all of the test-taking strategies that will help you pass your nursing examinations and the NCLEX-PN examination.

ORGANIZATION

The *Saunders Strategies for Success for the NCLEX-PN®* Examination contains 4 parts and 15 chapters. The chapters that describe the test-taking strategies include several sample questions that illustrate how to use the test-taking strategy. The sample questions represent all types of question formats including multiple choice, fill in the blank, multiple response, and prioritizing (ordered response); questions that contain a figure or illustration; and chart/exhibit questions. In addition to the sample questions in the chapters, 500 practice questions accompany this book; 205 practice questions are in the book. The software contains the 205 practice questions from the book along with an additional 295 practice questions. All of the practice questions are reflective of the framework and the content identified in the 2005 NCLEX-PN test plan. The practice questions in this book relate to each Client Needs category and each Integrated Process of the NCLEX-PN examination. The Client Needs categories include Safe, Effective Care Environment, Health Promotion and Maintenance, Psychosocial Integrity, and Physiological Integrity. The Integrated Processes include caring, clinical problem-solving process (nursing process), communication and documentation, and teaching and learning.

PART 1: The NCLEX-PN® Examination

Chapter 1 THE TEST PLAN

The information contained in this chapter focuses on how the test plan is developed and the components of the test plan. The Levels of Cognitive Ability, Client Needs categories, and the Integrated Processes are identified.

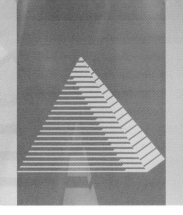

Chapter 2 THE EXAMINATION PROCESS

This chapter discusses several issues related to the examination process. These include computerized adaptive testing and how it works to determine competency; registration procedures for the NCLEX-PN examination; procedures for scheduling a test date; how to request special accommodations for testing; and procedures that take place at the test center. The procedure for processing examination results, candidate performance reports, and interstate endorsement are also discussed.

Chapter 3 CLIENT NEEDS

The National Council of State Boards of Nursing identifies four Client Needs categories in the NCLEX-PN examination. This chapter identifies these Client Needs and any subcategories, along with the percentage of test questions and the content addressed in each category.

Chapter 4 INTEGRATED PROCESSES

The National Council of State Boards of Nursing identifies four Integrated Processes that are fundamental to the practice of nursing and are integrated throughout the categories of Client Needs. This chapter reviews these Integrated Processes and illustrates how they are incorporated into examination questions.

Chapter 5 TYPES OF QUESTIONS ON THE EXAMINATION

This chapter reviews the types of questions that may be administered on the NCLEX-PN examination. These include multiple choice, fill in the blank, multiple response, prioritizing (ordered response); questions that contain a figure or illustration; and chart/exhibit questions.

PART 2: Strategies for Success

Chapter 6 NONACADEMIC PREPARATION: YOUR PATH TO SUCCESS

This chapter discusses the issue of test preparation from a nonacademic view and provides an emphasis on a holistic approach for your individual test preparation. This chapter identifies the components of a structured study plan and pattern, anxiety reduction techniques, and personal focus issues.

Chapter 7 HOW TO AVOID READING INTO THE QUESTION

One of the pitfalls that can cause a problem with answering a question correctly is "reading into the question." What this means is that you are considering issues beyond the information that is presented in the question. This chapter describes the strategies to use when answering a question to prevent this from happening.

Chapter 8 TRUE OR FALSE RESPONSE QUESTIONS

This chapter describes the differences between a true response question and a false response question. Key words or phrases that indicate whether the question is a true response question or a false response question are identified.

Chapter 9 QUESTIONS THAT REQUIRE PRIORITIZING

Many of the test questions in the examination will require you to use the skill of prioritizing nursing actions. Prioritizing questions will address content in any nursing area. These types of questions can be difficult because when a question requires prioritization, all of the options may be correct and you will need to determine the correct order of action. This chapter describes the test-taking strategies that you can use to assist in answering prioritizing questions correctly. Also included are the strategies for determining the need to notify the registered nurse and/or physician.

Chapter 10 MANAGING AND DELEGATING CARE, AND CLIENT CARE ASSIGNMENT QUESTIONS

Some of the test questions relate to the nurse's responsibilities regarding delegating care and assignment-making and the supervisory role of these responsibilities. This chapter reviews the guidelines and principles to use to perform these activities. Guidelines for time management are also reviewed because managing time efficiently is a key factor for completing activities and tasks within a definite time period.

Chapter 11 COMMUNICATION QUESTIONS

In the NCLEX-PN test plan, the National Council of State Boards of Nursing identifies the concept of communication as a component of one of the Integrated Processes. Therefore, you will be presented with questions that relate to the communication process. This chapter reviews the guidelines and techniques to use when answering questions that relate to the communication process.

Chapter 12 PHARMACOLOGY QUESTIONS

Pharmacology is one of the most difficult nursing content areas to master and feel comfortable with. The NCLEX-PN test plan addresses pharmacological and parenteral therapies in the Physiological Integrity category and identifies 9% to 15% as the percentage of test questions that will possibly appear on your examination. Therefore, it is important for you to spend ample time reviewing pharmacology in preparation for this examination. This chapter provides you with the guidelines and strategies to use to answer pharmacology questions correctly.

Chapter 13 ADDITIONAL PYRAMID STRATEGIES

This chapter reviews additional helpful strategies that will assist in answering a test question correctly. Also included in this chapter are strategies that are useful for answering questions that relate to medication and intravenous calculations, questions that relate to laboratory values, and questions that relate to client positioning.

PART 3: Additional Tips for Test-Takers

Chapter 14 TIPS FOR REPEAT TEST-TAKERS

This chapter provides information about the tips and strategies that will help prepare to retake the NCLEX-PN examination if necessary. Some of these tips and strategies address the procedure for self-assessment, developing a remediation plan, the steps in a remediation plan, and planning a retake date.

Chapter 15 TIPS FOR INTERNATIONAL NURSES

This chapter is written specifically for the international or foreign-educated nurse who wants to take the NCLEX-PN examination. This chapter provides the information regarding the processes that will need to be pursued to become a licensed practical/vocational nurse in the United States.

PART 4: Practice Test

Part IV includes a 205-question practice test that contains questions representative of the NCLEX-PN test plan. Multiple-choice questions and questions in the alternate test question format are included in this test.

SPECIAL FEATURES OF THE BOOK

PYRAMID POINTS

Pyramid Points are the bullets that are placed at specific areas throughout the chapters. The Pyramid Points provide you with immediate recognition of content that is important in preparation for the NCLEX-PN examination.

PRACTICE TEST QUESTIONS

The chapters in this book contain several practice questions that illustrate specific test-taking strategies. In addition to the practice questions integrated into the chapters, there is a 205-question practice test in the book, and the software that accompanies the book contains a total of 500 questions (205 questions from the practice test and 295 additional questions).

ALTERNATE FORMAT TEST QUESTIONS

In additional to multiple-choice questions, alternate format test questions are included in both the practice test located in Part 4 and on the accompanying software.

ANSWER SECTION FOR PRACTICE TEST QUESTIONS

The answer sections for each practice test question in Part 4 and on the accompanying software include the correct answer, rationale, test-taking strategy, question categories, and reference source. The structure for the answer section is unique and provides the following information.

The Rationale: The rationale provides you with the significant information regarding both correct and incorrect options.

Test-Taking Strategy: The test-taking strategy provides you with the logical path in selecting the correct option and assists you in selecting an answer to a question on which you must guess. Specific suggestions for review are identified in the test-taking strategy.

Question Categories: Each question is identified based on the categories used by the NCLEX-PN test plan. Additional content categories are provided with each question to assist you in identifying areas in need of review. The categories identified with each practice question include Level of Cognitive Ability, Client Needs, Integrated Process, and the specific nursing Content Area. All categories are identified by their full names so that you do not need to memorize codes or abbreviations.

Reference: A reference, including a page number, is provided so you can easily find the information that you need to review in your undergraduate nursing textbooks.

SOFTWARE

Packaged in this book you will find a CD-ROM containing NCLEX-PN review software. This software contains 500 practice questions in the multiple-choice format or in the alternate question format. This Windows- and Macintosh-compatible program offers two testing modes for review.

Study—all questions in a specific selected content area. The answer, rationale, test-taking strategy, question categories, and reference source appear after answering each question.

Examination—75 randomly chosen questions from the entire pool of 500 questions. The answer, rationale, test-taking strategy, question categories, reference source, and results appear after you answer all 75 questions.

CONTENT AREAS ON THE SOFTWARE

When you use the software, you will be able to select practice questions based on a Client Needs area or a content area. The Client Needs areas include Safe, Effective Care Environment, Health Promotion and Maintenance, Psychosocial Integrity, and Physiological Integrity. The content areas are shown in the following box.

CONTENT AREAS

- Fundamental Skills
- Maternity/Antepartum
- Maternity/Intrapartum
- Maternity/Postpartum
- Child Health
- Mental Health
- Delegating/Prioritizing
- Leadership/Management
- Pharmacology
- Adult Health/Eye
- Adult Health/Ear
- Adult Health/Neurological
- Adult Health/Musculoskeletal
- Adult Health/Immune
- Adult Health/Gastrointestinal
- Adult Health/Endocrine
- Adult Health/Renal
- Adult Health/Oncology
- Adult Health/Respiratory
- Adult Health/Cardiovascular
- Adult Health/Integumentary

HOW TO USE THIS BOOK

Saunders Test-Taking Strategies for Success for the NCLEX-PN® Examination is especially designed to help you with your successful journey to the peak of the *Saunders Pyramid to Success*, becoming a licensed practical/vocational nurse. This book focuses on test-taking strategies that will help you pass your nursing examinations and the NCLEX-PN examination. You should begin your process through the *Saunders Pyramid to Success* by reading all of the chapters in this book to learn the strategies that you can use to answer test questions. Next, answer the questions in the practice test located in Part 4. Finally, use the software that accompanies this book and answer these practice questions.

When using the software, it is best to begin by selecting the Study Mode because you will receive immediate feedback regarding the answer, rationale, test-taking strategies, question codes, and reference source. Therefore, you are provided with immediate information about your strengths and weaknesses. Once you have answered the practice test question, read the rationale and the test-taking strategy. The rationale provides you with the significant information regarding both the correct and incorrect options. The test-taking strategy offers you the logical path to selecting the correct option. The strategy also identifies content area that you need to review if you had difficulty with the question. Use the reference source listed to easily find the information that you need to review.

It is very important to identify your strengths and weaknesses with regard to nursing content areas. It is also important to strengthen any weak areas in order to be successful on the NCLEX-PN examination. There are several products in Saunders Pyramid to Success that can be used to strengthen any weak areas. These additional products in *Saunders Pyramid to Success* can be obtained by calling 1-800-426-4545 or visiting www.elsevierhealth.com. These products are described below.

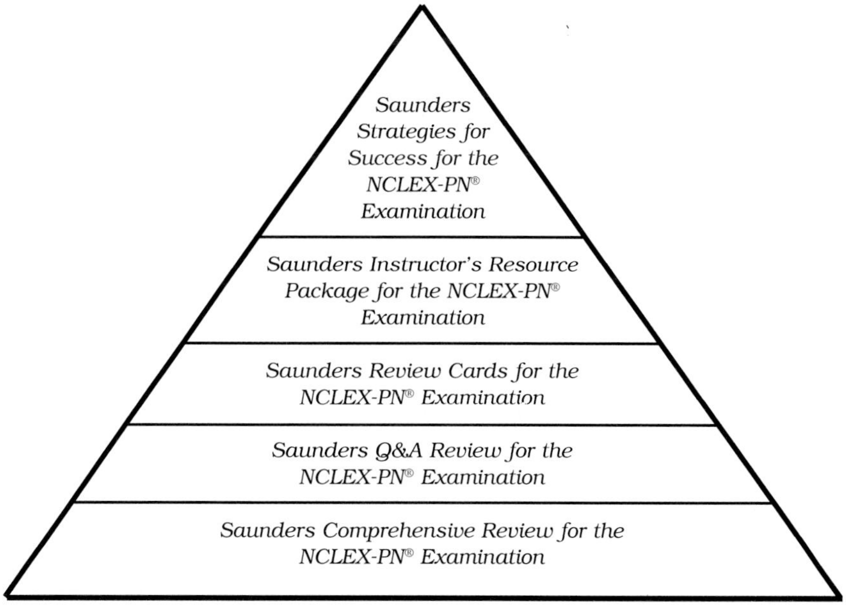

Saunders Comprehensive Review for the NCLEX-PN® Examination

This is an excellent resource to use while you are in nursing school as well as in preparation for the NCLEX-PN examination. This book contains 20 units and 66 chapters, and each chapter is designed to identify specific components of nursing content. The book and accompanying software contains more than 3500 practice questions and includes alternate format questions.

Saunders Q&A Review for the NCLEX-PN® Examination

This book and accompanying software provides you with more than 3000 practice questions based on the NCLEX-PN test plan. The chapters are uniquely designed and are based on the NCLEX-PN examination test plan framework including Client Needs and Integrated Processes. Alternate format questions are included. With practice questions uniquely focused on the Client Needs and the Integrated Processes, you can assess your level of competence.

Saunders Review Cards for the NCLEX-PN® Examination

This product provides you with more than 900 practice test questions, including multiple-choice questions and the new alternate test items, such as fill-in-the-blank, multiple response, prioritizing (ordered response), and figure or illustration questions. The practice question is located on one side of the review card. The reverse side of the review card contains the correct answer, rationale, and question categories, for the practice question on the front of the card.

Saunders Instructor's Resource Package for the NCLEX-PN® Examination

A final component of the *Saunders Pyramid to Success* is the *Saunders Instructor's Resource Package for the NCLEX-PN® Examination.* This manual and CD-ROM accompany the Saunders program of NCLEX-PN review products. Be sure to ask your nursing program director and nursing faculty about this CD-ROM and its use for a review course or a self-paced review in your school's computer laboratory.

Good luck with your journey through the *Saunders Pyramid to Success.* I wish you continued success throughout your nursing program and in your new career as a licensed practical/vocational nurse!

Linda Anne Silvestri, MSN, RN

To All Nursing Students and Graduates,

Taking a nursing examination can be a very anxiety provoking situation because you must pass your nursing examinations in order to pass nursing courses and ultimately become a graduate nurse. Taking the NCLEX-PN® examination is just as anxiety provoking because you must pass the NCLEX examination in order to become a licensed practical/vocational nurse and begin your career.

It is critically important that you learn how to take an examination. You must use your nursing knowledge and what you learned from your clinical experiences to help you with testing. However, you also need to become skillful with test-taking strategies to pass examinations. Becoming skillful with testing takes time and practice; that's why it is important to develop, refine, and master these skills early on, when you begin your nursing education. Mastering these test-taking skills will bring you success!

I am excited and pleased to be able to provide you with the *Saunders Pyramid to Success* products that will prepare you for taking tests during your nursing program and prepare you for the NCLEX-PN examination. I want to thank all of my former nursing students that I have assisted in preparing for NCLEX examinations for their willingness to offer ideas regarding their needs in preparing for licensure. Student ideas have certainly added a special uniqueness to all of the products available in *Saunders Pyramid to Success.*

This publication provides you with all of the test-taking strategies that will help you with testing. Once you have practiced these strategies and mastered the skill of successful test-taking, the examination experience will be a more comfortable one.

So, let's get started and begin our journey through the *Pyramid to Success* and let's master the skill of test-taking!

Sincerely,

Linda Anne Silvestri MSN, RN

Linda Anne Silvestri, MSN, RN

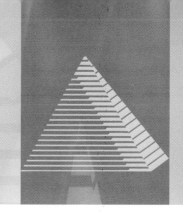

Acknowledgements

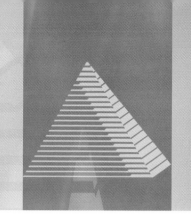

Sincere appreciation and warmest thanks is extended to the many individuals who in their own way have contributed to the publication of this book.

First, I want to thank all of my nursing students at the Community College of Rhode Island in Warwick, who approached me in 1991 and persuaded me to assist them in preparing to take the NCLEX examination. Their enthusiasm and inspiration led to the commencement of my professional endeavors in conducting NCLEX-RN® and NCLEX-PN® review courses for nursing students. I also thank the numerous nursing students who have attended my review courses for their willingness to share their needs and ideas. Their input has certainly added a special uniqueness to this publication.

I wish to acknowledge all of the nursing faculty who taught in my NCLEX-RN and NCLEX-PN review courses. Their commitment, dedication, and expertise have certainly assisted nursing students in achieving success with the NCLEX examination. I want to acknowledge Laurent W. Valliere for his commitment and dedication in assisting my nursing students to prepare for the NCLEX from a nonacademic point of view. Additionally, I thank my assistant, Dianne Ventrice, for all of her support and help in preparing this publication.

I sincerely acknowledge and thank two very important individuals from Elsevier Health Sciences. I thank Nancy O'Brien, managing editor, for all of her assistance and ideas with creating this publication. I also thank Charlene Ketchum, associate developmental editor, for her continual assistance, enthusiasm, and support as I prepared this publication and for all of her assistance in maintaining organization and assisting me in completing this publication.

I also want to acknowledge all of the staff at Elsevier Health Sciences for their tremendous assistance throughout the preparation and production of this publication. A special thank you to all of them.

I thank all of the special people in the production department, Jeff Patterson, publishing services manager; Jeanne Genz, project manager; and Jyotika Shroff, designer whose consistent editing assisted in finalizing this publication.

I sincerely thank Bob Boehringher, director of nursing marketing, and Andrew Eilers, marketing manager, whose support, hard work, and special creativity assisted with this publication.

I would also like to acknowledge Patricia Mieg, educational sales representative, who encouraged me to submit my ideas about the *Pyramid to Success* to the Saunders Company.

I want to acknowledge my parents, who opened my door of opportunity in education. I thank my mother, Frances Mary, for all of her love, support, and assistance as I continuously worked to achieve my professional goals. I thank my father, Arnold Lawrence, who always provided insightful words of encouragement. My memories of his love and support will always remain in my heart.

I also thank my sister, Dianne Elodia, my brother, Lawrence Peter, and my niece, Gina Marie, who were constantly supportive, giving, and helpful during my research and preparation of this publication.

I sincerely thank Dr. JoAnn Mullaney from Salve Regina University in Newport, Rhode Island. As a colleague and friend, she has always encouraged and supported me through my professional endeavors.

I also need to thank Salve Regina University for the opportunity to educate nursing students in the baccalaureate nursing program and for its support during my research and writing of this publication. I would like to especially acknowledge my colleagues, Dr. Sandra Solem, Dr. Ellen McCarty, Dr. JoAnn Mullaney, Dr. Jane McCool, Dr. Peggy Matteson, and Dr. Bethany Sykes for all of their support and encouragement.

I wish to acknowledge the Community College of Rhode Island who provided me the opportunity to educate nursing students in the associate degree of nursing program, and a special thank you to Patricia Miller, MSN, RN, and Michelina McClellan, MS, RN, from Baystate Medical Center, School of Nursing, in Springfield, Massachusetts, who were my first mentors in nursing education.

Lastly, a very special thank you to all my nursing students, past, present and future. You light up my life! And your curiosity, enthusiasm to learn, and desire to become successful is so inspiring.

Linda Anne Silvestri, MSN, RN

Table of Contents

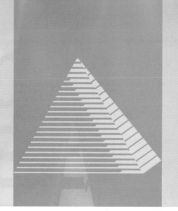

"Sleep....Get 8 hours the night before and eat a healthy and satisfying breakfast. Use breathing techniques and try to relax after every question."

—April Oland Childs,
Salve Regina University, Newport, RI

"I have always found, while studying a chapter...I first outline the chapter with its subtitles. This helps me to define the different content within the chapter. If it's done before the classroom lecture, it also helps to follow along when the teacher is going through with the chapter and all the information in the chapter seems to be sounding alike. It may take a little time, but each chapter usually fits on one piece of paper, and then as I am studying for the test, I can fill in little notes to help me to keep all the different diseases, systems, or procedures separate in my mind and just at a glance!"

—Rhonda Lee Singer, Lebanon County Career and Technology Center, Lebanon, PA

Part 1

The NCLEX-PN® Examination

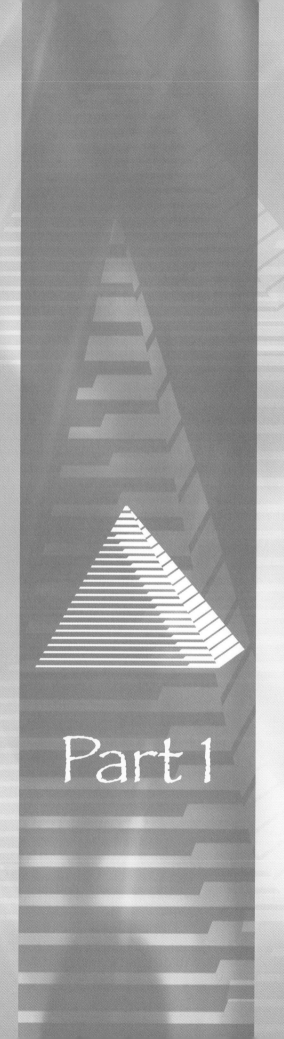

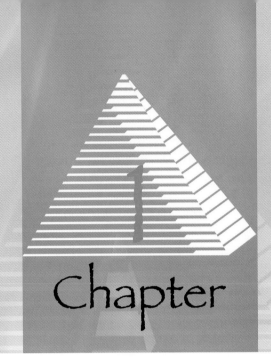

Chapter 1 The Test Plan

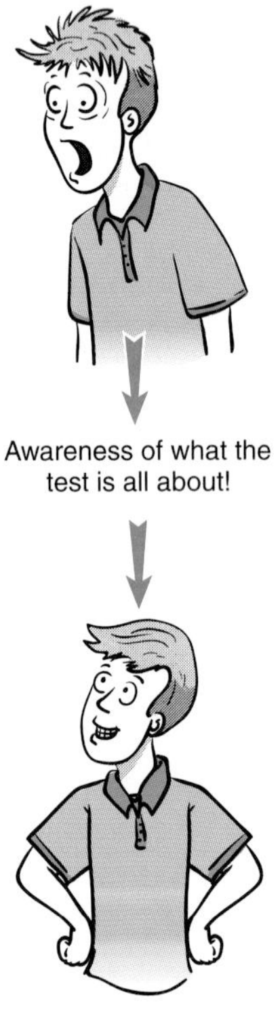

Awareness of what the test is all about!

An important strategy for success for the National Council Licensure Examination for Licensed Practical/Vocational Nurses (NCLEX-PN®) is to become as familiar as possible with the NCLEX-PN test plan. A significant amount of anxiety can occur in a candidate (test-taker) facing the challenge of this examination. Knowing the format and general content of the examination will assist in alleviating your fear and anxiety.

This chapter focuses on how the test is developed and the components of the test plan. Some of this information was obtained from the National Council of State Boards of Nursing (NCSBN) website (www.ncsbn.org) and from the *Test Plan for the National Council Licensure Examination for Practical/Vocational Nurses* (effective date: April 2005), National Council of State Boards of Nursing, Chicago, 2004. Additional information regarding the test and its development can be obtained by accessing the NCSBN website or by writing to the NCSBN (see following box for NCSBN contact information).

NATIONAL COUNCIL OF STATE BOARDS OF NURSING CONTACT INFORMATION

National Council of State Boards of Nursing
111 E. Wacker Drive, Suite 2900
Chicago, IL 60601
Website: www.ncsbn.org

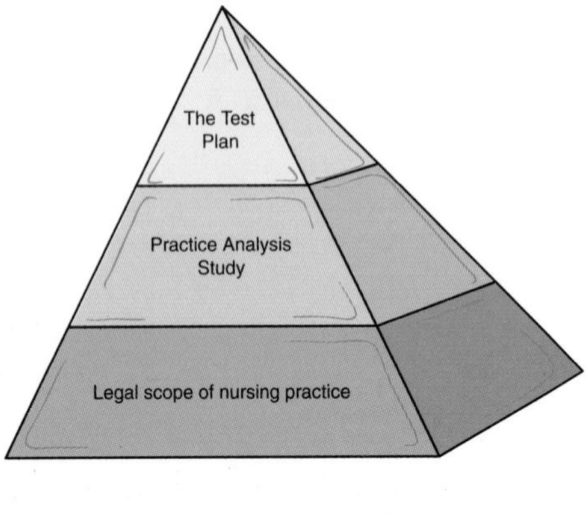

HOW IS THE TEST PLAN DEVELOPED?

The test plan for the NCLEX-PN examination is developed by NCSBN. As an initial step in the test development process, NCSBN considers the legal scope of nursing practice as governed by state laws and regulations, including the nurse practice acts, and uses these laws to define the areas on the examination that will assess the competence of a candidate (test-taker) for nurse licensure.

NCSBN also conducts a Practice Analysis study to determine the framework for the test plan for NCLEX-PN. The participants of this study include newly licensed practical and vocational nurses. The participants are provided a list of nursing activities and are asked about the frequency of performing these specific activities, their impact on maintaining client safety, and the setting where the activities were performed. The analysis of the data obtained from this study guides the development of a framework for entry-level nurse performance that incorporates specific client needs and the processes fundamental to the practice of nursing. The NCLEX-PN test plan is derived from this framework. Because nursing practice continues to change, this study is conducted every 3 years. The results of this study, most recently conducted in 2003, provided the structure for the test plan implemented in April of 2005.

WHO WRITES THE QUESTIONS?

Question (item) writers are selected by the National Council of State Boards of Nursing after an extensive application process. The writers are registered nurses who are responsible for teaching basic students in the clinical area. Question writers voluntarily submit an application to become a writer and must meet specific established criteria designated by the National Council in order to be accepted as a participant in the process.

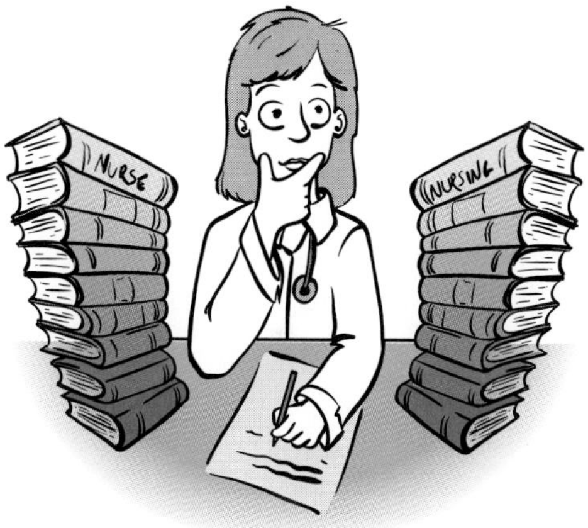

WHAT ARE THE COMPONENTS OF THE TEST PLAN?

The content of NCLEX-PN reflects the activities that a newly licensed entry-level licensed practical/vocational nurse must be able to perform in order to provide clients with safe and effective nursing care. The questions are written to address the Levels of Cognitive Ability, Client Needs, and Integrated Processes as identified in the test plan developed by the NCSBN (see following box).

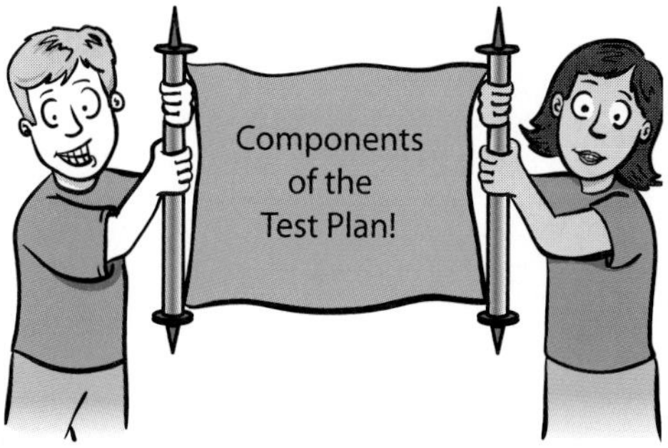

EXAMINATION QUESTIONS

Each examination question addresses:

A Level of Cognitive Ability

A Client Needs category

An Integrated Process

Levels of Cognitive Ability

The examination for licensure as a licensed practical/vocational nurse may include questions at the cognitive levels of knowledge, comprehension, application, and analysis. However, the majority of questions address the application and analysis level. To understand the differences in the four cognitive levels, read the following sample questions.

LEVELS OF COGNITIVE ABILITY

Knowledge
Comprehension
Application
Analysis

Sample Question

Level of Cognitive Ability: Knowledge

A nurse reviews the laboratory results of a client's blood glucose level. The nurse knows that which of the following is a normal level?

1. 40 mg/dL
2. 100 mg/dL
3. 180 mg/dL
4. 220 mg/dL

Answer: 2

In a knowledge-type question, you need to simply recall data. In this sample question, recalling the normal blood glucose level is all that is needed to answer correctly. Remember, the normal blood glucose level ranges from 70 to 110 mg/dL.

Sample Question

Level of Cognitive Ability: Comprehension

A hospitalized client with type 1 diabetes mellitus complains of hunger and nervousness and the nurse notes that the client is diaphoretic. The nurse understands that the client is most likely experiencing:

1. anxiety related to the hospitalization.
2. signs related to an infection.
3. a hyperglycemic reaction.
4. a hypoglycemic reaction.

Answer: 4

In a comprehension-type question, you need to understand the basis for the information presented in the question and draw inferences from that information. In this question, you need to understand that the client's signs and symptoms are a result of the diagnosis and treatment for type 1 diabetes mellitus and that the signs and symptoms relate to hypoglycemia. Remember, hunger, nervousness, and sweating are signs of hypoglycemia. Relate the "three Ps"—polyuria, polydipsia, and polyphagia—to hyperglycemia.

Sample Question

Level of Cognitive Ability: Application
A client is experiencing a hypoglycemic reaction. The nurse administers which best item to the client to treat the reaction?
1. Water
2. Diet soda
3. Milk
4. One sugar-free cookie

Answer: 3
In an application-type question, you will be asked about an intervention, a nursing action, a decision, or a problem that needs to be solved. In this sample question you are asked to select the best item for treating a hypoglycemic reaction. Remember, if a hypoglycemic reaction occurs, the client should be given an item that contains 10 to 15 g of carbohydrate.

Sample Question

Level of Cognitive Ability: Analysis
The nurse administers 10 units of Regular insulin at 7:00 AM to a client with type 1 diabetes mellitus. The nurse monitors the client most closely for a hypoglycemic reaction during which hours?
1. 9:00 AM to 10:00 AM
2. 1:00 PM to 7:00 PM
3. 9:00 AM to 3:00 PM
4. 11:00 AM to 12:00 noon

Answer: 1
In an analysis-type question, you are required to consider and examine possibly several concepts in the question in order to answer the question correctly. In this question, it is necessary to know that regular insulin is short-acting insulin, that it peaks in 2 to 3 hours, and that a hypoglycemic reaction is most likely to occur during peak time. Remember, the peak time of the insulin is the most likely time for a hypoglycemic reaction to occur.

Client Needs

The NCSBN identifies a test plan framework based on Client Needs. The NCSBN identifies four major categories of Client Needs, and some of these categories are further divided into subcategories. The Client Needs categories include Safe, Effective Care Environment, Health Promotion and Maintenance, Psychosocial Integrity, and Physiological Integrity. Table 1-1 identifies these Client Needs categories, any subcategories, and the associated percentage of test questions. Chapter 3, titled Client Needs, explains each Client Need category, lists the content most likely to be addressed on the examination, and provides sample questions for each category or subcategory.

Table 1-1

CLIENT NEEDS CATEGORIES, SUBCATEGORIES, AND PERCENTAGE (%) OF QUESTIONS

Categories/Subcategories	Questions
Safe, Effective Care Environment	
Coordinated care	11%-17%
Safety and infection control	8%-14%
Health Promotion and Maintenance	7%-13%
Psychosocial Integrity	8%-14%
Physiological Integrity	
Basic care and comfort	11%-17%
Pharmacological therapies	9%-15%
Reduction of risk potential	10%-16%
Physiological adaptation	12%-18%

Integrated Processes

The NCSBN identifies four processes that are fundamental to the practice of nursing. These processes are a component of the test plan and are integrated throughout the four categories of Client Needs: Safe, Effective Care Environment, Health Promotion and Maintenance, Psychosocial Integrity, and Physiological Integrity. The Integrated Processes identified by the NCSBN include caring, clinical problem-solving process (nursing process including data collection, planning, implementation, and evaluation), communication and documentation, and teaching and learning (see the following box). Chapter 4, Integrated Processes, explains each Integrated Process and provides sample questions for each.

INTEGRATED PROCESSES

- Caring
- Clinical problem-solving process (nursing process)
- Communication and documentation
- Teaching and learning

REFERENCES

DeWit, S. (2005). *Fundamental concepts and skills for nursing* (2nd ed). Philadelphia: Saunders.

Linton, A. & Maebius, N. (2003). *Introduction to medical-surgical nursing* (3rd ed). Philadelphia: Saunders.

National Council of State Boards of Nursing, Inc. *Test Plan for the National Council Licensure Examination for Licensed Practical/Vocational Nurses* (effective Date: April 2005) National Council of State Boards of Nursing, Chicago, 2004.

National Council of State Boards of Nursing, Inc. online: Available at www.ncsbn.org.

Chapter 2

The Examination Process

A significant amount of anxiety can occur in a candidate (test-taker) taking the National Council Licensure Examination for Practical/Vocational Nurses (NCLEX-PN®) examination. Knowing what you will encounter during the process of testing will assist in alleviating your fear and anxiety.

COMPUTERIZED ADAPTIVE TESTING (CAT): HOW DOES IT WORK?

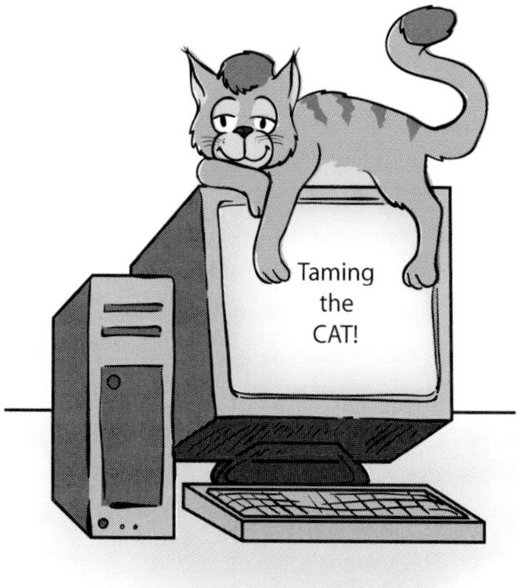

The abbreviation CAT stands for "computerized adaptive testing." This means that the examination is created as you answer each question. All of the test questions are categorized on the basis of the test plan structure and the level of difficulty of the question. As you answer a question, the computer will determine your competency on the basis of the answer that you selected. If you selected a correct answer, the computer scans the question bank and selects a more difficult question for your next question. If you selected an incorrect answer, the computer scans the question bank and selects an easier question for your next question. Table 2-1 illustrates how this process works. This process continues until the test plan requirements, based on the test plan structure, are met and a reliable pass or fail decision is made.

When a test question is presented on the computer screen, it must be answered or the test will not move on. This means that you will not be able to skip questions, go back and review questions, or go back and change answers. Remember, in a CAT examination, once an answer is recorded, all subsequent questions administered depend, to an extent, on the answer selected for that question. Skipping and returning to earlier questions is not compatible with the logical methodology of a computerized adaptive test. The inability to skip questions or go back to change answers will not be a disadvantage to you. Actually, you will not fall into that trap of changing a correct answer to an incorrect one with CAT.

Table 2-1

COMPUTER SELECTION OF TEST QUESTIONS

Question	Level of Difficulty	Test-Taker Response
1	Easy	Correct
2	Medium	Correct
3	Difficult	Correct
4	Difficult	Incorrect
5	Medium	Incorrect
6	Easy	Correct
7	Medium	Incorrect
8	Easy	Correct
9	Medium	Correct
10	Difficult	Correct

The test questions will continue to be selected in this way until a reliable pass or fail decision is made.

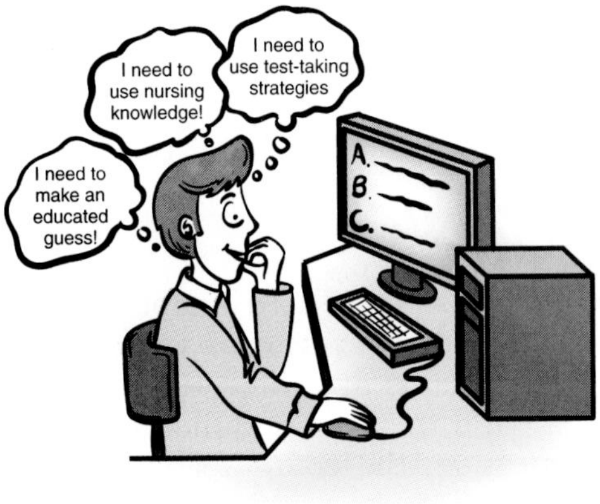
I need to use nursing knowledge!
I need to use test-taking strategies
I need to make an educated guess!
A.
B.
C.

If you are faced with a question that contains unfamiliar content, you may need to make an educated guess to answer. There is no penalty for guessing on this examination. Remember, with the majority of the questions, the answer will be right there in front of you. If you need to guess, use your nursing knowledge to its fullest extent, as well as all of the test-taking strategies that you have learned in this book.

You do not need any computer experience to take this examination. You will be provided with a keyboard tutorial at the start of the examination that will instruct you on the use of the on-screen optional calculator, the use of the mouse, and how to record an answer. In addition to the traditional four-option multiple-choice questions, the tutorial also provides instructions on how to respond to different question formats. A proctor is always present to assist in explaining the use of the computer to ensure your full understanding of how to proceed.

KEYBOARD TUTORIAL

- How to use the computer
- How to use the on-screen optional calculator
- How to use the mouse
- How to record an answer
- How to respond to different question formats

REGISTERING FOR THE EXAMINATION: WHAT DO YOU NEED TO DO?

The initial step in the registration process is to submit an application to the state board of nursing in the state in which you intend to obtain licensure. You need to obtain information from the board of nursing regarding the specific registration process because the process may vary from state to state. In most states, you may register for the examination through the Internet, by mail, or by telephone. The NCLEX candidate website (see following box) provides information regarding what you will need to register to take this examination.

NCLEX CANDIDATE WEBSITE: www.vue.com/nclex

It is very important that you follow the registration instructions and complete the registration forms precisely and accurately. Registration forms not properly completed, or not accompanied by the proper fees in the required method of payment, will be returned to you and will delay testing.

There is a fee for taking the examination, and you may have to pay additional fees to the board of nursing in the state in which you are applying. You will be sent a confirmation indicating that your registration was received. If you do not receive a confirmation within 4 weeks of submitting your registration, you should contact the candidate services.

AUTHORIZATION TO TEST (ATT) FORM: WHAT DO YOU NEED IT FOR?

Once your eligibility to test has been determined by the board of nursing in the state in which licensure is requested, your registration form is processed and an authorization to test (ATT) form will be sent to you. You cannot make an appointment until the board of nursing declares eligibility and you receive an ATT form.

The ATT form contains important information including your test authorization number, candidate identification number, and an expiration date. Note the expiration date on the form because you must test by this date. You also need to take your ATT form to the test center on the day of your examination. You will not be admitted to the examination if you do not have it.

HOW DO YOU SCHEDULE A TESTING DATE?

The examination will take place at a Pearson Professional Center; an appointment can be made through the Internet or by telephone. First-time test-takers will be offered an appointment within 30 days of the call to schedule an appointment, and repeat test-takers will be offered an appointment within 45 days. You can schedule an appointment at any Pearson Professional Center; a confirmation of your appointment will be sent to you. You do not have to take the examination in the same state in which you are seeking licensure.

If for any reason you need to cancel or reschedule your appointment to test, you can make the change on the candidate website (www.vue.com/nclex) or by calling candidate services. The change needs to be made one full business day (24 hours) before your scheduled appointment.

If you fail to arrive for the examination or do not cancel or reschedule your testing appointment without providing appropriate notice, you will forfeit your examination fee, and your ATT will be invalidated. This information will be reported to the board of nursing in the state in which you have applied for licensure, and you will be required to re-register and pay the testing fees again.

It is important that you arrive at the testing center at least 30 minutes before the test is scheduled to begin. If you arrive late, you may be required to forfeit your examination appointment. If it is necessary for the appointment to be forfeited, you will need to re-register for the examination and pay an additional fee. The board of nursing will be notified that you did not test.

Arrive at the test center at least 30 minutes before the test is scheduled!

A few days before your scheduled date of testing, take the time to drive to the testing center to determine its exact location, the length of time required to arrive to that destination, and any potential obstacles that might delay you, such as road construction, traffic, or parking sites.

WHAT DO YOU DO IF YOU NEED SPECIAL TESTING ACCOMMODATIONS?

A test-taker with needs who requires special testing accommodations should contact the board of nursing before submitting a registration form. The board of nursing will provide the procedures for the request. The board of nursing must authorize special testing accommodations. After board of nursing approval, the National Council of State Boards of Nursing (NCSBN) reviews the requested accommodations and must approve the request. If the request is approved, the testing appointment must be made by the NCLEX program coordinator, who can be contacted by calling NCLEX candidate services. Canceling or rescheduling an appointment must be done through the NCLEX program coordinator.

THE TESTING CENTER: WHAT CAN YOU EXPECT?

The testing center is designed to ensure complete security of the testing process. Strict candidate identification requirements have been established. To be admitted to the testing center, you must bring the ATT form, along with two forms of identification (ID). Both forms of identification must be signed, current or nonexpired, and one must contain a recent photograph of you. The name on the photograph identification must be the same as the name on the ATT form.

> **WHAT YOU MUST BRING TO THE TESTING CENTER**
> The ATT form
> Two forms of ID that are signed and current or nonexpired
> One ID must contain a recent photograph and the name on the ID must be the same as the name on the ATT form

A digital fingerprint, signature, and photograph will be taken at the test center, and accompany the NCLEX results to confirm your identity. If you leave the testing room for any reason, you will be required to have your fingerprint taken again to be readmitted to the room.

Personal belongings are not allowed in the testing room. Secure storage will be provided for you; however, storage space is limited, so you must plan accordingly. In addition, the testing center will not assume responsibility for your personal belongings. The test center waiting areas are generally small; therefore, friends or family members who accompany you are not permitted to wait in the testing center while you are taking the examination.

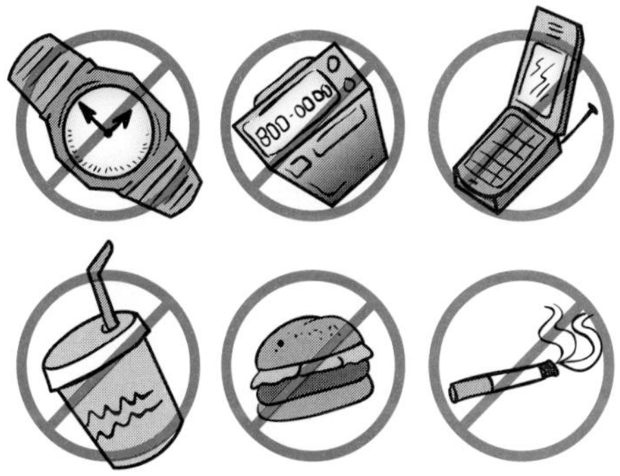

Once you have completed the admission process and a brief orientation, the proctor will escort you to your assigned computer. You will be seated at an individual table area with an appropriate workspace that includes computer equipment, appropriate lighting, an erasable note board, and a marker. No items, including unauthorized scratch paper, are allowed into the testing room. Electronic devices such as watches, beepers, or cell phones are not allowed in the testing room. Eating, drinking, or the use of tobacco is not allowed in the testing room.

You will be observed at all times by the test proctor while taking the examination. Additionally, all test sessions are video and audio recorded. Pearson Professional Centers have no control over the sounds made by typing on the computer. If these sounds are distracting, raise your hand to summon the proctor. Earplugs are available upon request.

You must follow the directions given by the test center staff and must remain seated during the test, except when authorized to leave. If you feel that you have a problem with the computer, need an additional note board, need to take a break, or need the test proctor for any reason, you must raise your hand.

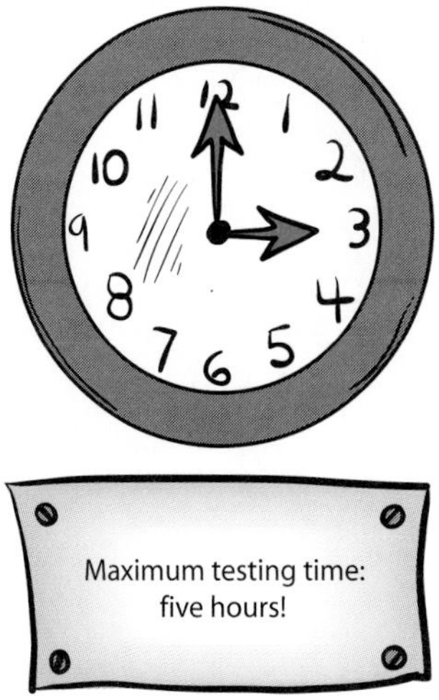
Maximum testing time: five hours!

HOW MUCH TESTING TIME DO YOU HAVE?

The maximum testing time is 5 hours, and this period includes the tutorial, two preprogrammed optional breaks, and any unscheduled breaks that you may take. The first preprogrammed optional break takes place after 2 testing hours, and the second preprogrammed optional break after 3½ hours of testing. The computer screen will notify you of the time for these breaks. When you return from taking a break, you will be required to provide a fingerprint to be readmitted to the testing room.

HOW MANY QUESTIONS ARE IN THE EXAMINATION?

The minimum number of questions that you need to answer is 85. Of these 85 questions, 60 are operational (scored) questions and 25 are pretest (unscored) questions. The maximum number of questions in the test is 205. Of the total number of questions that you need to answer, 25 are pretest (unscored) questions.

The pretest questions may be presented as scored questions on future examinations. These pretest questions are not identified as such, that is, you do not know which questions are the pretest (unscored) questions. Therefore, it is important to answer every question as if it were scored.

Minimum number of questions in the test is 85.
Maximum number of questions in the test is 205.

WHAT HAPPENS WHEN THE EXAM IS COMPLETED?

Once the test is completed, you will complete a brief computer-delivered questionnaire about your testing experience. After this questionnaire is completed, you need to raise your hand to summon the test proctor. The test proctor will collect and inventory all note boards and then permit you to leave.

HOW ARE THE RESULTS PROCESSED?

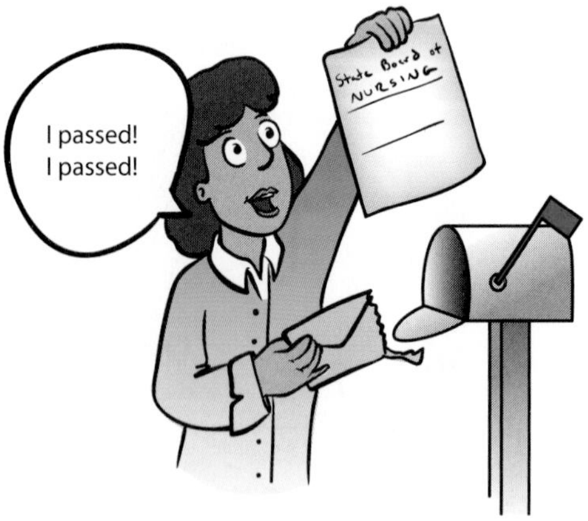

Every computerized examination is scored twice; once by the computer at the testing center and then again after the examination is transmitted to Pearson Professional Centers. No results are released at the test center. The board of nursing will mail your results to you approximately 1 month after taking the examination.

In some states, candidates may be able to access "unofficial" results 2 business days after taking the examination via the NCLEX Candidate website or through the Quick Results line. The website is www.pearsonvue.com/nclex and the NCLEX Quick Results line is 1-900-776-2539 (1-900-77-NCLEX). There is a fee for obtaining your "unofficial" results and it is important to remember that the results are "unofficial" and do not authorize you to practice as a licensed nurse.

You should not telephone Pearson Professional Centers, the NCSBN, candidate services, or the state board of nursing for results.

HOW IS A PASS OR FAIL DECISION MADE?

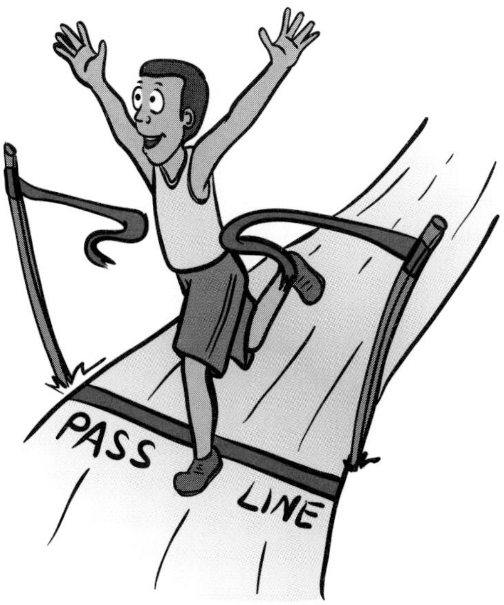

All of the examination questions are categorized by test plan area and level of difficulty. This is important to keep in mind when considering how a pass or fail decision is made by the computer, because a pass or fail decision is not based on a percentage of correctly answered questions. After the minimum number of questions have been answered (85 questions), the computer compares the test-taker's ability level to the standard required for passing, which is set by the NCSBN. If the test-taker is clearly above the passing standard, then the test-taker passes the examination. If the test-taker is clearly below the passing standard, then the test-taker fails the examination. If the computer is not able to clearly determine if the test-taker has passed or failed because the test-taker's ability is close to the passing standard, then the computer continues asking questions. After each question, the test-taker's ability is determined, and when it becomes clear on which side of the passing standard that the test-taker falls (above the standard or below the standard), the examination ends. If the test-taker is administered the maximum number of questions (205 questions), the computer will make a pass or fail decision by recomputing the test-taker's final ability level, based on every question answered, and comparing it with the passing standard. If the ability level is above the passing standard, the test-taker passes (Figure 2-1). If it is not above the passing standard, the test-taker fails (Figure 2-2).

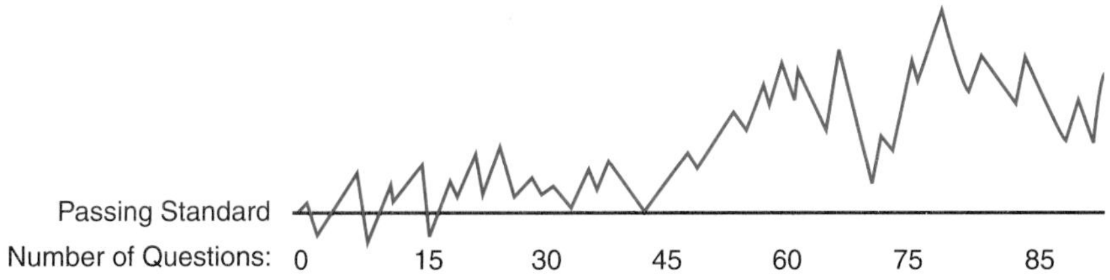

Figure 2-1 A test-taker that has passed.

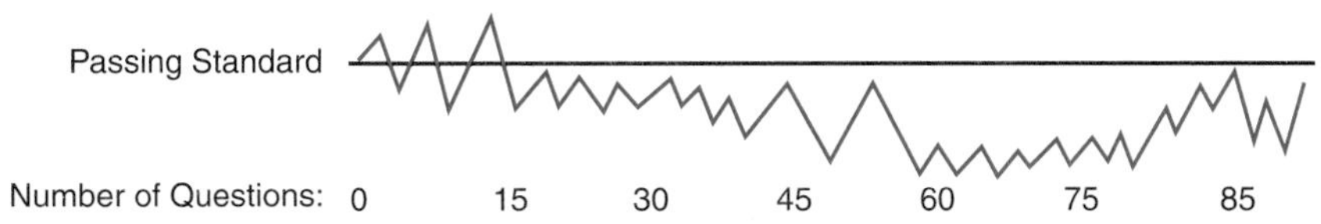

Figure 2-2 A test-taker that has failed.

HOW IS A PASS OR FAIL DECISION MADE IF YOU RUN OUT OF TIME?

If the examination ends because you have run out of time, the computer may not have enough information to make a clear pass or fail decision. If this is the situation, the computer will review the test-taker's performance during testing. If the test-taker's ability was consistently above the passing standard, the test-taker passes.

WHO RECEIVES A CANDIDATE PERFORMANCE REPORT?

A candidate performance report is provided to a test-taker who failed the examination. This report provides test-takers with information about their strengths and weaknesses in relation to the test plan and provides a guide for studying and retaking the examination. The test-taker must wait 45 to 91 days (based on board of nursing policy) before retaking the examination.

WHAT IS INTERSTATE ENDORSEMENT?

Because the NCLEX-PN examination is a national examination, you can apply to take the examination in any state. Once licensure is received, you can apply for interstate endorsement (a license from another state). The procedures and requirements for interstate endorsement may vary from state to state, and these procedures can be obtained from the state board of nursing in the state in which endorsement is sought.

REFERENCES

National Council of State Boards of Nursing, Inc. *Test Plan for the National Council Licensure Examination for Licensed Practical/Vocational Nurses* (effective date: April 2005) National Council of State Boards of Nursing, Chicago, 2004.

National Council of State Boards of Nursing, Inc. online: Available at www.ncsbn.org

Pearson Professional Centers website: www.pearsonvue.com/nclex

Chapter 3

Client Needs

In the test plan implemented in April 2005, the National Council of State Boards of Nursing (NCSBN) has identified a test plan framework based on Client Needs.

The NCSBN identifies four major categories of Client Needs, some of which are further divided into subcategories. The Client Needs categories include Safe, Effective Care Environment, Health Promotion and Maintenance, Psychosocial Integrity, and Physiological Integrity.

CLIENT NEEDS CATEGORIES

- Safe, Effective Care Environment
- Health Promotion and Maintenance
- Psychosocial Integrity
- Physiological Integrity

Some of the information contained in this chapter was obtained from the National Council of State Boards of Nursing, Inc. *Detailed Test Plan for the National Council Licensure Examination for Licensed Practical/Vocational Nurses* (effective date: April 2005) National Council of State Boards of Nursing, Chicago, 2004, and the website for the NCSBN: www.ncsbn.org.

SAFE, EFFECTIVE CARE ENVIRONMENT

The Safe, Effective Care Environment category includes two subcategories: Coordinated Care and Safety and Infection Control. Coordinated Care (11%-17%) addresses content that tests the knowledge, skill, and ability required to enhance the care delivery setting to protect clients, families, significant others, visitors, and health care personnel. Safety and Infection Control (8%-14%) addresses content that tests the knowledge, skill, and ability required to protect clients, families, significant others, visitors, and health care personnel from health and environmental hazards.

SAFE, EFFECTIVE CARE ENVIRONMENT

Coordinated care = 11% to 17% of the questions

Safety and infection control = 8% to 14% of the questions

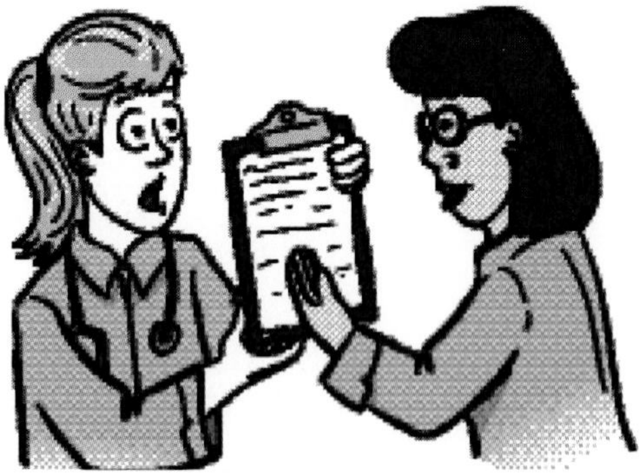

Coordinated Care

In the subcategory Coordinated Care, content may include the following*:

Advance directives
Client advocacy
Client care assignments
Client rights, including confidentiality and informed consent
Consultation with other health care team members
Continuity of care
Ethical and legal issues and responsibilities
Management and supervision concepts
Performance improvement
Prioritizing
Referrals and resource management

An example of a question that addresses this subcategory is provided below.

Question: Coordinated Care

A client scheduled for surgery tells the nurse that he signed an informed consent but was never told about the risks of the surgery. The nurse serves as the client's advocate by:

1. writing a note on the front of the client's record so that the surgeon will see it when the client arrives in the operating room.
2. documenting in the client's record that the client was not told about the risks of the surgery.
3. notifying a registered nurse and requesting that the surgeon be contacted and asked to explain the surgical risks to the client.
4. reassuring the client that the risks are minimal and unlikely to occur.

Answer: 3

Test-Taking Strategy: Use therapeutic communication techniques to eliminate option 4. From the remaining options, focus on the words "never told about the risks of the surgery." A nurse serves as a client advocate by protecting the rights of clients to be informed and to participate in decisions regarding care. The only option that ensures that the client will be informed of the surgical risks is option 3.

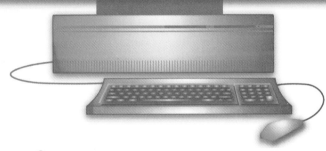

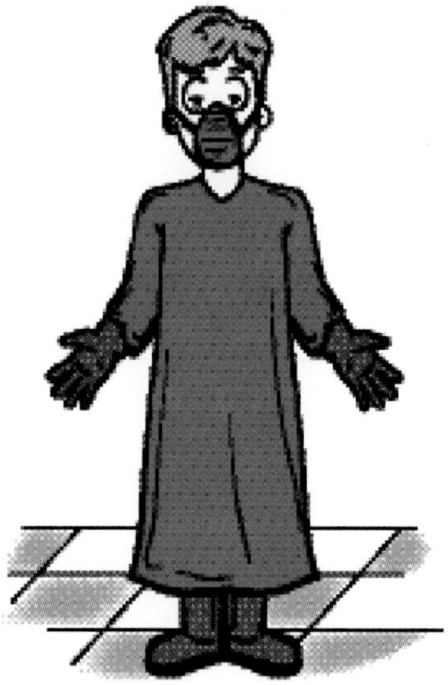

Safety and Infection Control

In the subcategory, Safety and Infection Control, content may include the following*:

- Handling hazardous and infectious material
- Internal and external disaster plans
- Medical and surgical asepsis
- Preventing accidents and preventing errors
- Preventing injuries and home safety
- Reporting accidents or errors and documenting on incident reports
- Restraints and safety devices
- Safe use of equipment
- Security plans
- Standard, transmission-based, and other precautions

An example of a question that addresses this subcategory is provided below.

Question: Safety and Infection Control

A licensed practical nurse (LPN) employed in an emergency department (ED) receives a telephone call from the police department and is told that several victims involved in a train accident will be brought to the ED. The LPN immediately informs the registered nurse and then plans to take which initial action?

1. Call as many nurses as possible at home to have them come to the hospital to care for the victims.
2. Follow the directions outlined in the hospital's disaster preparedness plan (emergency response plan).
3. Ask the housekeeping and laundry department to deliver an extra cart of linen that contains several blankets.
4. Call the operating room and inform them that they may be receiving numerous victims that require surgery.

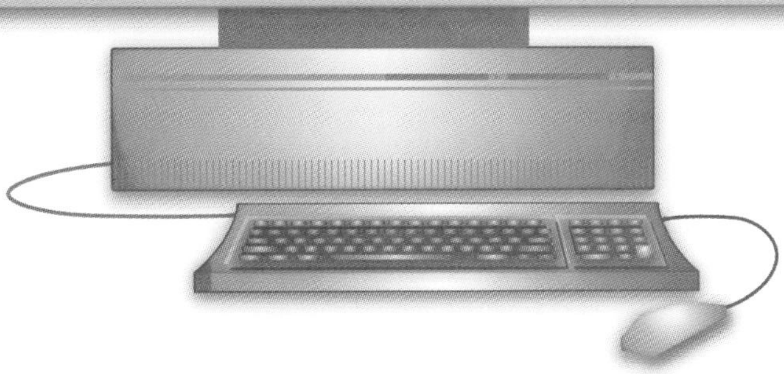

Answer: 2

Test-Taking Strategy: If a nurse is notified that several victims of a disaster will be arriving to the emergency department, the nurse would immediately plan to activate the emergency response plan by notifying a registered nurse and/or supervisor and by following the directions in the plan. Also, note that option 2 is the umbrella (global) option and once this action is implemented, the others will follow.

HEALTH PROMOTION AND MAINTENANCE

The Health Promotion and Maintenance category (7%-13%) addresses the principles related to growth and development. This Client Needs category also addresses content that tests the knowledge, skill, and ability required to assist the client, family members, and/or significant other to prevent health problems, to recognize alterations in health, and to develop health practices that promote and support wellness.

HEALTH PROMOTION AND MAINTENANCE

Health Promotion and Maintenance = 7% to 13% of the questions

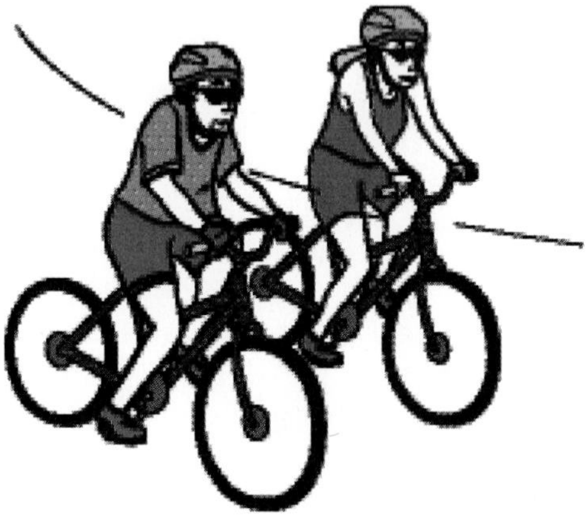

In the Health Promotion and Maintenance category, content may include the following*:

- Data collection techniques
- Disease prevention
- Family planning, family interaction patterns, and human sexuality
- Growth and development, developmental stages and transitions, and the aging process
- Maternity (antepartum, intrapartum, postpartum) and newborn care
- Expected body image changes
- Health promotion and screening programs
- High-risk behaviors
- Immunizations
- Lifestyle choices
- Principles of teaching/learning
- Self-care

An example of a question that addresses the Health Promotion and Maintenance category is provided below.

Question: Health Promotion and Maintenance

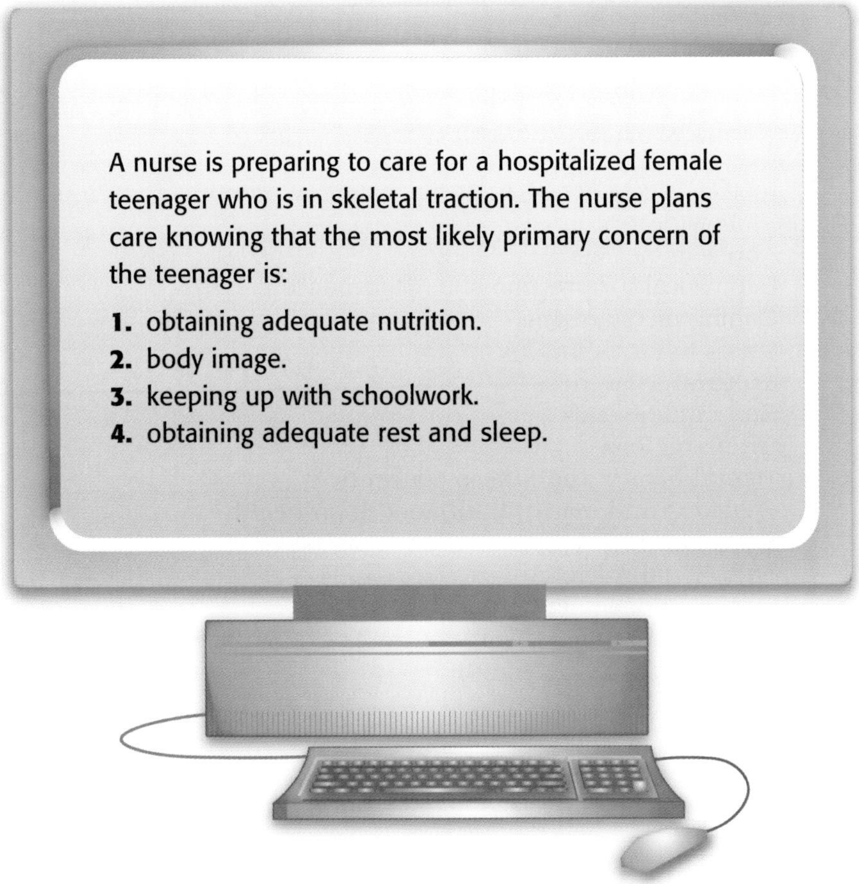
A nurse is preparing to care for a hospitalized female teenager who is in skeletal traction. The nurse plans care knowing that the most likely primary concern of the teenager is:
1. obtaining adequate nutrition.
2. body image.
3. keeping up with schoolwork.
4. obtaining adequate rest and sleep.

Answer: 2

Test-Taking Strategy: Note the key word "primary," and focus on the client, a teenager. Think about the psychosocial development of the teenager (adolescent) to direct you to option 2. Remember, body image is of particular importance to an adolescent.

PSYCHOSOCIAL INTEGRITY

The Psychosocial Integrity category (8%-14%) addresses content that tests the knowledge, skill, and ability required to provide care that assists to promote and support the emotional, mental, and social well-being of the client.

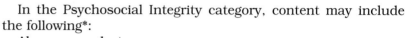

PSYCHOSOCIAL INTEGRITY

Psychosocial Integrity = 8% to 14% of the questions

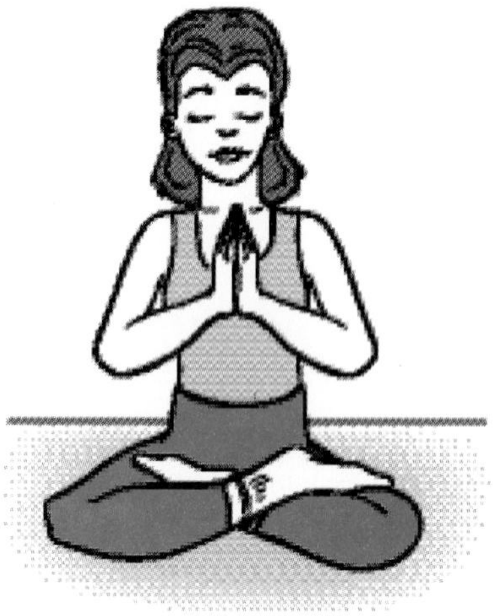

In the Psychosocial Integrity category, content may include the following*:

- Abuse or neglect
- Behavioral interventions
- Coping mechanisms
- Crisis intervention
- Cultural awareness
- End of life issues
- Grief and loss
- Mental health and illness concepts
- Religious and spiritual influences on health
- Sensory and perceptual alterations
- Situational role changes
- Stress management
- Substance-related disorders
- Suicide/violence precautions
- Support systems
- Therapeutic communication techniques
- Therapeutic environment
- Unexpected body image changes

An example of a question that addresses the Psychosocial Integrity category is provided below.

Question: Psychosocial Integrity

A male child is brought to the school nurse's office because of complaints of abdominal pain. On data collection, the nurse notes the presence of several bruises on the child's abdomen and back and several cigarette burn marks. The nurse suspects child abuse and plans for which priority action?

1. Calling the parents to ask them how the child's bruises and burn marks occurred
2. Removing the child from the abusive situation to prevent further injury
3. Documenting the bruises noted on the child
4. Asking the child how long his parents have been abusing him

Answer: 2

Test-Taking Strategy: Use Maslow's Hierarchy of Needs theory. Remember that physiological needs are the priority and if a physiological need does not exist, then safety is the priority. This will direct you to option 2. In the case of suspected child abuse, the priority is to remove the child from the abusive situation to prevent further injury. Additionally, all cases of suspected child abuse must be reported to local authorities.

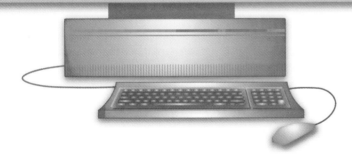

PHYSIOLOGICAL INTEGRITY

The Physiological Integrity category includes four subcategories: Basic Care and Comfort, Pharmacological Therapies, Reduction of Risk Potential, and Physiological Adaptation. Basic Care and Comfort (11%-17%) addresses content that tests the knowledge, skill, and ability required to provide comfort and assistance to the client in the performance of activities of daily living. Pharmacological Therapies (9%-15%) addresses content that tests the knowledge, skill, and ability required to administer medications and to monitor clients receiving parenteral therapies. Reduction of Risk Potential (10%-16%) addresses content that tests the knowledge, skill, and ability required to prevent complications or health problems related to the client's condition, or any prescribed treatments or procedures. Physiological Adaptation (12%-18%) addresses content that tests the knowledge, skill, and ability required to participate in providing care to clients with acute, chronic, or life-threatening conditions.

PHYSIOLOGICAL INTEGRITY

- Basic Care and Comfort = 11% to 17% of the questions
- Pharmacological Therapies = 9% to 15% of the questions
- Reduction of Risk Potential = 10% to 16% of the questions
- Physiological Adaptation = 12% to 18% of the questions

Basic Care and Comfort

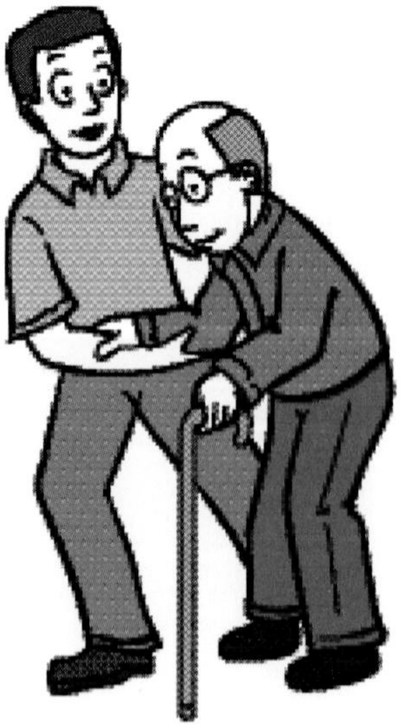

In the Basic Care and Comfort subcategory, content may include the following*:

- Alternative and complementary therapies
- Assistive devices
- Elimination
- Hygiene
- Mobility and immobility
- Nonpharmacological comfort interventions
- Nutrition and oral hydration
- Palliative/comfort care
- Rest and sleep

An example of a question that addresses this subcategory is provided below.

Question: Basic Care and Comfort

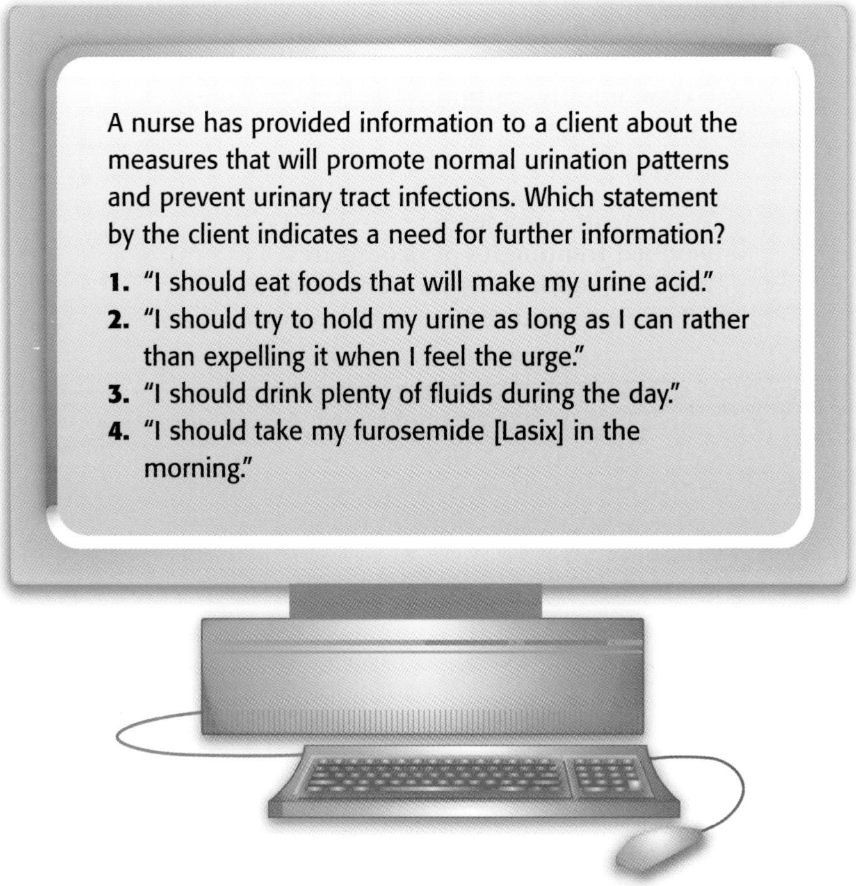
A nurse has provided information to a client about the measures that will promote normal urination patterns and prevent urinary tract infections. Which statement by the client indicates a need for further information?
1. "I should eat foods that will make my urine acid."
2. "I should try to hold my urine as long as I can rather than expelling it when I feel the urge."
3. "I should drink plenty of fluids during the day."
4. "I should take my furosemide [Lasix] in the morning."

Answer: 2

Test-Taking Strategy: Use the process of elimination and note the words "a need for further information." These words indicate a false response question and that you need to select the incorrect client statement. Focusing on the issue, *to prevent urinary tract infections*, and recalling that urinary stasis can lead to infection will direct you to option 2. Remember, the client should be instructed to urinate at regular intervals and when the urge to void is felt.

Pharmacological Therapies

In the Pharmacological Therapies subcategory, content may include the following*:

- Blood transfusions
- Counting narcotics/controlled substances
- Discontinuing an intravenous line
- Dosage calculations
- Intravenous therapy and parenteral fluids
- Medication administration
- Medication routes
- Monitoring intravenous sites and flow rates
- Pharmacological agents, actions, expected effects, side effects, and adverse effects
- Pharmacological pain management
- Phoning in client prescriptions to the pharmacy

An example of a question that addresses this subcategory is provided below.

Question: Pharmacological Therapies

Cyclosporine (Sandimmune) oral solution is prescribed for a client who had a kidney transplant. The nurse provides information to the client about the medication and tells the client that which of the following is most important to monitor?

1. Apical heart rate
2. Peripheral pulses
3. Platelet count
4. Temperature

Answer: 4

Test-Taking Strategy: Use the process of elimination. Eliminate options 1 and 2 first because they are similar. From the remaining options, note the key words "most important." Recalling that infection is an adverse effect will direct you to option 4. Remember, common adverse effects of cyclosporine are nephrotoxicity, infection, hypertension, tremor, and hirsutism.

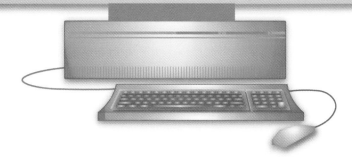

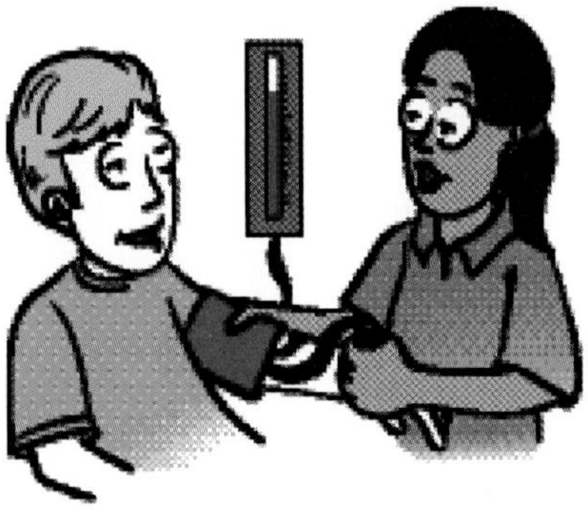

Reduction of Risk Potential

In the Reduction of Risk Potential subcategory, content may include the following*:

- Diagnostic tests and laboratory values
- Potential for alterations in body systems
- Potential for complications of diagnostic tests and surgical and nonsurgical treatments and procedures
- System specific data collection techniques
- Therapeutic procedures
- Vital signs

An example of a question that addresses this subcategory is provided below.

Question: Reduction of Risk Potential

A nurse assists a physician with performing a liver biopsy on a client. Following the procedure, the nurse assists the client to which position?

1. Prone
2. On the right side
3. On the left side
4. Left Sims'

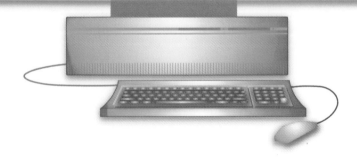

Answer: 2

Test-Taking Strategy: Use knowledge regarding anatomy and the anatomical location of the liver to answer the question. Recalling that the liver is located on the right side of the upper abdomen will direct you to option 2. Remember following a liver biopsy, the client is positioned on the right side for a minimum of 2 hours to splint the puncture site and prevent bleeding.

Physiological Adaptation

In the Physiological Adaptation subcategory, content may include the following*:

- Alterations in body systems
- Basic pathophysiology
- Fluid and electrolyte imbalances
- Infectious diseases
- Medical emergencies
- Radiation therapy
- Unexpected responses to therapy

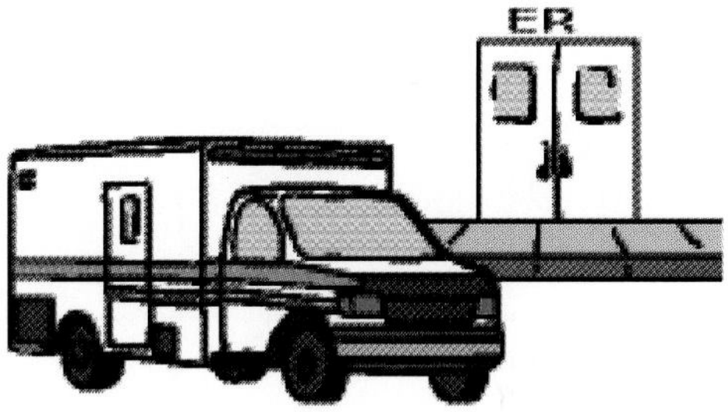

An example of a question that addresses this subcategory is provided below.

Question: Physiological Adaptation

A nurse is reviewing the medical records of the four clients that she will be caring for. The nurse determines that which client is at risk for deficient fluid volume?

1. A client on long-term corticosteroid therapy
2. A client with congestive heart failure
3. A client with syndrome of inappropriate antidiuretic hormone
4. A client with a nasogastric tube attached to suction

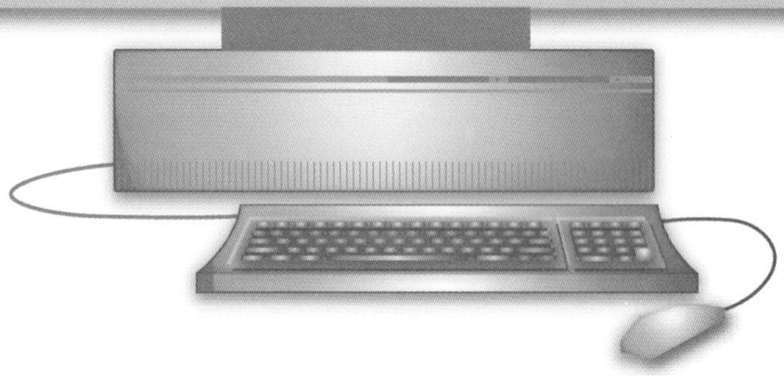

Answer: 4

Test-Taking Strategy: Focus on the issue, *the client at risk for deficient fluid volume.* Think about the pathophysiology associated with each condition identified in the options. The only client that loses fluid is the client with a nasogastric tube attached to suction.

REFERENCES

DeWit, S. (2005). *Fundamental concepts and skills for nursing* (2nd ed). Philadelphia: Saunders.
Hodgson, B. & Kizior, R. (2005). *Saunders nursing drug handbook 2005.* Philadelphia: Saunders.
Linton, A. & Maebius, N. (2003). *Introduction to medical-surgical nursing* (3rd ed). Philadelphia: Saunders.
National Council of State Boards of Nursing, Inc. *Test Plan for the National Council Licensure Examination for Licensed Practical/Vocational Nurses* (effective date: April 2005), National Council of State Boards of Nursing, Chicago, 2004.
National Council of State Boards of Nursing, Inc. online: Available at www.ncsbn.org
Potter, P. & Perry, A. (2005). *Fundamentals of nursing* (6th ed). St. Louis: Mosby.

Chapter 4 Integrated Processes

The National Council of State Boards of Nursing (NCSBN) identifies four processes that are fundamental to the practice of nursing. These processes are a component of the test plan and are integrated throughout the four categories of Client Needs that include Safe Effective Care Environment, Health Promotion and Maintenance, Psychosocial Integrity, and Physiological Integrity. The Integrated Processes are caring, clinical problem-solving process (nursing process including data collection, planning, implementation, and evaluation), communication and documentation, and teaching and learning.

INTEGRATED PROCESSES

- Caring
- Clinical problem-solving process
- Communication and documentation
- Teaching and learning

CARING

Caring is the essence of nursing and is basic to any helping relationship. Caring is central to every encounter that a nurse may have with a client. Through caring, the nurse humanizes the client. Treating the client with respect and dignity is a true expression of caring. In the technological environment of health care, emphasizing the client's individuality counteracts any potential process of depersonalization. Caring is an Integrated Process of the test plan for NCLEX-PN®. This means that this concept is nuclear to all Client Needs components of the test plan.

On NCLEX-PN, the concept of caring is primary. It is very easy for you to become involved with looking at a question from a technological viewpoint; you need to think about the concept of caring when reading a test question and when selecting an option. Remember that this examination is all about nursing, and that nursing is caring!

A sample question is provided below.

Question: Integrated Process/Caring

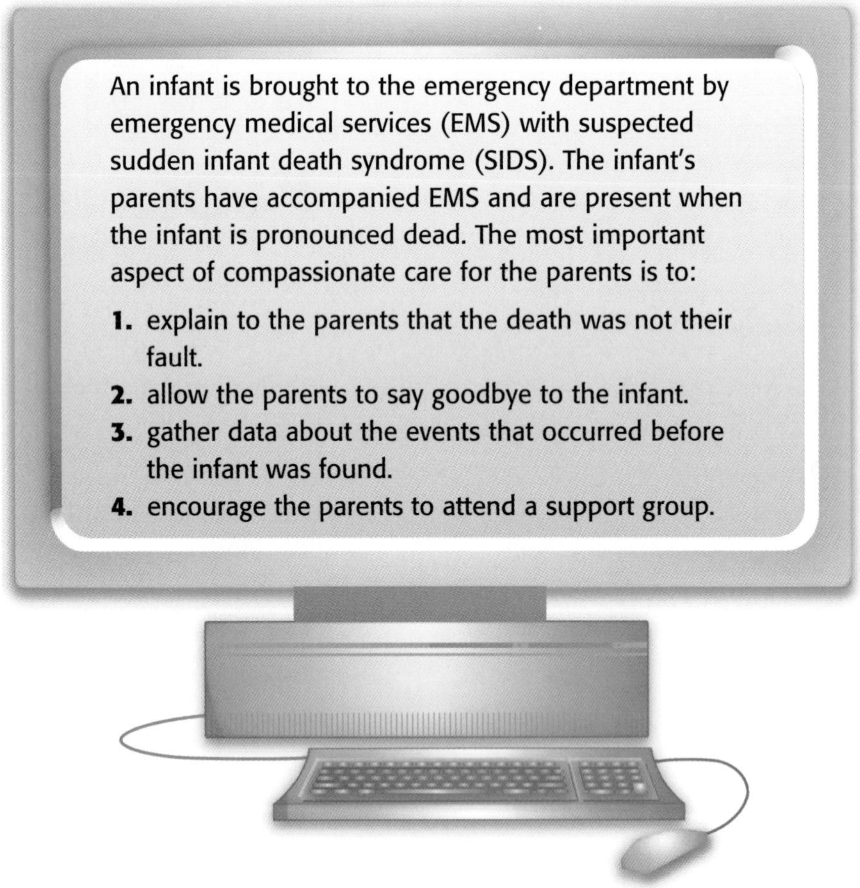
An infant is brought to the emergency department by emergency medical services (EMS) with suspected sudden infant death syndrome (SIDS). The infant's parents have accompanied EMS and are present when the infant is pronounced dead. The most important aspect of compassionate care for the parents is to:
1. explain to the parents that the death was not their fault.
2. allow the parents to say goodbye to the infant.
3. gather data about the events that occurred before the infant was found.
4. encourage the parents to attend a support group.

Answer: 2

Test-Taking Strategy: Focus on the issue, *compassionate care.* This will direct you to option 2 because it is the only option that addresses the issue. The nurse gathers data about the events that occurred before the infant was found, asks factual questions that avoid placing guilt on the parents, and encourages the parents to attend a support group; however, these interventions are not specifically related to the aspect of compassionate care. Remember that the concept of caring is primary, and that nursing is caring!

CLINICAL PROBLEM-SOLVING PROCESS (NURSING PROCESS)

The steps of the clinical problem-solving process (nursing process) include data collection, planning, implementation, and evaluation. These steps are extremely useful when answering questions that require you to prioritize. Following the steps of the clinical problem-solving process will guide you to the correct option.

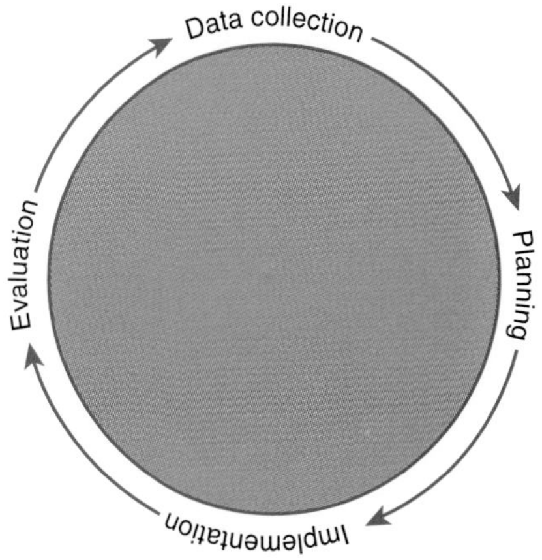

Data Collection

Data collection is the first step of the clinical problem-solving process (nursing process). In the process of data collection, the nurse participates in a systematic method of establishing a database regarding the client. This step includes gathering information relative to the client, communicating information gained in data collection, and contributing to the formulation of nursing diagnoses. The database provides the foundation for the remaining steps of the clinical problem-solving process.

Data collection begins with the first contact with the client. During all successive contacts, the nurse continues to collect information that is significant to the needs of the client. With each contact, the nurse uses all of the senses to gather data about the client.

During the process of data collection, the nurse collects data about the client from a variety of sources. The client is the primary source of data. Family members or significant others are secondary sources of data, and these sources may supplement or verify information provided by the client. Data may also be obtained from the client's record through the medical history, laboratory results, and diagnostic reports. Medical records from previous admissions may also provide additional client data. The nurse may also consult with other health care team members who had contact with the client.

The information collected by the nurse includes both subjective and objective data. Subjective data include the information that the client states and are based on the client's opinion. Objective data are the observable, measurable pieces of information about the client. Objective data include measurements such as vital signs or laboratory findings, and information obtained from observation of the client. Objective data also include clinical manifestations such as the signs and symptoms of an illness or disease.

> Subjective data include the information given by the client.
> Objective data are the observable, measurable pieces of information about the client.

In the process of data collection, the nurse is responsible for recognizing significant findings in the client, determining the need for additional information, reporting findings to relevant members of the health care team, and documenting findings thoroughly and accurately.

The nurse contributes to the formulation of nursing diagnoses by assisting in organizing relevant health care data and by assisting in determining significant relationships between data and client needs and problems.

When answering a test question, if the question requires you to prioritize, remember that data collection is the first step of the clinical problem-solving process. If a question is asking to identify the initial or first action, and a data collection action is presented in one of the options, then that option is most likely the correct one. However, a possible exception to this guideline is if the question presents an emergency situation. If the question addresses an emergency situation, read the information carefully. In an emergency situation, an intervention rather than the collection of data may be the priority!

Data collection is the first step of the clinical problem-solving process (nursing process).

If you are asked to identify the initial or first action, follow the steps of the nursing process; if a data collection action is presented as one of the options, that option is most likely correct.

If the question addresses an emergency situation, read carefully; an intervention may be the priority.

A sample question is provided below.

Question: Integrated Process: Nursing Process/Data Collection

A postoperative client asks a nurse for pain medication. The nurse should take which action first?

1. Ask the client how long it has been since the last dose of pain medication was administered.
2. Gather data from the client about the pain.
3. Prepare the prescribed dose of pain medication.
4. Ask the client if the last dose of the medication was effective.

Answer: 2

Test-Taking Strategy: Use the steps of the clinical problem-solving process (nursing process) and remember that data collection is the first step. This will assist in eliminating option 3 because this option relates to implementing rather than collecting data. From the remaining options, focus on the word "first." Option 1 can be eliminated because the nurse would not ask the client how long it has been since the last dose of pain medication; the nurse would check the client's medication record for this information. Although option 4 is an appropriate action it does not focus on the issue of the question, *that the client asks for pain medication.* Also, note the relationship between the issue and option 2.

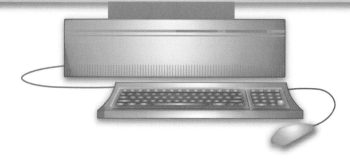

Planning

Planning is the second step of the clinical problem-solving process. In this step, the nurse provides input into plan development, participates in setting goals for meeting the client's needs, and participates in designing strategies to achieve these goals.

This step involves the functions of setting priorities, assisting in determining goals and outcome criteria for goals of care, assisting in developing the plan of care, collaborating with other health team members, and communicating the plan of care. Setting priorities assists the nurse to organize and plan care that solves the most urgent problems. Priorities may change as the client's level of wellness changes. Both actual and risk for (potential) problems should be considered when establishing priorities.

Once priorities are established, the client and nurse mutually decide on the expected goals. The goals serve as a guide in the selection of nursing interventions and in determining the criteria for evaluation of goal achievement. Before implementing nursing actions, the nurse should assist in establishing mechanisms to determine goal achievement and the effectiveness of nursing interventions. Unless criteria have been predetermined, it is difficult to know whether the goal is achieved and the problem is resolved. It is important for the nurse to identify health or social resources available to the client and to collaborate with other health care team members when planning the delivery of care. The nurse needs to communicate the plan of care, review the plan of care with the client, and document the plan of care thoroughly and accurately.

When answering a test question, keep in mind that actual problems are usually more important than risk for (potential) problems. However, read the question carefully because, at times, risk for (potential) problems may take precedence over actual problems. Also, remember that the examination that you will take is a nursing examination, not a medical examination. Therefore, the answer to the question most likely involves something that is included in the nursing care plan rather than the medical plan, unless the question specifically asks you what prescription (medical order) is anticipated.

Planning is the second step of the clinical problem-solving process (nursing process).

Planning involves setting priorities, assisting in determining goals and outcome criteria for goals of care, assisting in developing the plan of care, collaborating with other health team members, and communicating the plan of care.

A sample question is provided below.

Question: Integrated Process: Nursing Process/Planning

A nurse is reviewing the nursing diagnoses written in a nursing care plan for a client with chronic obstructive pulmonary disease. The nurse determines that which nursing diagnosis is the priority?

1. Ineffective Role Performance related to role loss
2. Disturbed Thought Processes related to sleep deprivation
3. Anxiety related to loss of control during dyspneic episodes
4. Imbalanced Nutrition: Less Than Body Requirements related to dyspnea and fatigue

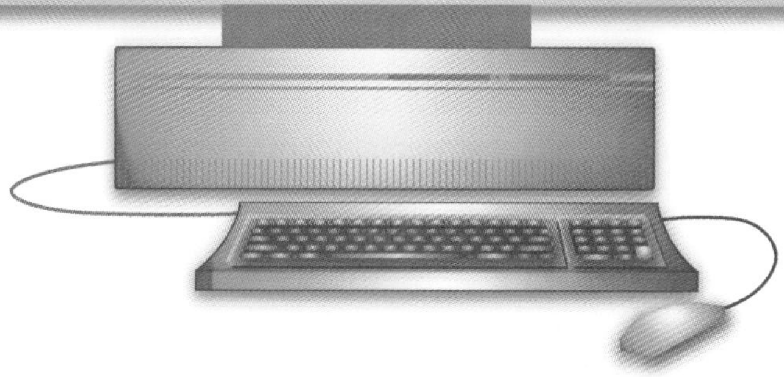

Answer: 4

Test-Taking Strategy: Note the key word "priority." Maslow's Hierarchy of Needs theory can be used as a guide to answer this question. (Refer to Chapter 9 for information about Maslow's Hierarchy of Needs theory.) According to Maslow's theory, physiological needs are the priority. This will direct you to option 4. Options 1, 2, and 3 are psychosocial needs and are a lesser priority than physiological needs. Remember physiological needs are the priority.

Implementation

Implementation is the third step of the clinical problem-solving process (nursing process) and includes initiating and completing nursing actions required to accomplish the defined goals. This step is the action phase that involves assisting with organizing and managing client care; providing care to achieve established goals; and communicating and documenting the nursing interventions and client responses.

This step also includes the role of encouraging the client to follow the prescribed treatment plan and assisting the client to maintain optimal functioning. Additionally the process of implementation includes monitoring client care administered by unlicensed nursing personnel, and reinforcing teaching on principles, procedures, and techniques required for the maintenance and promotion of health.

During implementation, the nurse uses intellectual skills, interpersonal skills, and technical skills. Intellectual skills involve problem solving and making judgments. Interpersonal skills involve the ability to communicate, listen, and convey compassion. Technical skills relate to the performance of treatments, procedures, and the use of necessary equipment when providing care to the client.

INTELLECTUAL SKILLS

Problem solving

Making judgments

INTERPERSONAL SKILLS

Ability to communicate

Ability to listen

Ability to convey compassion

TECHNICAL SKILLS

Performing treatments and procedures

Using the necessary equipment when providing care to the client

The implementation step concludes when the nurse's actions are completed and these actions, including their effects and the client's response, are communicated and documented.

The client presented in the test question is your only assigned client. When you are selecting an option, remember that you are caring for one and only one client, unless the question indicates that you are caring for multiple clients. For example, if a question asks for the best nursing action for a client who is anxious about surgery, which is scheduled later in the day, do not be reluctant to select the option that addresses staying with the client until the time of surgery. Remember, this is your only assigned client so implement what is best for the client!

You need to answer the question from a textbook and ideal perspective, rather than a reality one. Remember, always follow the textbook guidelines and principles when carrying out procedures and performing interventions!

Answer the question, remembering that you have all the time needed and the resources and supplies needed readily available at the client's bedside. For example, if a question addresses a client with cardiac disease who experiences chest pain, remember that you have all of the supplies if needed for that client (such as nitroglycerin and a blood pressure machine) readily available and that you will not need to waste time obtaining these supplies from other hospital areas.

Implementation is the third step of the clinical problem-solving process (nursing process).
The client in the test question is your only assigned client.
The client in the test question is the only client you need to be concerned about.
Answer the question from a textbook and ideal perspective, rather than a reality one.
Answer the question, remembering that you have all the time, resources, and supplies needed and readily available at the client's bedside.

A sample question is provided below.

Question: Integrated Process: Nursing Process/ Implementation

A nurse is assisting in monitoring a client following a cardiac catheterization procedure. The client suddenly complains of a feeling of wetness at the injection site. The nurse quickly checks the site and discovers that the client is bleeding. The best initial nursing action is to:

1. apply firm pressure to the site using a sterile gauze pad.
2. apply firm pressure to the site using a bath towel.
3. ask the client to place pressure on the site.
4. check the client's blood pressure.

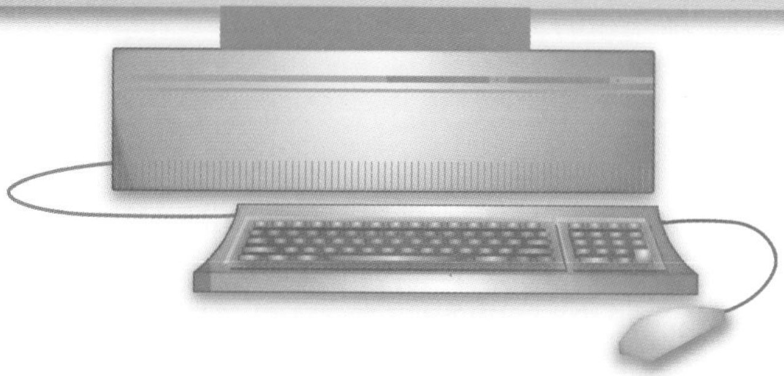

Answer: 1

Test-Taking Strategy: Note the key words "best initial nursing action." These words may indicate that more than one or all of the options are correct and that you need to prioritize the actions. Option 3 can be eliminated because the nurse would not ask a client to apply pressure to the site in this situation; this is the nurse's responsibility. Although option 4 is correct, it is not the initial action. From the remaining options, select option 1 because using a sterile gauze pad to apply pressure is the best action to prevent an infection. Remember that all of your needed supplies are readily available at the client's bedside.

Evaluation

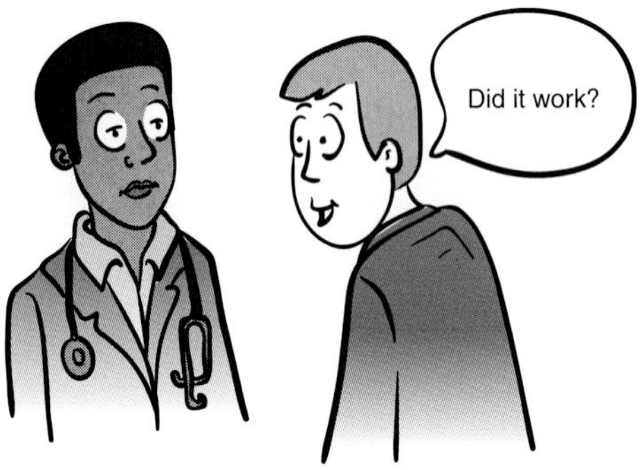

Evaluation is the fourth and final step of the clinical problem-solving process (nursing process). Evaluation is a way of measuring client progress toward meeting goals.

Although evaluation is the final step of the nursing process, it is an ongoing and integral component of each step. The process of data collection is reviewed to determine if sufficient information was obtained, and if the information obtained was specific and appropriate. The plan and expected outcomes are examined to determine whether they are realistic, achievable, time-referenced, measurable, and effective. Interventions are examined to determine their effectiveness in achieving the expected outcomes.

Since evaluation is an ongoing process, it is vital to all steps of the clinical problem-solving process (nursing process). It is the continuous process of comparing actual outcomes with expected ones, and it provides the means for determining the need to modify the plan of care. Inherent in this step of the nursing process are the communication of evaluation findings and the process of documenting and reporting the client's response to treatment, care, and teaching to relevant members of the health care team.

Evaluation questions may be written to compare actual outcomes of care with the expected outcomes, how the nurse should monitor or make a judgment concerning a client's response to therapy or to a nursing action, or to determine a client's understanding of the prescribed treatment measures. Evaluation questions are frequently written in a false response format. For example, the question may ask for a client statement that indicates inaccurate information related to the issue of the question.

Evaluation is the fourth step of the clinical problem solving process (nursing process).
Evaluation is a continual process of comparing actual outcomes with expected ones.
Evaluation provides the means for determining the need to modify the plan of care.

A sample question is provided below.

Question: Integrated Process: Nursing Process/Evaluation

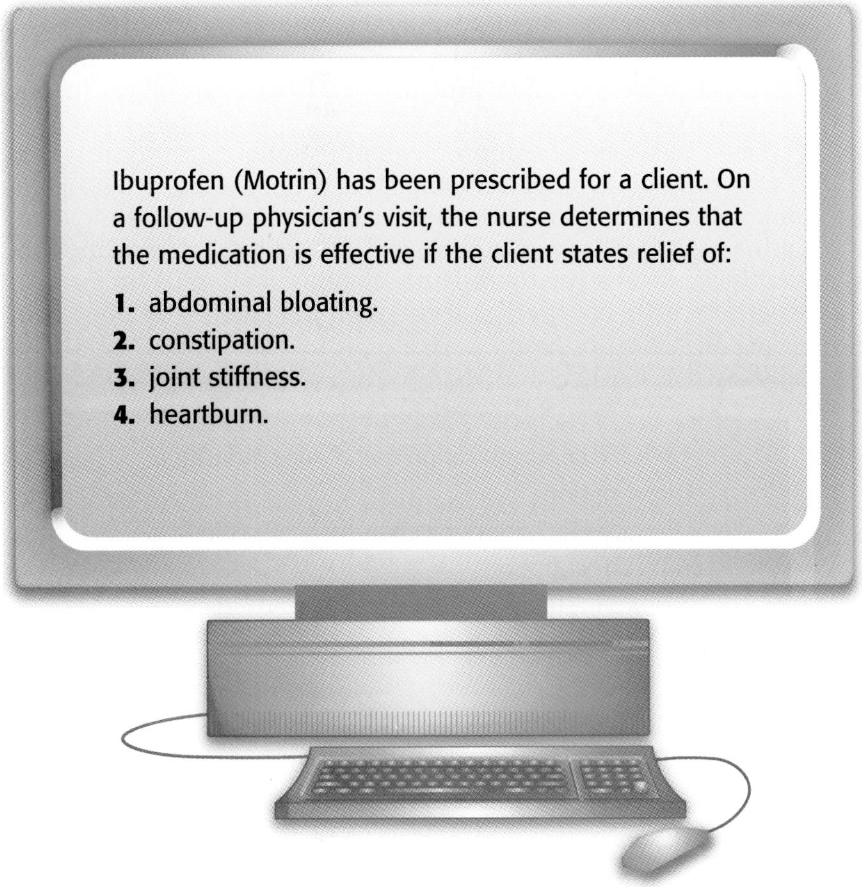
Ibuprofen (Motrin) has been prescribed for a client. On a follow-up physician's visit, the nurse determines that the medication is effective if the client states relief of:
1. abdominal bloating.
2. constipation.
3. joint stiffness.
4. heartburn.

Answer: 3

Test-Taking Strategy: Medication questions can be difficult to answer correctly if you are unfamiliar with the medication. Knowing that ibuprofen is a nonsteroidal antiinflammatory medication that may be used to treat rheumatoid disorders will assist in answering the question. If you did not know this, use the process of elimination, noting that options 1, 2, and 4 are similar in that they all relate to the gastrointestinal system. Options that are similar are incorrect!

COMMUNICATION AND DOCUMENTATION

Communication

The process of communication occurs as the nurse interacts with a client or the client's family member or significant others. Communication-type test questions are integrated throughout the NCLEX-PN test plan and may address a situation in any health care setting.

Use of therapeutic communication techniques is key to an effective nurse-client relationship. When answering a test question, select the option that identifies use of a therapeutic communication technique and avoid selecting an option that identifies use of a nontherapeutic communication technique. Always select the option that focuses on the client's feelings, concerns, anxieties, or fears.

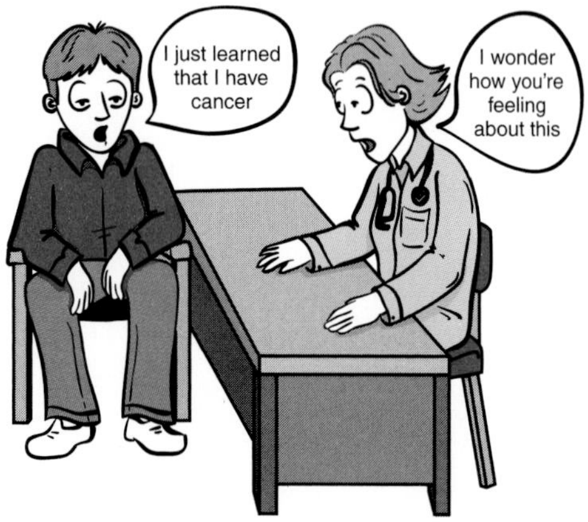
I just learned that I have cancer
I wonder how you're feeling about this

Therapeutic communication techniques indicate a correct option.
Nontherapeutic communication techniques indicate an incorrect option.
If an option reflects a client's feelings, anxieties, or concerns, select that option.

A sample question is provided below.

Question: Integrated Process: Communication

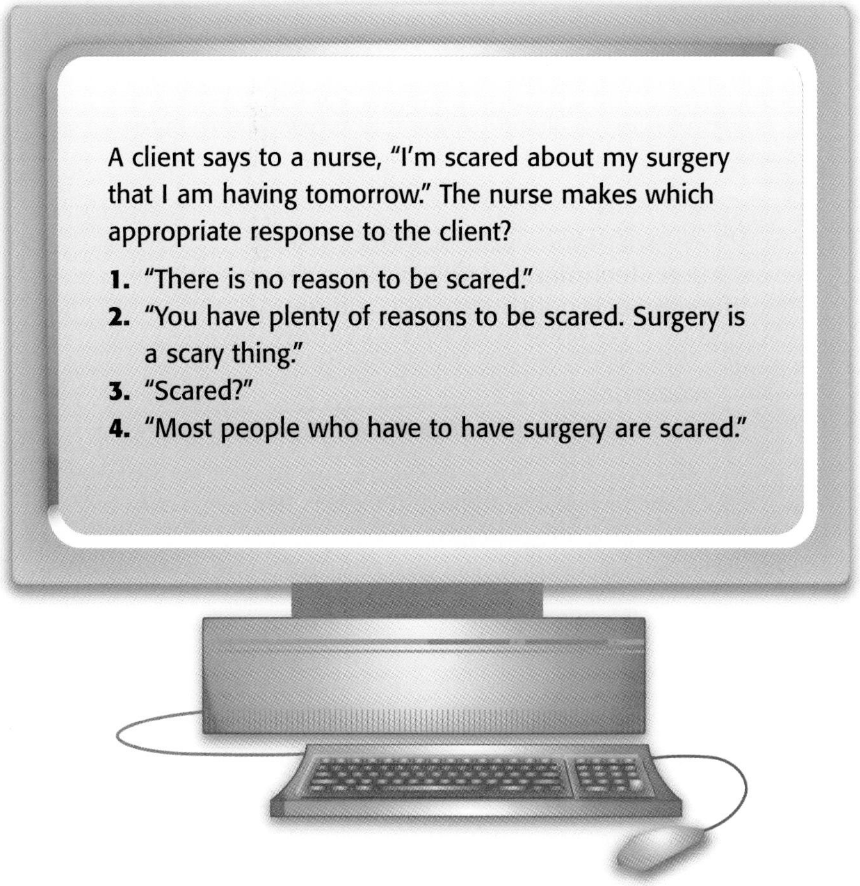
A client says to a nurse, "I'm scared about my surgery that I am having tomorrow." The nurse makes which appropriate response to the client?
1. "There is no reason to be scared."
2. "You have plenty of reasons to be scared. Surgery is a scary thing."
3. "Scared?"
4. "Most people who have to have surgery are scared."

Answer: 3

Test-Taking Strategy: Use therapeutic communication techniques to direct you to option 3. In option 3 the nurse uses the therapeutic technique of reflection to encourage the client to further discuss the scared feelings. Options 1, 2, and 4 are examples of nontherapeutic communication techniques. Option 1 uses false reassurance. Option 2 will escalate the client's fear about surgery. Option 4 belittles the client's expressed feelings. Remember, therapeutic communication techniques indicate a correct option.

Documentation

Documentation is a critical component of a nurse's responsibility. The process of documentation serves many purposes and provides a comprehensive representation of the client's health status and the care given by all members of the health care team. There are many methods for documenting, but the responsibilities surrounding this practice remain the same.

The ethical and legal responsibilities related to documentation and the specific guidelines and principles related to both narrative and computerized documentation systems are important areas to review.

A sample question is provided below.

Question: Integrated Process: Documentation

A nurse discovers that she needs to make a correction to a written entry in a client's chart. The nurse would appropriately:

1. contact the nursing supervisor to cosign the correction.
2. remove the page, recopy the data to a new page, and add the correct entry.
3. draw a single line through the entry that needs correction followed by his or her (the nurse's) initials.
4. erase the entry that needs correction and add the correct entry.

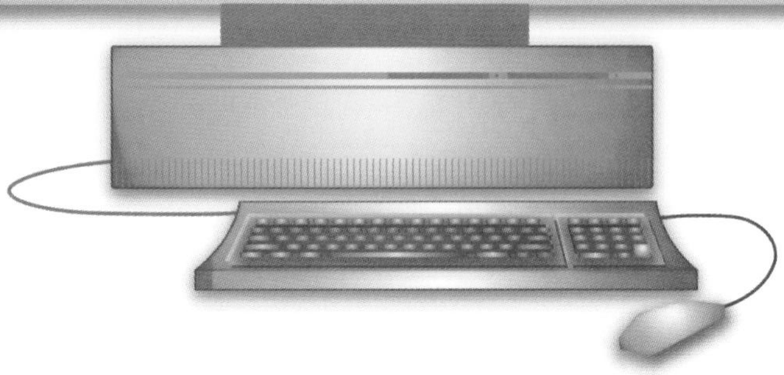

Answer: 3

Test-Taking Strategy: Use guidelines and principles related to documentation to answer this question. This will direct you to option 3. There are no useful reasons for options 1 and 2. The nurse would never erase an entry made in a client's chart. Remember to review the guidelines and principles related to both narrative and computerized documentation systems.

TEACHING and LEARNING

Client and family education is a primary nursing responsibility. The licensed practical or vocational nurse may need to teach a client about self-care needs related to activities of daily living or may need to reinforce a teaching plan initiated by the registered nurse. Remember that determination of the client's readiness and the client's motivation to learn is the initial step in the teaching and learning process. Always use the principles related to teaching and learning theory to answer a question related to teaching and learning. Frequently, these types of questions ask what the nurse would teach the client or what observation by the nurse indicates that the client needs teaching.

> If a test question addresses client teaching, remember that client motivation and client readiness to learn is the *first* priority.

A sample question related to teaching and learning is presented following the content identifying teaching and learning principles.

Teaching and Learning Principles

There are many teaching and learning principles that a nurse should use, including the following:

- The nurse needs to determine the client's readiness and motivation to learn and the client's learning needs.
- The nurse needs to collect data about the client's existing knowledge of the information to be presented and plan teaching on that knowledge.
- The ability to learn depends on the client's physical and cognitive abilities.
- The nurse needs to consider the client's health beliefs and how they will influence the client's willingness to learn.
- The nurse needs to consider the client's age, developmental level, and educational level, and use teaching strategies based on these factors.
- Learning objectives facilitate the teaching process and identify what the client is to learn.
- The client should be an active participant in the teaching and learning process.
- The nurse should include the client's spouse, significant other, or another family member in the learning process if appropriate.

Continued

TEACHING TOOLS

Pamphlets, booklets, brochures
Diagrams, graphs, charts, pictures
Slides, audiotapes, videotapes, television
Physical objects
Programmed instruction
Computer instruction

- The nurse should use a combination of teaching methods (cognitive, affective, and psychomotor) and teaching tools to improve client attentiveness and involvement.
- The nurse should allow ample time for the client to understand the material taught.
- The nurse should evaluate a client's learning by observing the client's performance of the behavior.

Question: Integrated Process: Teaching and Learning

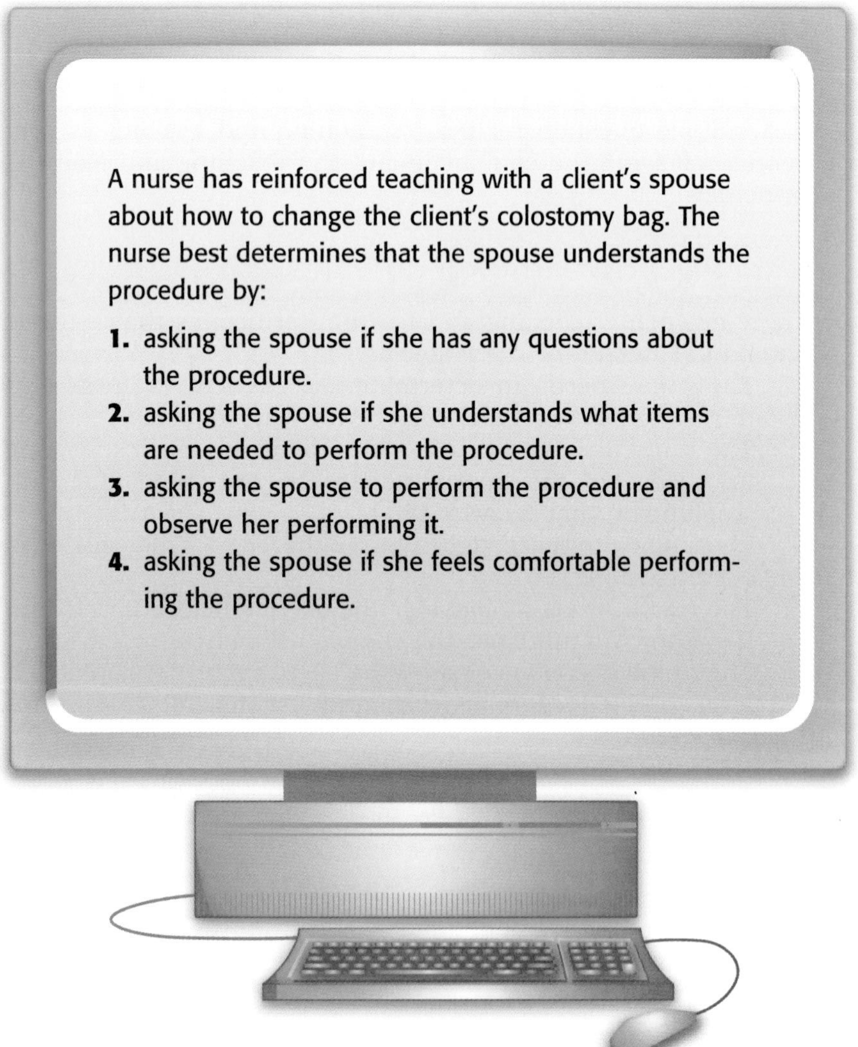

A nurse has reinforced teaching with a client's spouse about how to change the client's colostomy bag. The nurse best determines that the spouse understands the procedure by:

1. asking the spouse if she has any questions about the procedure.
2. asking the spouse if she understands what items are needed to perform the procedure.
3. asking the spouse to perform the procedure and observe her performing it.
4. asking the spouse if she feels comfortable performing the procedure.

Answer: 3

Test-Taking Strategy: Note the key word "best" in the stem of the question and focus on the issue, *the spouse's ability to perform a procedure.* The nurse would best evaluate learning by observing the performance of the behavior. Although options 1, 2, and 4 are questions that the nurse would ask, they do not evaluate the spouse's ability to perform the procedure. Remember, use teaching and learning principles when answering these questions.

REFERENCES

DeWit, S. (2005). *Fundamental concepts and skills for nursing* (2nd ed). Philadelphia: Saunders.

Hodgson, B. & Kizior, R. (2005). *Saunders nursing drug handbook 2005.* Philadelphia: Saunders.

Linton, A. & Maebius, N. (2003). *Introduction to medical-surgical nursing* (3rd ed). Philadelphia: Saunders.

National Council of State Boards of Nursing, Inc. *Test Plan for the National Council Licensure Examination for Licensed Practical/ Vocational Nurses* (effective date: April 2005), National Council of State Boards of Nursing, Chicago, 2004.

National Council of State Boards of Nursing, Inc. online: Available at www.ncsbn.org

Potter, P. & Perry, A. (2005). *Fundamentals of nursing* (6th ed). St. Louis: Mosby.

Chapter 5

Types of Questions on the Examination

The types of questions that may be administered to you when you take this examination include multiple choice, fill in the blank, multiple response, prioritizing (ordered response), questions that contain a figure or illustration (hot spots), and a chart/exhibit type of question.

TYPES OF QUESTIONS ON THE EXAMINATION

- Multiple choice
- Fill in the blank
- Multiple response
- Prioritizing (ordered response)
- Figure or illustration (hot spots)
- Chart/exhibit

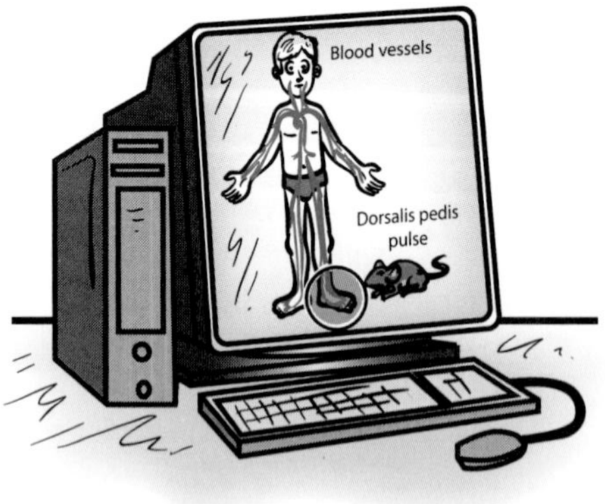

Some questions, such as those that present a figure or illustration, may require you to use the computer's mouse. For example, you may be presented with a figure that displays the arterial vessels of an adult client. In this figure, you may be asked to point and click (using the mouse) on the area (represented by a circle and also known as the hot spot) where the dorsalis pedis pulse can be felt.

The National Council of State Boards of Nursing (NCSBN) provides specific directions for you to follow with these questions. Be sure to read these directions as they appear on the computer screen.

Follow the directions that appear with a question carefully!

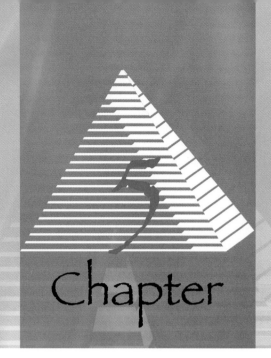

MULTIPLE CHOICE QUESTIONS

Most of the questions that you will be asked to answer will be in the multiple choice format. These questions will provide you with data about a particular client situation and four answers or options. You are probably familiar with this type of question.

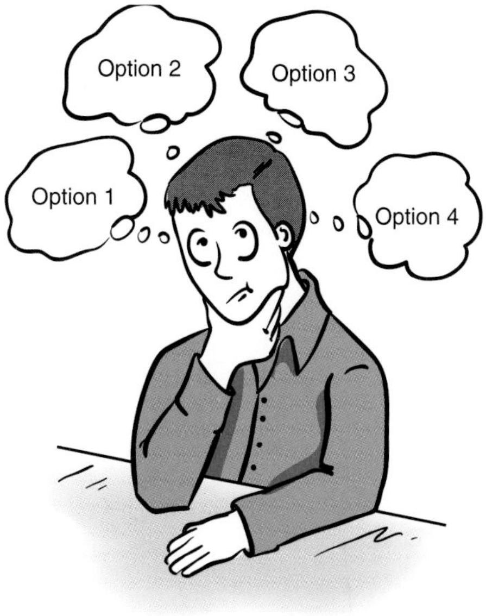

> Most questions will be in a multiple choice format!

Below is an example of a multiple choice question.

Types of Questions: Multiple Choice

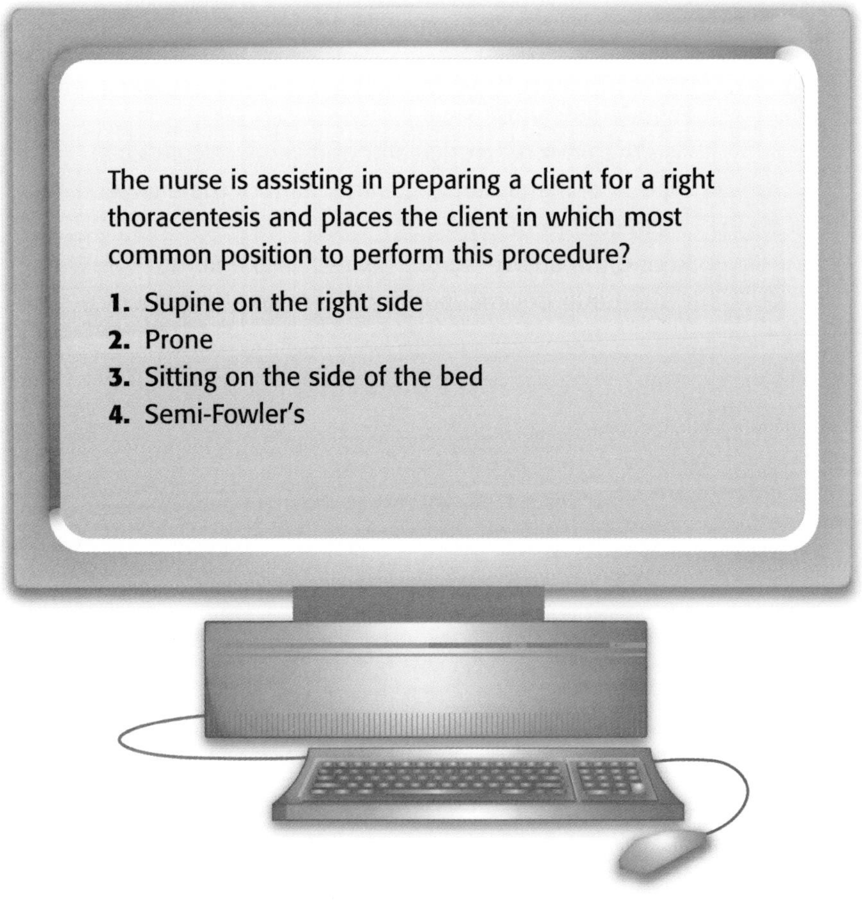

The nurse is assisting in preparing a client for a right thoracentesis and places the client in which most common position to perform this procedure?

1. Supine on the right side
2. Prone
3. Sitting on the side of the bed
4. Semi-Fowler's

Answer: 3

Test-Taking Strategy: First, think about what this procedure entails. If you are not sure, use medical terminology skills recalling that *thora-* relates to the lung and *-centesis* relates to removal of fluid. Visualize this procedure and note that the client will have a right thoracentesis. Also, recall that gravity allows fluid to accumulate in the lower thoracic cavity. This will help you to eliminate options 1, 2, and 4.

FILL-IN-THE BLANK QUESTIONS

Most of these types of questions will ask you to perform a medication calculation, calculate an intravenous flow rate, or calculate an intake or output record on a client. You will need to type in your answer. When answering these types of questions, two things are very important. First, follow the directions on the computer screen. In a medication calculation question, the directions may indicate to type in only the numeric component of the answer if the question requires a calculation. In other words, if the answer to a question is 2.5 mL, type only 2.5 if the directions indicate to do so. In an intravenous flow rate question, the directions may indicate to round the answer to the nearest whole number or the tenth decimal position. For example, if the answer is 21.4 drops per minute, type the answer as 21. Second, use the on-screen calculator for your calculations; then use the erasable note board provided to you for testing to recalculate and verify your answer.

FILL-IN-THE-BLANK QUESTIONS

- Follow directions!
- Use the on-screen calculator and verify calculations.
- Type in only the numeric component of the answer if directed to do so.
- Round the answer to the nearest whole number or the tenth decimal position if directed to do so.

Below are examples of fill-in-the blank questions.

Types of Questions: Fill in the Blank

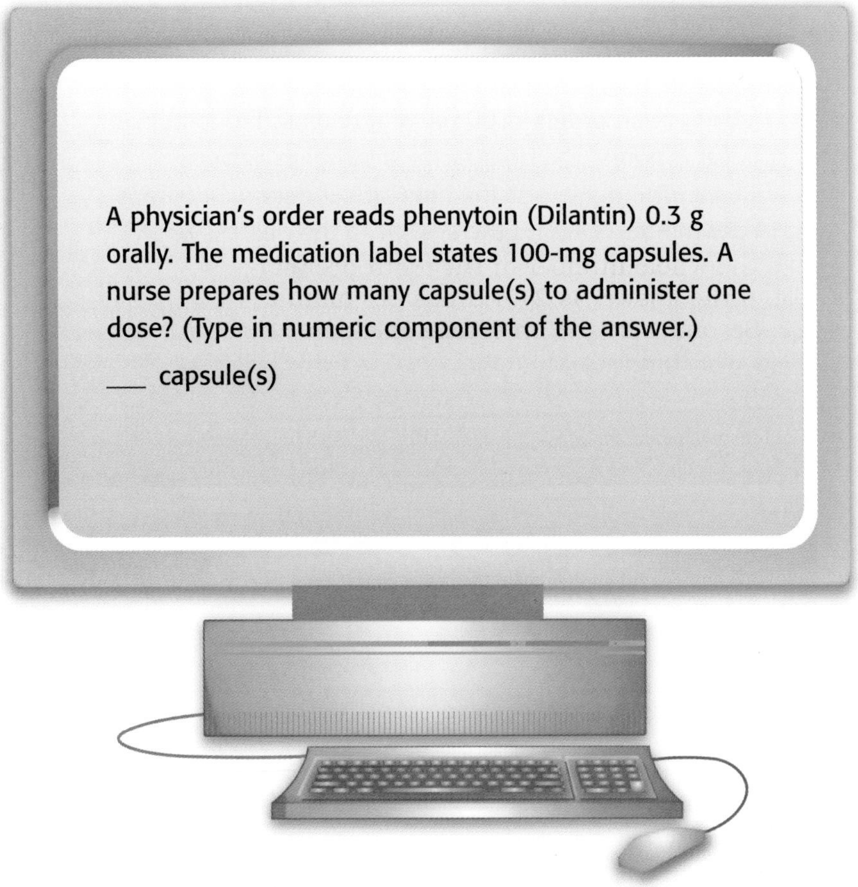
A physician's order reads phenytoin (Dilantin) 0.3 g orally. The medication label states 100-mg capsules. A nurse prepares how many capsule(s) to administer one dose? (Type in numeric component of the answer.)
___ capsule(s)

Answer: 3

Test-Taking Strategy: Read the information in the question and the directions and note that it is necessary to convert 0.3 gram (g) to milligram (mg). In the metric system, to convert larger (g) to smaller (mg) multiply by 1000 or move the decimal 3 places to the right. Therefore, 0.3 g = 300 mg. The nurse would prepare 3 capsules. Remember to use the on-screen calculator and verify your answer. As directed, type in the numeric component of the answer.

Types of Questions: Fill in the Blank

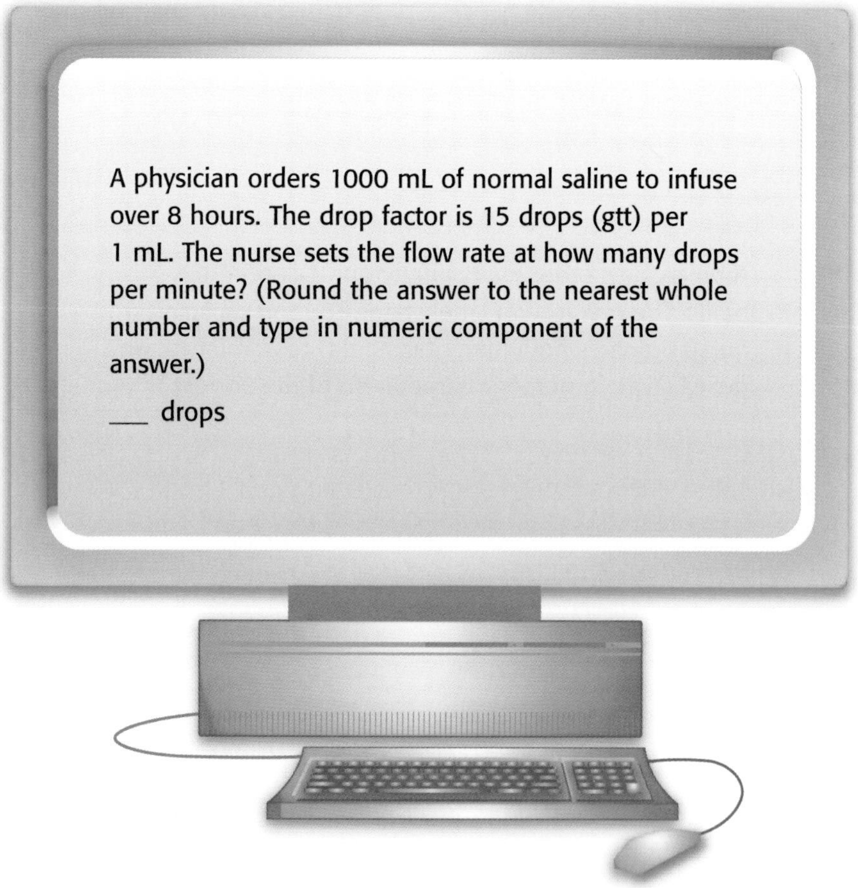

A physician orders 1000 mL of normal saline to infuse over 8 hours. The drop factor is 15 drops (gtt) per 1 mL. The nurse sets the flow rate at how many drops per minute? (Round the answer to the nearest whole number and type in numeric component of the answer.)
___ drops

Answer: 31

Test-Taking Strategy: Read the information in the question and the directions. Using the IV flow rate formula yields a result of 31.2 drops per minute. Rounding to the nearest whole number yields 31. Remember to use the on-screen calculator and verify your answer. As directed, type in the numeric component of the answer.

Types of Questions: Fill in the Blank

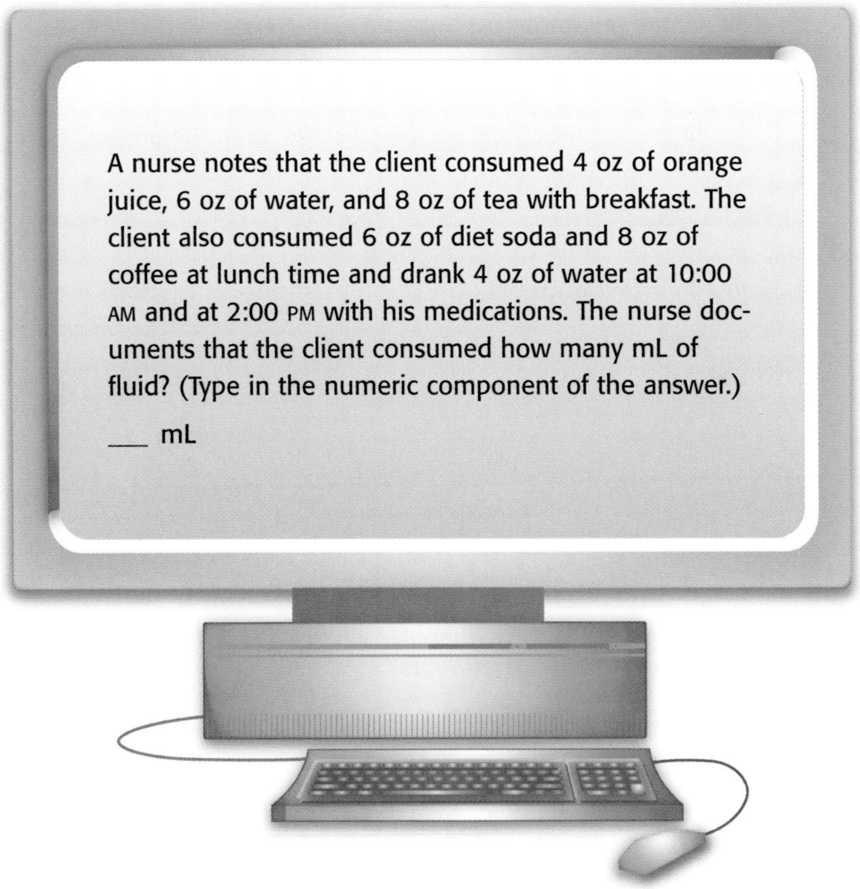
A nurse notes that the client consumed 4 oz of orange juice, 6 oz of water, and 8 oz of tea with breakfast. The client also consumed 6 oz of diet soda and 8 oz of coffee at lunch time and drank 4 oz of water at 10:00 AM and at 2:00 PM with his medications. The nurse documents that the client consumed how many mL of fluid? (Type in the numeric component of the answer.)
___ mL

Answer: 1200

Test-Taking Strategy: Focus on the information in the question and note that the client consumed a total of 40 ounces. Next note that the question requires determining the amount of mL consumed. Recall that 1 ounce equals 30 mL and multiply 40 ounces by 30 mL to yield 1200 mL. Remember to use the on-screen calculator and verify your answer. As directed, type in the numeric component of the answer.

MULTIPLE RESPONSE QUESTIONS

In this type of question, you will be asked to select or check all of the options, such as nursing interventions, that relate to the information in the question. There is no partial credit given for correct selections. You need to do exactly as the question asks, select *all* that apply.

MULTIPLE RESPONSE QUESTIONS

All correct options *only* must be selected in order for the answer to be correct.

If not all of the correct options are selected, then the answer is incorrect.

If any incorrect options are selected, then the answer is incorrect.

Below is an example of a multiple response question.

Types of Questions: Multiple Response

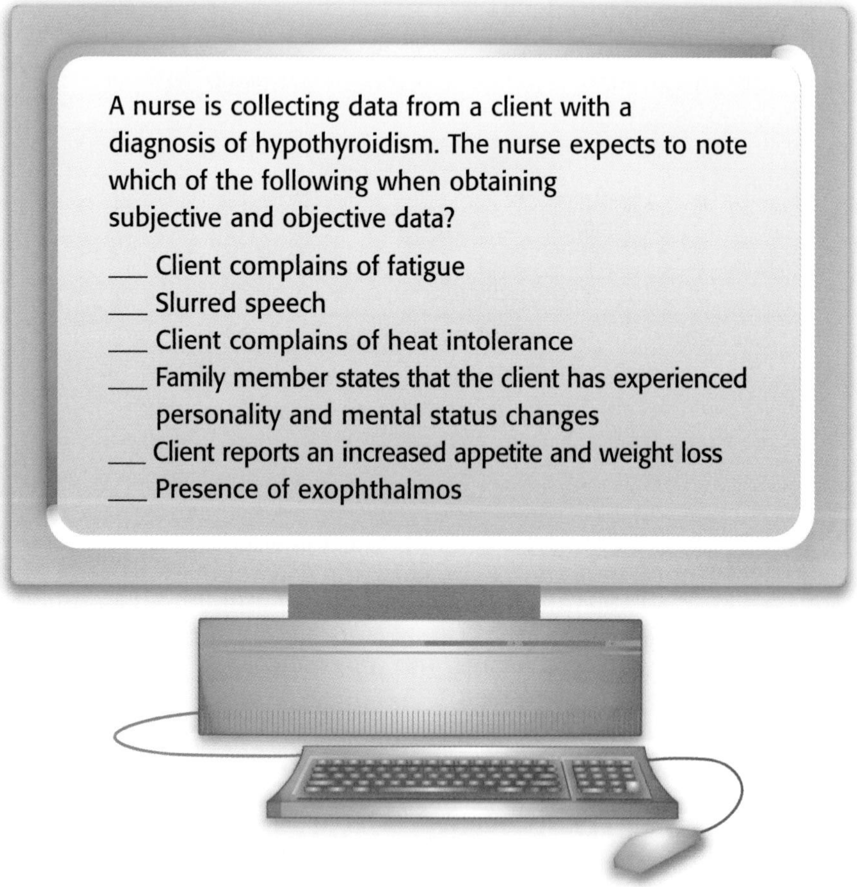
A nurse is collecting data from a client with a diagnosis of hypothyroidism. The nurse expects to note which of the following when obtaining subjective and objective data?
___ Client complains of fatigue
___ Slurred speech
___ Client complains of heat intolerance
___ Family member states that the client has experienced personality and mental status changes
___ Client reports an increased appetite and weight loss
___ Presence of exophthalmos

Answer:

X Client complains of fatigue
X Slurred speech
___ Client complains of heat intolerance
X Family member states that the client has experienced personality and mental status changes
___ Client reports an increased appetite and weight loss
___ Presence of exophthalmos

Test-Taking Strategy: Focus on the issue, *data collection findings in a client with a diagnosis of hypothyroidism (insufficient circulating thyroid hormone).* Recalling the action of the thyroid hormone and that hypothyroidism has a systemic effect that slows bodily processes will assist in selecting the correct options.

PRIORITIZING (ORDERED-RESPONSE) QUESTIONS

These questions may ask you to number or use the computer mouse to drag and drop your nursing actions in order of priority. Information is presented in a question and based on the data, you need to determine what you will do first, second, third, and so forth.

Below is an example of a prioritizing (ordered response) question.

Types of Questions: Prioritizing (Ordered Response)

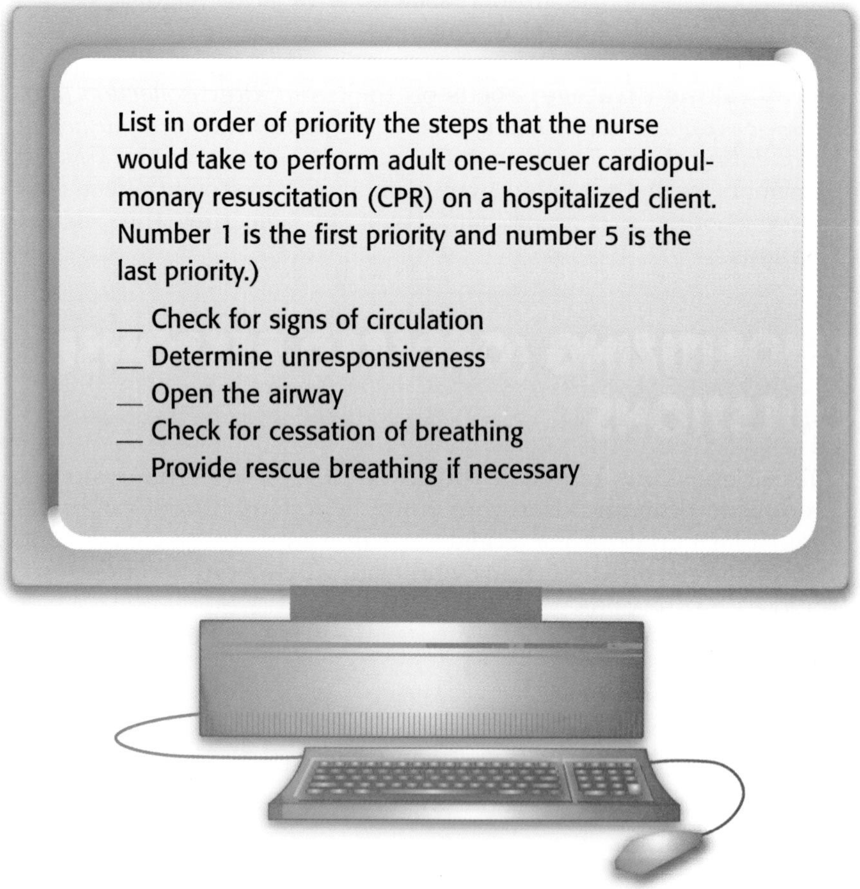
List in order of priority the steps that the nurse would take to perform adult one-rescuer cardiopulmonary resuscitation (CPR) on a hospitalized client. Number 1 is the first priority and number 5 is the last priority.)
__ Check for signs of circulation
__ Determine unresponsiveness
__ Open the airway
__ Check for cessation of breathing
__ Provide rescue breathing if necessary

Answer: 5, 1, 2, 3, 4

Test-Taking Strategy: First remember that determining unresponsiveness is a component of data collection and is the first step. From this point, use the ABCs—airway, breathing, and circulation—to determine the order of the remaining options.

FIGURE OR ILLUSTRATION

This type of question will provide you with a figure or illustration and will ask you to answer the question based on it. The question could contain a chart, table, or a figure or illustration. In this type of question, you may also be asked to use the computer mouse and point and click on a specific area (circle or hot spot) in the visual. Remember, a figure or illustration may appear in any type of question, including a multiple-choice question. Below is an example of a figure or illustration question.

Types of Questions: Figure or Illustration

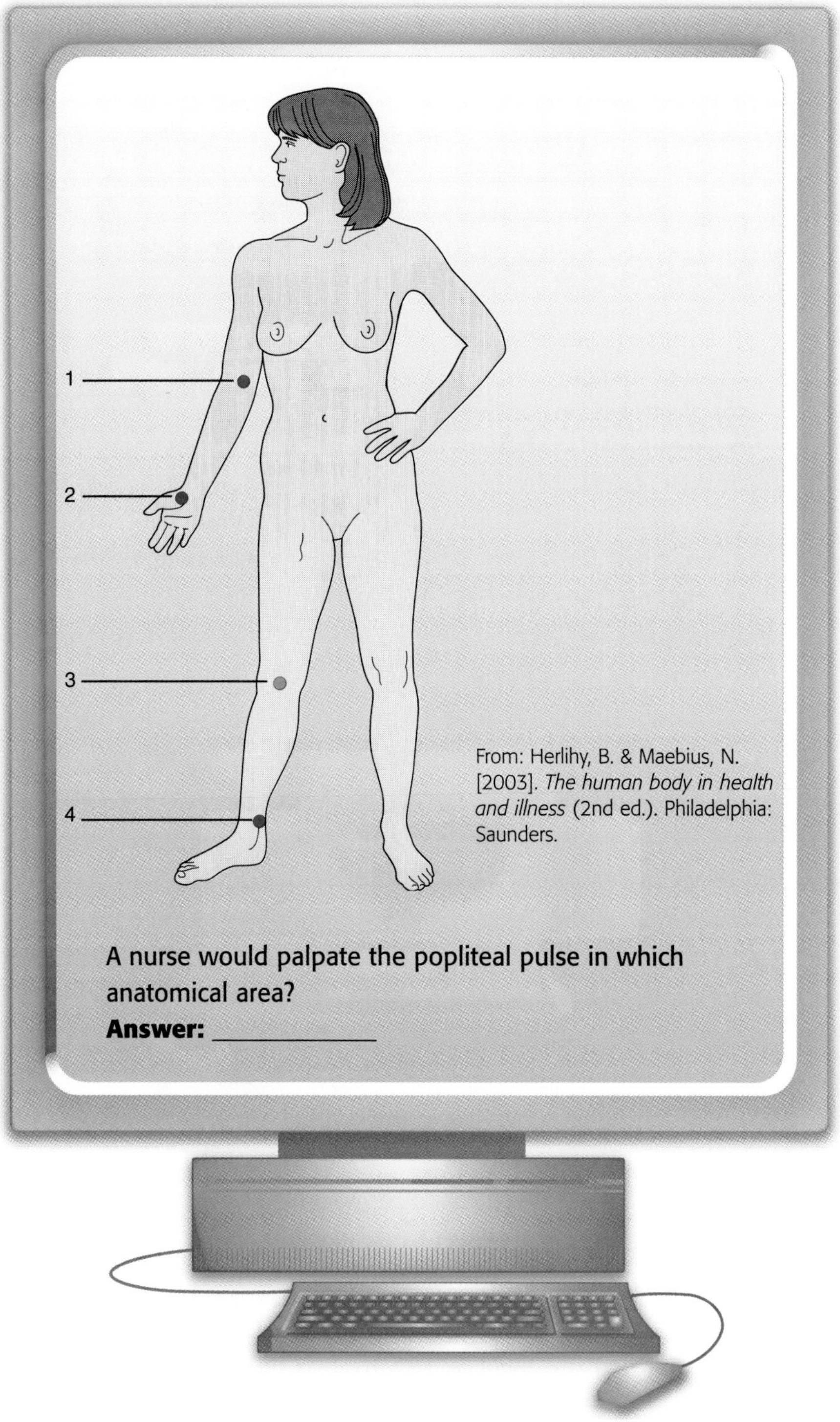
1
2
3
4
From: Herlihy, B. & Maebius, N. [2003]. *The human body in health and illness* (2nd ed.). Philadelphia: Saunders.
A nurse would palpate the popliteal pulse in which anatomical area?
Answer: ___________

Answer: 3

Test-Taking Strategy: Focus on the issue, *palpating the popliteal pulse.* Recalling that the popliteal pulse is located behind the knee will assist in answering the question correctly. Option 1 identifies the anatomical area for palpating the brachial pulse. Option 2 identifies the area for palpating the radial pulse. Option 4 identifies the area for palpating the posterior tibial pulse.

CHART/EXHIBIT

In this type of question, you will be presented with a question and a chart/exhibit. You will need to refer to the information in the chart/exhibit in order to answer the question. A sample question is presented below.

Types of Questions: Chart/Exhibit

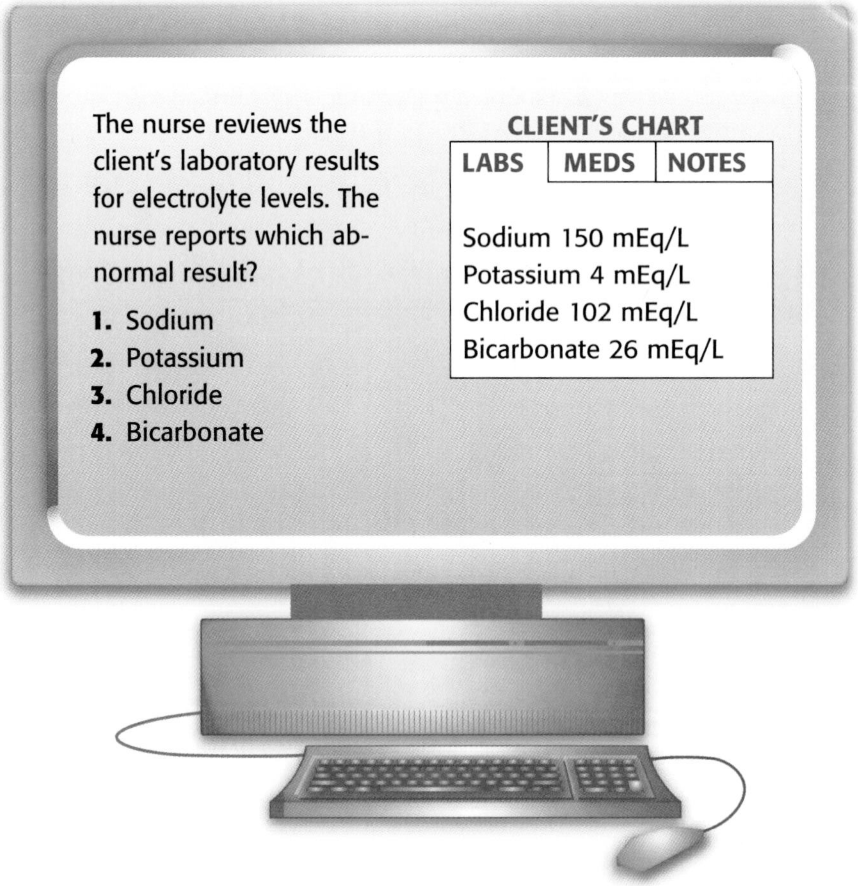
The nurse reviews the client's laboratory results for electrolyte levels. The nurse reports which abnormal result?
1. Sodium
2. Potassium
3. Chloride
4. Bicarbonate
CLIENT'S CHART
LABS
MEDS
NOTES
Sodium 150 mEq/L
Potassium 4 mEq/L
Chloride 102 mEq/L
Bicarbonate 26 mEq/L

Answer: 1

Test-Taking Strategy: In this question you are provided with the client's chart and laboratory results. You need to refer to the laboratory results in order to answer the question. On the NCLEX-PN examination, you will need to use the computer mouse and click on the appropriate tab noted on the client's chart. In this question you would click on the Laboratory tab. The normal sodium level is 135 to 145 mEq/L; normal potassium is 3.5 to 5.1 mEq/L; chloride 98 to 107 mEq/L; and bicarbonate 22 to 29 mEq/L.

REFERENCES

Chernecky, C. & Berger, B. (2004). *Laboratory tests and diagnostic procedures* (4th ed). Philadelphia: Saunders.

DeWit, S. (2005). *Fundamental concepts and skills for nursing* (2nd ed). Philadelphia: Saunders.

Hodgson, B. & Kizior, R. (2005). *Saunders nursing drug handbook 2005.* Philadelphia: Saunders.

Linton, A. & Maebius, N. (2003). *Introduction to medical-surgical nursing* (3rd ed). Philadelphia: Saunders.

National Council of State Boards of Nursing, Inc. *Test Plan for the National Council Licensure Examination for Licensed Practical/ Vocational Nurses* (effective date: April 2005), National Council of State Boards of Nursing, Chicago, 2004.

National Council of State Boards of Nursing, Inc. online: Available at www.ncsbn.org.

Potter, P. & Perry, A. (2005). *Fundamentals of nursing* (6th ed). St. Louis: Mosby.

"I found using flash cards to review before the boards helpful. Carry them with you and review any chance you get. I also went with 2 classmates the two nights before the exam and relaxed, reviewed, and stayed in a quiet hotel away from family and interruptions. I felt this made a huge difference even though it was hard to sleep the night before the exam. We used the time to study and also quizzed each other. Very helpful. The boards are hard to study for, but I think reviewing the basics is key."

—Michele Superba, Greenfield Community College, Greenfield, MA

"Keep several NCLEX review books scattered throughout the house. I had one in the kitchen for "quizzing while cooking," one in the living room in front of the television for quizzing during commercials, and one next to my bed so I could do my "obligatory 100 questions per night." I also had a set of NCLEX review cards that I split up into several stacks and stashed in various bags/purses so I would always have them with me when out and about."

—Charlene, University of Southern Indiana, Evansville, IN

Part 2

Strategies for Success

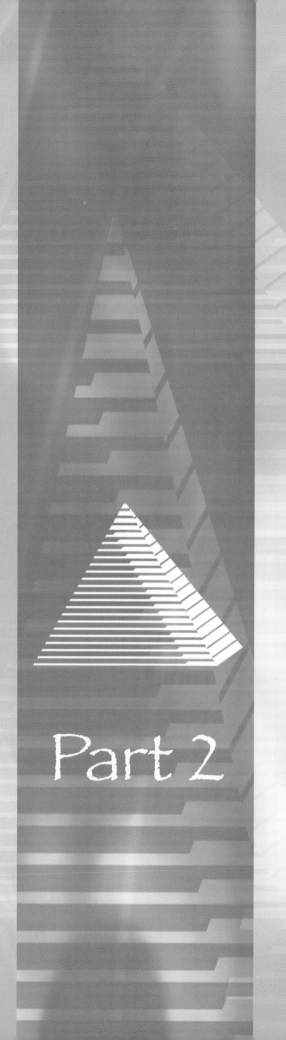

Chapter 6 Nonacademic Preparation: Your Path to Success

The NCLEX-PN® examination is an important one because receiving that nursing license means that you can begin your career as a licensed practical/vocational nurse.

A positive attitude, a structured study plan for preparation, and controlling anxiety in your path to success will ensure achievement in reaching the peak of the pyramid to success.

REACHING THE PEAK OF THE PYRAMID
- A positive attitude
- A structured study plan for preparation
- Controlling test anxiety

HOW CAN YOU MAINTAIN A POSITIVE ATTITUDE?

The first step in maintaining a positive attitude is to think about the accomplishments that you have achieved. You have been successful in your nursing program and you have graduated. It is also important to avoid any negative thoughts about yourself and your ability to pass the NCLEX-PN examination. Confidence in yourself and your ability is critical. So keep thinking about accomplishments.

Whenever you begin to doubt yourself and your ability to pass the NCLEX-PN examination you need to change those negative feelings into positive ones. You may be asking yourself, "How can I do this?" Always remember that you can accomplish anything if you believe in yourself. Whenever you feel doubt about your abilities, stop whatever you are doing, stand up, brush yourself off with your hands, and repeat to yourself, "I am getting rid of these negative feelings! I am confident in myself and *yes*, I can do this!"

Another way to maintain a positive attitude is with the use of visuals. Draw a picture of yourself and below the picture write your name and the letters LPN or LVN after it. Make several copies of the picture and post the pictures in several places that you frequent, such as on your mirror, on your refrigerator, in your car, and in your other special places. And remember to place a copy in front of you when you study for this examination. Smile whenever you look at these signs because smiling will keep you happy and help to make you feel good about yourself.

Remember you can accomplish anything if you have confidence and believe in yourself!

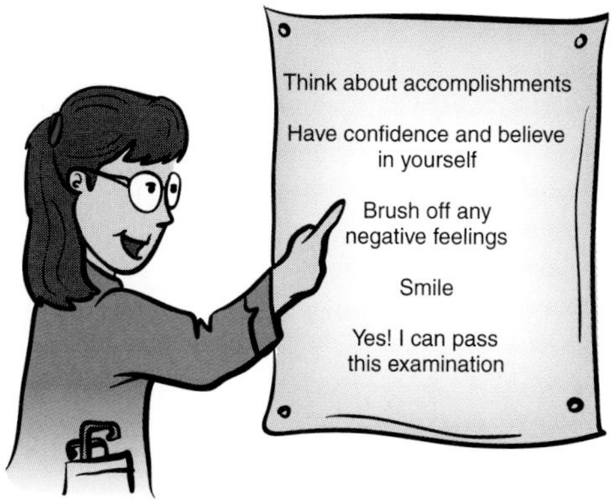

HOW DO YOU DEVELOP A STRUCTURED STUDY PLAN FOR PREPARATION?

When Should You Schedule a Date for the Examination?

An important decision to make is deciding on a date for taking the NCLEX-PN examination. Once you have a date in mind or planned, you can develop your structured study plan. You may ask, "When should I schedule my date? How do I know when I will be ready?" Readiness to take this examination is highly individual. Your readiness may be very different from someone else's. What you need to remember is that your nursing education has focused on preparing you for this examination. Now, what you need to do is to review nursing content in a structured and focused way in preparation for this examination. There are two things to keep in mind as you are trying to decide on a date for taking the NCLEX-PN examination. First, remember that review and preparation are necessary. Second, you want to take the examination soon after graduation while all of the nursing knowledge is still fresh in your mind. Focus on your needs and your strengths and weaknesses and plan to take this examination within 1 and no later than 2 months after graduation.

SCHEDULING A DATE FOR THE EXAM

- Review and prepare
- Focus on your strengths and weaknesses
- Schedule an examination date within 1 to 2 months after graduation

How Do You Start to Develop a Study Plan?

The first task is to decide what study patterns worked best for you in the past, and remain with these patterns. If you have always studied alone and this has always been successful, continue with this pattern and avoid joining a study group. If you have been most successful with studying in a group, then plan to prepare for this examination with your study partners. Remember, it is best not to plan study sessions that are different than what has brought you success in the past.

The next step is to get a calendar and name it, for example, "My Special NCLEX Calendar." On the calendar, mark your long-term goal, which should be the date of your examination. On all of the days preceding your date for the examination, mark your short-term goals, which will be your daily study times. There may be days that you will not be able to devote study time because of personal and family commitments. On these days, place an X. On all of the remaining days, write in your study times and plan to schedule at least 5 study days each week. Remember, you need some days for rest, relaxation, and fun!

How Long and When Should You Schedule Each Study Session?

The length of the study session will depend on you and your ability to focus and concentrate. What you need to think about is quality rather than quantity when you are deciding on a realistic amount of time for each session. Plan to schedule at the very least, 2 hours of quality time daily. If you can spend more than 2 hours, then by all means do so.

You may be asking, "What do you mean by quality time?" Quality time means spending uninterrupted quiet time at your study session. This may mean that you will have to isolate yourself for these study sessions. Think again about what has worked for you during nursing school when you studied for examinations, and select a study place that has worked for you in the past. If you have a special study room at home that you have always used, then plan your study sessions in that special room. If you have always studied at a library, then plan your study sessions at the library. If you plan to study at home, make the time spent studying uninterrupted and a quiet time. Sometimes it is difficult to balance your study time with your family obligations and possibly a work schedule, but if you can, plan your study time when you know that you will be at home alone. Try to eliminate anything that may be distracting during your study time. For example, unplug your telephone so that you will not be disturbed. If you have small children, plan your study time during their naptime or during their school hours.

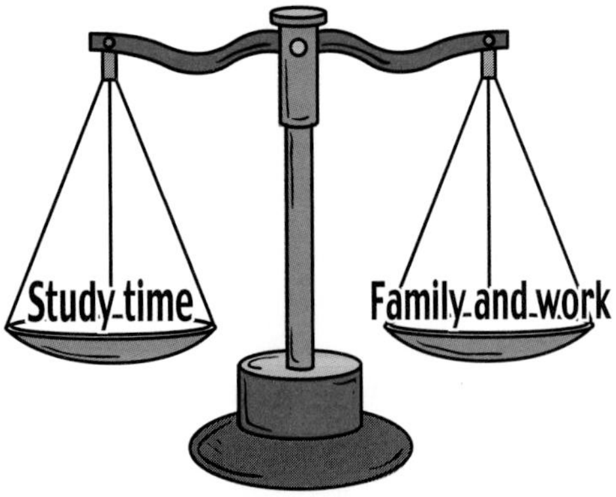

Another consideration in planning your study session is the time of the session. Some individuals find that they are more alert and will retain more if they study in the morning, whereas others may find that afternoon or evening hours are best for retaining information. So depending on your needs, plan your sessions accordingly. Remember this examination is all about *you*, so plan to meet *your* needs and stick to *your* plan!

What Do You Use to Study?

This examination consists entirely of questions that you need to answer. Therefore, the very best way to prepare is to study from a question and answer perspective. Also, recall that this examination is administered on a computer, so using a computer to study is extremely beneficial. Obtain a notebook, name it, for example, "My Special NCLEX Notes," and keep it next to your computer when you are studying. As you study, write down the specific topics that you may have difficulty with. These are the areas that you may need to review further. There are several resources available that you can use depending on your needs. The *Saunders Comprehensive Review for the NCLEX-PN® Examination* is one valuable tool that contains both content and practice questions. Its accompanying CD-ROM contains more than 3500 practice questions, thus providing you with questions on a computer. The questions are presented in multiple-choice format and in the alternate test question format that is used in the NCLEX-PN examination. When using this CD-ROM, it is best to access the *Study Mode* because you are given important information immediately after answering the question. This information includes the correct answer, rationale for the correct and incorrect options, the test-taking strategy for answering the question, content area to review if you answered the question incorrectly, and the reference source. As you study, if you have difficulty with a specific topic, write it in your "Special NCLEX Notes" and be sure to review the topic. Do not attempt to prepare for this examination by studying all of your class notes that you have from nursing school because they are much too detailed and you will become overwhelmed. And do not prepare for this examination by planning to read all of your nursing textbooks. You have already read them and you need to use them along with your review book as a resource if necessary for difficult information.

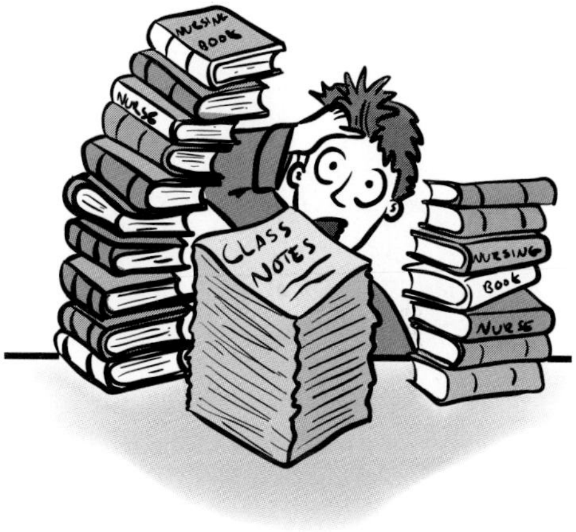

Additional resources to use for studying include the *Saunders Q & A Review for the NCLEX-PN® Examination,* which also provides you with more than 3000 practice questions on its CD-ROM different from those in the *Saunders Comprehensive Review for the NCLEX-PN® Examination,* and the Saunders Review Cards for the NCLEX-PN® Examination, which provides you with more than 900 practice test questions, including multiple-choice questions and the new alternate test items, such as fill-in-the-blank, multiple-response, prioritizing (ordered response), and image (hot spot) questions. The practice question is located on one side of the review card. The reverse side of the review card contains the correct answer, rationale, and question categories for the practice question on the front of the card. These additional resources can be obtained online at the Elsevier website (see following box).

> Review books can be obtained at the Elsevier website in the Nursing Review and Testing Section: www.elsevierhealth.com.

HOW CAN YOU CONTROL TEST ANXIETY?

How Will Anxiety Affect You?

Preparing to take the NCLEX-PN examination can produce a great deal of anxiety. You may be thinking that NCLEX-PN is the most important examination that you will ever have to take, and that it reflects the culmination of everything that you have worked so hard for. NCLEX-PN is an important examination because receiving that nursing license means that you can begin your career as a licensed practical or vocational nurse. Some anxiety about the examination can be helpful because it keeps your senses and thinking processes alert and sharp. However, a great deal of anxiety can be detrimental because it can block your thinking processes.

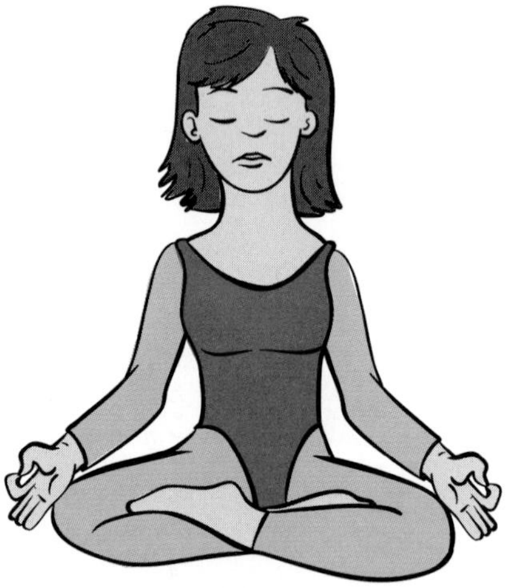

What Will Eliminate Some of the Anxiety?

An important component to eliminate some of the anxiety is to be as prepared as possible for this examination. Maintaining a positive attitude and discipline with following your structured study plan will certainly help.

Another way to eliminate some anxiety is to be comfortable with where the testing center is located. A test drive to the testing center a few days before the examination is beneficial. Note the time of your examination and drive to the testing center as if you were planning to take the examination. Time the drive and note the amount of traffic or road construction, parking facilities, or whatever else that may delay you. You will most likely have some anxiety on the day of your examination and the last thing that you need is traffic delays or other situations that may obstruct you and increase your anxiety. On the test drive, when you arrive at the test facility, you may want to walk into it and become familiar with the lobby and the surroundings. This may help to alleviate some of the peripheral nervousness associated with entering an unknown building. Do whatever it takes to keep your anxiety under control.

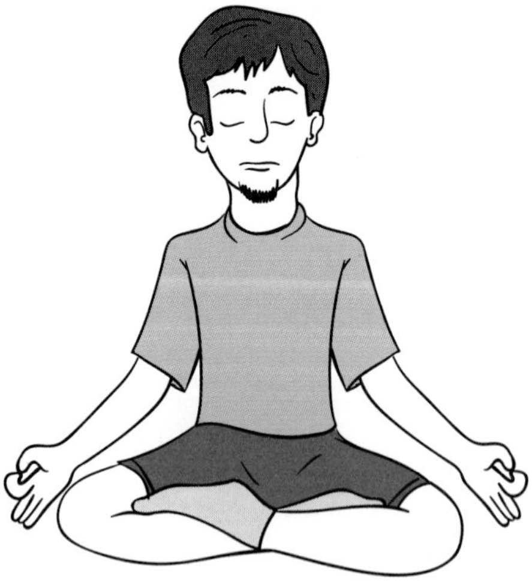

What Can You Do When You Become Anxious?

Breathing exercises are extremely helpful in alleviating anxiety and can be used at any time, including during your testing. These exercises will help not only to relax you but also oxygenate your body. During your clinical experience as a nursing student you most likely cared for a client whose oxygenation level was being monitored by pulse oximetry. If the client's pulse oximetry was low, and you instructed the client to take some slow deep breaths, you would note that the oxygenation level increased. This same effect will occur if you take slow deep breaths. You want to decrease the anxiety, relax, and have your body and brain as oxygenated as possible on the day of the examination.

During the time before the examination if you become anxious or are having difficulty sleeping at night, sit or lie in a comfortable position, close your eyes, relax, inhale deeply, hold your breath to a count of four, exhale slowly, and, again, relax. Repeat this breathing exercise several times until you begin to feel relaxed and free from anxiety. During the examination, if you find that you are becoming anxious, distracted, and are having difficulty focusing, sit back, close your eyes, and perform your breathing exercises to help relax you and get oxygen moving through your body. Remember, you want oxygen in your brain on the day of the examination!

What Is Positive Pampering and Why Is It Important?

Positive pampering means that you will take care of yourself from a holistic perspective. It will help to maintain an academic and nonacademic balance as you prepare for this examination and will help to alleviate some anxiety. You need to care for yourself by including physical activity, a balanced diet, and fun and relaxation in your preparation plan.

POSITIVE PAMPERING

- Physical activity
- Balanced diet
- Fun
- Relaxation

Just as you have developed a schedule for study, you need a schedule that includes some fun and some form of physical activity. It is your choice—aerobics, running, weight lifting, bowling, a movie, a massage, going to the beach, or whatever makes you feel good. Time spent away from the hard study schedule and devoted to some form of fun and physical exercise pays its rewards 100-fold. You will feel more energetic with a schedule that includes these activities.

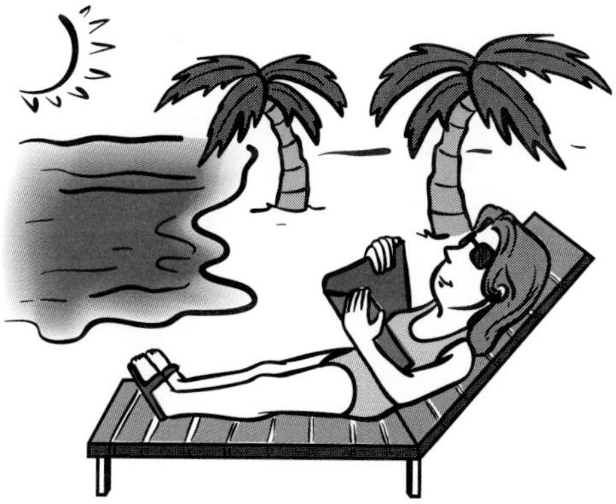

Establish healthy eating habits if you have not already done so. Eat lighter and well-balanced meals and eat more frequently. Include complex carbohydrates in your diet for energy. Avoid caffeine because it will make you jittery and anxious, and avoid eating fatty foods because they will slow you down and make you feel sleepy.

Pamper yourself to maintain balance!

What Should You Do on the Day before the Examination?

On the day before the examination you may become anxious and immediately think, "I am not ready!" Stop whatever you are doing and reflect on all that you have accomplished. Smile, brush off those negative feelings, do your breathing exercises, and look at all of the pictures of yourself that read your name with the letters LPN or LVN after it.

Your goal on the day of the examination is to maintain your positive attitude and control anxiety that you may experience. You need to rest your body and your mind. The mind is like a muscle—if it is overworked, it has no strength or stamina. Therefore, on the day before the examination, put your review books back in the bookshelf and spend the day doing activities that you enjoy and will relax you. Positive pampering is important on the day before the examination and you need to treat yourself to what you enjoy the most. At bedtime do the breathing exercises and listen to soothing music to help you relax and fall asleep and know that you have prepared yourself well for the challenge of tomorrow.

What Should You Do on the Day of the Examination?

ON THE DAY OF THE EXAMINATION

Think positive
Groom yourself for success
Maintain confidence and belief in yourself
Meet the challenges of the day
Become a licensed practical or vocational nurse
YES!

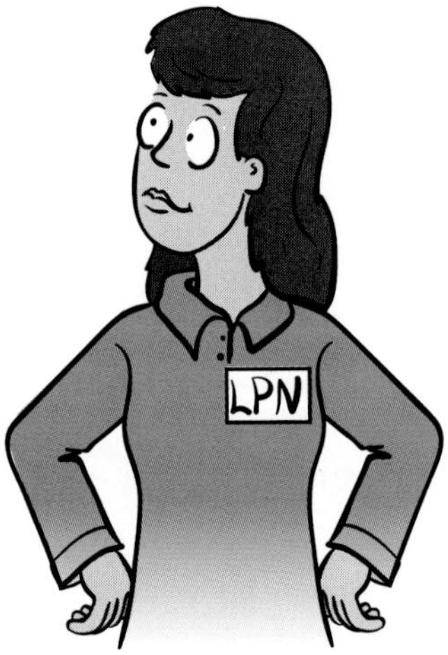

On the day of the examination, think positive! When you wake up and get out of bed, say, "Yes," brush off any negative feelings, and look at your picture with your name and LPN or LVN after it. You are absolutely ready to succeed, and all that you have accomplished is about to propel you to the level of licensed practical or vocational nurse. Allow yourself plenty of time, eat a healthy breakfast, and groom yourself for success. Remain confident and believe in yourself that you are ready to meet the challenges of the day and overcome any obstacle that may face you. Soon, today will be history, and soon you will receive the envelope on which you will read your name with the words "licensed practical or vocational nurse" after it.

Chapter 7

How to Avoid Reading into the Question

One of the pitfalls that can cause a problem with answering a question correctly is "reading into the question." What this means is that you are considering issues beyond the information that is presented in the question. There are some strategies that you can use to prevent this from happening when you are answering a question. Some of these include identifying the parts of a question, reading carefully and looking for key words or phrases, identifying the issue of the question and what the question is asking, using the process of elimination, and avoiding the "what if?" syndrome.

> Identify the parts of a question.
> Read carefully.
> Look for key words or phrases.
> Identify the issue.
> Use the process of elimination.
> Avoid asking yourself "What if?"

PARTS OF A QUESTION

What Are the Parts of a Question?

Except for the fill-in-the-blank questions, prioritizing (ordered response) questions, and some figure/illustration or chart/exhibit questions, the question will contain a case situation, a question stem, and the options.

> **QUESTION PARTS**
> Case situation
> Question stem
> Options

Fill-in-the-blank questions contain a case situation and a question stem but do not contain options. Fill-in-the blank questions will require you to perform a medication calculation, calculate an intravenous flow rate, or calculate an intake and output. Because you need to type in the answer for these types of questions, it makes sense that options are not provided.

In a prioritizing (ordered response) question, several items are presented, such as nursing interventions. In this type of question you do not need to select options; rather you will be required to list the items presented via a drag-and-drop feature on the computer, such as nursing interventions, in order of priority. Remember, in a prioritizing (ordered-response) question, all of the items listed will be correct.

Some of the figure/illustration or chart/exhibit questions do not provide options and you may need to use the computer mouse to point and click on the correct answer to the question.

It is important for you to identify the parts of a question as you read it because it will help you sort out the facts and determine what the question is asking.

What Is the Case Situation?

The case situation is the "heart" of the question. It provides you with the information that you need to think about to answer the question.

What Is a Question Stem?

The question stem is a statement that generally follows the case situation and asks you something very specific about the information in the case situation.

What Are the Options?

The options are all of the answers presented with the question. In a multiple-choice question, there are four options and you must select one. In a multiple response question, there are several options and you must select all options that apply to the case situation and the question stem.

A figure/illustration or a chart/exhibit question may be presented in a multiple-choice format. For example, you may be given a question with a figure of the lungs, a case situation and question stem related to auscultating breath sounds, and four options in which only one option is correct. Or, you may given a question with a figure and asked to use the computer mouse to click on the correct option. For example, the question may contain a figure of the human body, a case situation, and a question stem. On the figure you may note small circles sometimes called "hot spots" and will be asked to click on the circle that indicates the correct answer to the question.

Examples of the various types of questions that may appear in the examination, and the parts of the question are provided below. The answers to these sample questions and the test-taking strategy are also provided.

Parts of a Question: Multiple Choice

Case Situation: The nurse is reviewing the laboratory results of a client who is receiving magnesium sulfate and notes that the magnesium level is 7 mEq/L.
Question Stem: Based on this laboratory result, the nurse *most likely* expects to note which of the following in the client?
Options:

1. No specific signs or symptoms because this value is a normal level
2. Tremors
3. Respiratory depression
4. Hyperactive reflexes

Answer: 3

Test-Taking Strategy: Read each option carefully. Use the process of elimination and note the key words "most likely." Knowing that the level identified in the question is elevated will assist in eliminating option 1. Next, eliminate options 2 and 4 because they are similar. Remember, use nursing knowledge, focus on the information in the case situation, identify what the question is asking (the issue), note the key words, read carefully, and use the process of elimination.

Parts of a Question: Fill in the Blank

Case Situation: The physician prescribes an intravenous (IV) solution of 1000 mL 0.9% normal saline to infuse in 10 hours. The drop factor for the IV tubing is 15 drops (gtt) per mL.
Question Stem: The nurse sets the flow rate of the infusion at how many drops per minute?

Answer: 25

Test-Taking Strategy: Note the key words "sets the flow rate." Focus on the information in the question and that 1000 mL of fluid is to infuse in 10 hours and the drop factor is 15. Use the computer on-screen calculator and the formula for calculating an IV infusion to answer the question. Verify your answer. Remember, use nursing knowledge, focus on the information in the case situation, identify what the question is asking (the issue), and note the key words.

Parts of a Question: Multiple Response

Case Situation: The nurse enters a hospitalized client's room and discovers that the client is having a tonic-clonic seizure.
Question Stem: Select all actions that the nurse would appropriately implement?
Options:

___ Check airway patency
___ Restrain the client's extremities loosely
___ Call a code
___ Protect the client from injury
___ Assist with inserting an intravenous access

Answer:

_X_ Check airway patency
___ Restrain the client's extremities loosely
___ Call a code
_X_ Protect the client from injury

Test-Taking Strategy: Read each option carefully. Use the process of elimination and note the key word "appropriately." In this type of question it is helpful to visualize the situation to assist in determining the nurse's actions. Remember, use nursing knowledge, focus on the information in the case situation, identify what the question is asking (the issue), note the key words, read carefully, and use the process of elimination.

Parts of a Question: Prioritizing (Ordered Response)

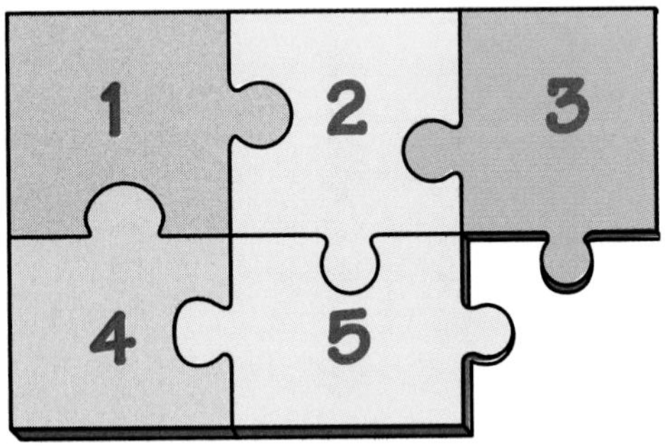

Case Situation: A nurse is preparing to change an abdominal dressing using sterile technique.

Question Stem: List in *order of priority* the actions that the nurse would take to perform this procedure. (Number 1 indicates the first action and number 5 indicates the last action.)

Options:

___ Don clean gloves and remove the old dressing
___ Set up a sterile field
___ Explain the procedure to the client
___ Don sterile gloves
___ Wash hands

Answer: 4, 3, 1, 5, 2

Test-Taking Strategy: Read each option carefully and note the key words, "order of priority." In this type of question it is helpful to visualize the situation to assist in determining the nurse's order of actions. Remember, use nursing knowledge, focus on the information in the case situation, identify what the question is asking (the issue), note the key words, and read carefully.

Parts of a Question: Figure/Illustration

Case Situation: The nurse is checking the apical heart rate on an adult client.

Question Stem: Using the computer mouse, click on the area where the nurse would place the stethoscope (Figure 7-1).

Answer: Answer is indicated by the area containing the X

Test-Taking Strategy: Note the key words, "apical heart rate." In this type of question it is helpful to visualize the position of the heart and to recall that the stethoscope is placed on the left fifth intercostal space at the midclavicular area. Remember, use nursing knowledge, focus on the information in the case situa-

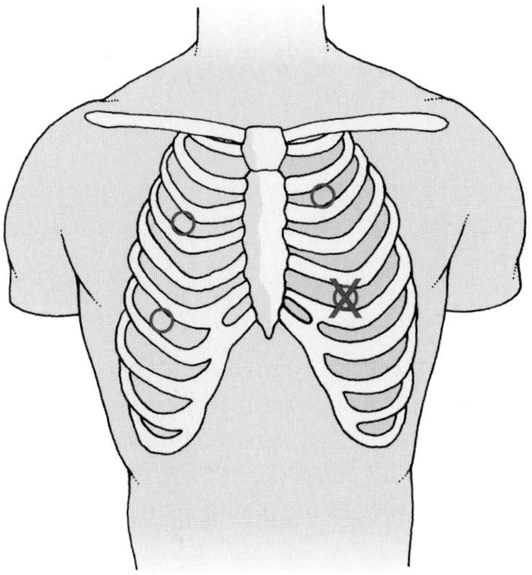

Figure 7-1 From: Ignatavicius, D. & Workman, M. [2006]. *Medical-surgical nursing: critical thinking for collaborative care,* 5th ed., Philadelphia: Saunders.

tion, identify what the question is asking (the issue), note the key words, and read carefully.

Parts of a Question: Chart/Exhibit
Case Situation: The nurse is preparing to administer digoxin (Lanoxin) 0.125 mg orally to a client.
Question Stem: The nurse withholds the medication and notifies a registered nurse if which recent laboratory level is noted in the client's chart?
Options:

1. Digoxin level
2. Potassium level
3. Sodium level
4. Chloride level

CLIENT'S CHART

LABS	MEDS	Diagnostic Tests

Digoxin level 1 ng/dL
Potassium level 3 mEq/L
Sodium level 140 mEq/L
Chloride level 102 mEq/L

Answer: 2

Test-Taking Strategy: In this question you are provided with the client's chart and laboratory results. You need to refer to the laboratory results in order to answer the question. On the NCLEX-PN examination, you will need to use the computer mouse and click on the appropriate tab noted on the client's chart. In this question you would click on the Laboratory tab. The normal sodium level is 135 to 145 mEq/L; normal potassium is 3.5 to 5.1 mEq/L; chloride 98 to 107 mEq/L; and the therapeutic digoxin level is 0.5 to 2.0 ng/dL.

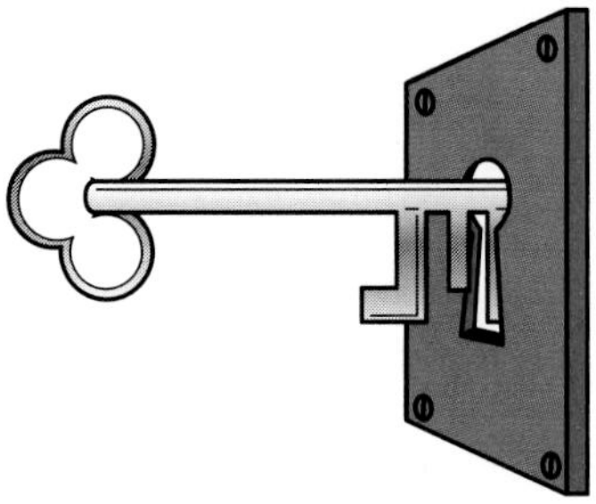

KEY WORDS OR PHRASES

Why Are Key Words or Phrases Important to Note?

Always read every word in the question carefully. As you read, look for key words or phrases in the case situation and stem of the question. Key words or phrases focus your attention on specific or critical points that you need to consider when answering the question.

Some key words or phrases may indicate that all of the options are correct, and that it will be necessary to prioritize in order to select the correct option. Remember, as you read the question, look for the key words or phrases; they will make a difference with regard to how you will answer the question.

KEY WORDS OR PHRASES

- Focus your attention on critical and specific points
- May indicate that there is only one option
- May indicate that you need to prioritize
- May indicate a true response question
- May indicate a false response question

What Are the Commonly Used Key Words or Phrases to Look For?

Common Key Words or Phrases That Indicate That There Is Only One Correct Option

Some of the key words or phrases used in a question indicate that there is only one correct option. Some of these include the following:

- Early sign
- Late sign
- Understands
- Goal has been achieved
- Adequately tolerating
- Avoid
- Needs reinforcement of the instructions
- Lack of understanding
- Goals have not yet been fully met
- Has not met the outcome criteria
- Ineffective
- Inadequate
- Unable to tolerate

Common Key Words or Phrases That Indicate the Need to Prioritize

There are also key words or phrases that may indicate that all of the options are correct, and that it will be necessary to prioritize in order to select the correct option. Some of these include the following:

Best
First
Initial
Immediately
Most likely or least likely
Most appropriate or least appropriate
Highest or lowest priority
Order of priority
At highest risk
At lowest risk
Best understanding

Common Key Words or Phrases That Indicate a True or False Response Question

Finally, there are key words or phrases that indicate that the question is a true-response or a false-response question. Key words or phrases used in these types of questions may indicate that there is only one correct option or may indicate the need to prioritize in order to select the correct option. (Additional information about true response and false response questions can be found in Chapter 8.)

Common key words or phrases that indicate a true response question include the following:

Early sign
Late sign
Best
First
Initial
Immediately
Most likely
Most appropriate
Highest priority
Order of priority
All nursing interventions that apply
Goal has been achieved
Adequately tolerating

Common key words or phrases that indicate a false response question include the following:

Least likely
Least appropriate
Least priority
Least helpful
At lowest risk
Avoid
Needs reinforcement of the instructions
Needs additional teaching

Lack of understanding
Goals have not yet been fully met
Has not met the outcome criteria
Ineffective
Inadequate
Unable to tolerate

Use of Key Words or Phrases in a Question

You may be asking, how are these key words or phrases used in a question? Let's look at some examples of question stems that contain key words.

Select all nursing interventions that apply in the care of the client.
Which statement by a client indicates an understanding of the instructions?
What is the initial nursing action?
Which of the following is an early sign of hypoxia?
List in order of priority the actions that the nurse would take?
Which of the following individuals is least likely to develop hypertension?
Which nursing diagnosis written in the care plan is of least priority?
The nurse would avoid which of the following actions?
The nurse determines that the client needs additional teaching if the client states which of the following?
The nurse determines that the treatment is ineffective if which if the following is noted?

THE ISSUE OF THE QUESTION

What Is the Issue of the Question?

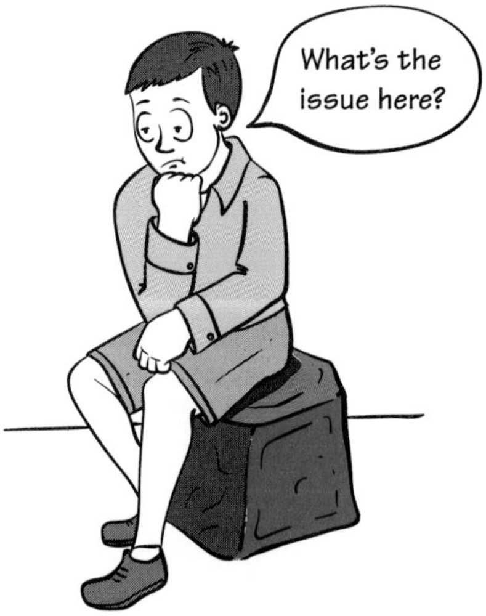

The issue of the question is the specific subject content that the question is asking. It is important to read every word in the question and note the key words or phrases; determine what the question is asking. Identifying the issue of the question will assist in eliminating the incorrect options and direct you to selecting the correct option.

What Are Some Examples of Question Issues?

There are hundreds of issues that you could be asked about when you take this examination. This is understandable especially when you think about all of the information that you needed to learn in nursing school. A test question may ask about any Client Needs area of the test plan for the NCLEX-PN examination, any content area of nursing, or anything that has to do with the role and responsibilities of the nurse. Therefore, the list of issues that could be tested is never ending. You may want to obtain a copy of the *Test Plan for the National Council Licensure Examination for Licensed Practical/Vocational Nurses* published by the National Council of State Boards of Nursing (NCSBN). This test plan identifies some of the content that will be tested on this examination and can be obtained at the NCSBN website at www.ncsbn.org.

Examples of issues that may be used in a test question are identified below. These examples are based on the Client Needs components of the test plan for the NCLEX-PN examination. (Refer to Chapter 3 for additional information about content in the Client Needs components of the test plan.)

"WILL IT EVER END?"

Test Question Issues*

Physiological Integrity

Basic Care and Comfort

Implementing alternative and complementary therapies
Using canes, walkers, crutches, or other assistive devices
Promoting and monitoring elimination patterns
Monitoring for complications of immobility
Promoting nutrition and therapeutic diets
Providing measures that promote comfort
Identifying personal hygiene issues

Pharmacological Therapies

Following the rights of medication administration
Monitoring for the action and expected effect of a medication
Monitoring for side effects of a medication
Monitoring for toxic or adverse effects of a medication
Identifying contraindications of a medication
Identifying interactions associated with a medication
Providing client teaching related to a medication or other health care area
Monitoring intravenous (IV) therapy
Monitoring for complications of an IV
Monitoring a transfusion of blood
Monitoring for complications of a blood transfusion
Administering medication via various routes including a gastrointestinal tube

Reduction of Risk Potential

Preparing a client for a diagnostic test, treatment, or procedure
Monitoring for complications of a diagnostic test, treatment, or procedure
Providing preprocedure and postprocedure care of a diagnostic test, treatment, or procedure
Caring for a client requiring surgery
Following procedures for taking vital signs
Recognizing alterations in the client
Monitoring laboratory results

Physiological Adaptation

Monitoring the client for a fluid or electrolyte imbalance

(Continued)

Providing interventions if a fluid and electrolyte imbalance exists
Providing interventions in the care of a client with an infectious disease
Responding to a medical emergency
Performing wound care and dressing changes
Providing care to a client with a tracheostomy
Providing care to a client on a ventilator
Identifying abnormalities on a client's cardiac monitor strip

Safe, Effective Care Environment

Coordinated Care

Acting as a client advocate
Providing information to a client on advance directives
Prioritizing nursing actions
Upholding client rights
Maintaining confidentiality
Describing informed consent requirements
Consulting with other members of the health care team
Identifying ethical and legal issues related to client care
Assigning client care to assistive personnel
Supervising client care tasks assigned to assistive personnel
Using resources appropriately
Participating in performance improvement (quality assurance) programs

Safety and Infection Control

Implements measures to prevent accidents and injuries
Implements measures to prevent an error
Implements emergency measures if a disaster occurs
Identifies the agency's emergency response plan
Assists with implementing a security plan
Handles hazardous and infectious materials safely
Provides a safe environment in the client's home
Maintains medical and surgical asepsis techniques
Implements standard/transmission-based and other precautions
Uses restraints and other safety devices correctly
Uses medical equipment safely
Completes incident and other reports
Documents care accurately following acceptable guidelines

Health Promotion and Maintenance

Identifies the stages of growth and development
Identifies expected body image changes that occur with the aging process
Promotes health and wellness and measures to prevent disease

(Continued)

Uses data collection techniques
Identifies health screening and health promotion programs
Identifies immunization schedules
Identifies high-risk behaviors and lifestyle choices that require intervention
Promotes self-care measures
Uses teaching and learning principles
Understands the concepts of human sexuality and the family
Provides antepartum, intrapartum, and postpartum care
Provides care to the newborn infant

Psychosocial Integrity

Uses therapeutic communication techniques
Identifies individual cultural, religious, and spiritual considerations of care
Identifies situations of client abuse and neglect and implements nursing responsibilities
Identifies substance abuse and addiction situations
Identifies client's coping mechanisms
Intervenes in a crisis
Assists the client with resolution of grief or loss
Identifies the client's end-of-life issues
Identifies stress management techniques and support systems
Cares for the client with a mental health disorder

Sample Question: The Issue of the Question

A client with metastatic cancer is receiving morphine sulfate to alleviate pain. The nurse monitors the client for which *adverse or toxic effect* of the medication?

Issue: In this question, note that the client is receiving *morphine sulfate* and that the question asks about an *adverse or toxic effect* of the medication. Therefore, the issue of this question is an *adverse or toxic effect of morphine sulfate.*

1. Dizziness
2. Sedation
3. Skeletal muscle flaccidity
4. Nausea

Answer: 3

Test-Taking Strategy: Read every word in the question and specifically determine what the question is asking. The question is asking about the adverse or toxic effect of morphine sulfate. Dizziness, sedation, and nausea are side effects of morphine sulfate that the client may experience, but are not adverse or toxic effects. Remember, focus on the information in the question and what the question is asking!

USING NURSING KNOWLEDGE AND THE PROCESS OF ELIMINATION

Why Nursing Knowledge Is So Important

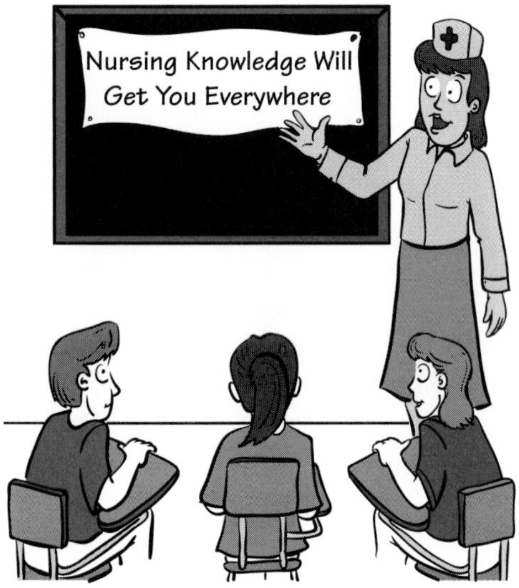

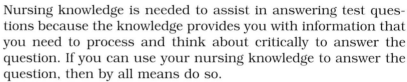

Nursing knowledge is needed to assist in answering test questions because the knowledge provides you with information that you need to process and think about critically to answer the question. If you can use your nursing knowledge to answer the question, then by all means do so.

On the NCLEX-PN examination, don't be surprised if you are given questions that contain content that you are totally unfamiliar with or are vaguely familiar with. This happens to many individuals who take this examination. When you are given a question that contains content that you are unfamiliar with, read the question carefully and focus on the issue. Sometimes you do not even need to know much about the content to answer the question. Additionally, with some of these unfamiliar questions, you are able to use nursing knowledge from a different content area to answer the question. The important thing is not to become alarmed and anxious if you receive a question with unfamiliar content. Sit back, take a deep breath, read carefully, focus on the issue, and use nursing knowledge from a different content area to answer the question.

What Do You Mean by Using the Process of Elimination?

The process of elimination is a course of action that involves reading each option presented with a question and removing the options that are incorrect and do not address the issue of the question. Using the process of elimination is extremely important when you are reading the options to a question and trying to determine the correct answer. Don't just hastily select an option because it sounds good. Always read every option carefully before selecting an answer.

Some students will read a question and before looking at the options, are able to determine a correct answer. This is a helpful strategy to use when answering a test question because you are using nursing knowledge to assist in answering the question correctly. The problem with this strategy is that you may have an answer to the question in mind and when you look at the options, your answer is not there. This can be very frustrating and anxiety provoking. Let's look at the following example.

A client who has type 1 diabetes mellitus complains of shakiness and hunger 2 hours after receiving a dose of regular insulin. The nurse determines that the client is having a hypoglycemic reaction and prepares to give the client which best item from the dietary kitchen to treat the reaction?

After you read this question, you will immediately think, "Orange juice! Yes, orange juice is the best item! I know the answer to this question." Then, you look at the options and find the following:

1. Milk
2. Diet soda
3. Sugar-free cookies
4. Sugar-free gelatin

Your answer, orange juice, is not there! So now what do you do? You need to use your nursing knowledge and think about what thought processes led you to identifying orange juice as the answer to the question. Remember that a food item that contains 10 to 15 g carbohydrate is used to treat a hypoglycemic reaction. Now, look at your options and use the process of elimination. In this question, you can eliminate options 2, 3, and 4 because these items do not contain carbohydrates.

What Do You Do if You Eliminate Two of the Options and Are Unsure of the Final Two?

As you use the process of elimination to eliminate the incorrect options, it is likely that you will be able to easily eliminate two of the four options in a multiple-choice question. Now what do you do with the last two options and how do you proceed to select the correct one? Follow these steps to help you when you are trying to decide which of the last two options is correct.

1. Read the question again.
2. Identify the case situation from the stem of the question.
3. Look for the key words or phrases.
4. Identify the issue of the question.
5. Ask yourself, "What is the question asking?"
6. Read the options again.
7. Make your final choice by focusing on what the question is asking, using nursing knowledge, and test-taking strategies.

What Is the "What if?" Syndrome?

The "What if?" syndrome occurs when you read a test question and instead of simply focusing on the information in the question you start asking yourself, "Well, what if?" You need to avoid asking yourself this question because this leads you right into the dreaded pitfall of "reading into the question." Read the question carefully, identify key words or phrases, and focus on the issue of the question. You may need to think critically to answer the question, but stay on track. Asking yourself, "What if?" moves you off track with regard to what the question is asking. Let's look at two questions and then examine the ways to avoid reading into them.

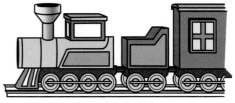

STAY ON TRACK!

Question: Avoiding the "What if?" Syndrome

A nurse is assisting in changing the tapes on a tracheostomy tube. The client coughs and the tube is dislodged. The *initial* nursing action is to:

1. cover the tracheostomy site with a sterile dressing to prevent infection.
2. ask the client to take deep breaths.
3. grasp the retention sutures to spread the opening.
4. call the respiratory therapy department to reinsert the tracheostomy tube.

You may immediately think, the tube is dislodged and I need someone to reinsert it! Read the question carefully. Note the key word "initial" and focus on the issue, that the client's tube is dislodged. The question is asking you for a nursing action, so that's what you need to look for as you eliminate the incorrect options. Use nursing knowledge and test-taking strategies to assist in answering the question.

Answer: 3

Test-Taking Strategy: Use the process of elimination and focus on the issue. Eliminate option 4 first because it will delay the immediate intervention needed. Eliminate option 1 because this action will block the airway. From the remaining options, eliminate option 2 because this action will not be helpful to maintain an open airway. If the tube is accidentally dislodged, the initial nursing action is to grasp the retention sutures and spread the opening. Additionally, use the ABCs—airway, breathing, and circulation—to direct you to the correct option.

Question: Avoiding the "What if?" Syndrome

A nurse is caring for a hospitalized client with a diagnosis of congestive heart failure who suddenly complains of shortness of breath and dyspnea. The nurse takes which *immediate* action?

1. Prepares to administer furosemide (Lasix)
2. Calls a respiratory therapist
3. Prepares to administer oxygen to the client
4. Elevates the head of the client's bed

You may immediately think the client has developed pulmonary edema, a complication of congestive heart failure, and needs a diuretic. Although pulmonary edema is a complication of congestive heart failure, there is no information in the question that indicates the presence of pulmonary edema. The question simply states that the client suddenly complains of shortness of breath and dyspnea. Read the question carefully. Note the key word "immediate" and focus on the issue, the client's complaint. The question is asking you for a nursing action, so that's what you need to look for as you eliminate the incorrect options. Use nursing knowledge and test-taking strategies to assist in answering the question.

Answer: 4

Test-Taking Strategy: Use the process of elimination and focus on the information in the question and on the issue. Note the key word, "immediate." Think about the client's complaint and look for the immediate nursing action. There are no data in the question that indicate that a respiratory therapist is needed. A physician's order is needed to administer oxygen. Furosemide is a diuretic and may or may not be prescribed for the client. Because there are no data in the question that indicate the presence of pulmonary edema, option 4 is correct.

REFERENCES

Chernecky, C. & Berger, B. (2004). *Laboratory tests and diagnostic procedures* (4th ed). Philadelphia: Saunders.

DeWit, S. (2005). *Fundamental concepts and skills for nursing* (2nd ed). Philadelphia: Saunders.

Hodgson, B. & Kizior, R. (2005). *Saunders nursing drug handbook 2005.* Philadelphia: Saunders.

Ignatavicius, D. & Workman, M. (2006). *Medical-surgical nursing: critical thinking for collaborative care* (5th ed). Philadelphia: Saunders.

Linton, A. & Maebius, N. (2003). *Introduction to medical-surgical nursing* (3rd ed). Philadelphia: Saunders.

National Council of State Boards of Nursing, Inc. *Test Plan for the National Council Licensure Examination for Licensed Practical/Vocational Nurses* (effective date: April 2005), National Council of State Boards of Nursing, Chicago, 2004.

National Council of State Boards of Nursing, Inc. online: Available at www.ncsbn.org.

Potter, P. & Perry, A. (2005). *Fundamentals of nursing* (6th ed). St. Louis: Mosby.

Chapter 8

True or False Response Questions

The questions presented on the NCLEX-PN® examination including multiple choice, fill in the blank, multiple response, figure/illustration questions, prioritizing (ordered response) questions, and chart/exhibit questions will be written as either a true response question or a false response question. The questions will primarily be written as a true response question; however, you need to be prepared for either type.

TRUE RESPONSE QUESTIONS

What Is a True Response Question?

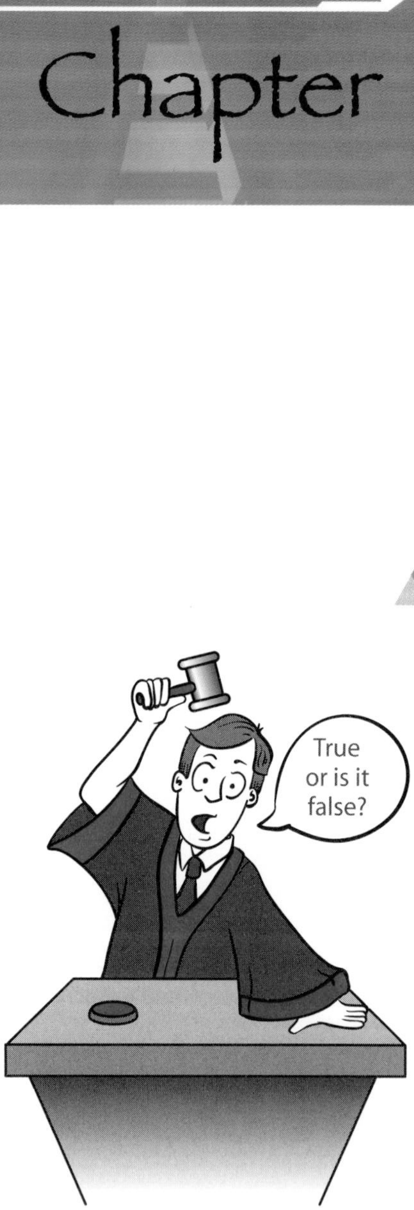

A true response question asks you to make a decision and select the option that is accurate or correct with regard to the data presented in the question. True response questions are primarily used on the NCLEX-PN examination. How will you know that the question is a true response one? Read the question carefully and focus on the stem of the question. The stem will contain key words or phrases that indicate that the question is a true response question.

> True response question: Select an option that is true or correct!

What Are the Key Words and Phrases Commonly Used in True Response Questions?

Remember to read the question carefully and focus on the stem of the question because the stem contains key words or phrases that indicate that the question is a true response question. Several examples of question stems and sample questions that indicate that the question is a true response question are listed below.

TRUE RESPONSE QUESTIONS: KEY WORDS

Early	First	Understands
Late	Immediately	Has been achieved
Most likely	Most appropriate	Adequately tolerating
Highest	Order of priority	
Best	All nursing interventions that apply	
Initial		

True Response Questions: Example Question Stems

What is the *earliest sign* of a change in level of consciousness?
Which of the following is a *late sign* of shock?
The nurse would *most likely* expect to note:
Which of the following individuals is at the *highest risk* for committing suicide?
A nurse palpates the carotid pulse at *which anatomical location*?
A nurse would *plan to order* what type of diet for the evening meal before the test?
A nurse *plans to administer* how many mL of medication?
What *best* action will the nurse implement?
Which action will the nurse do *first*?
What is the *initial* nursing action?
Based on these findings, the nurse *immediately:*
Which nursing action is *most appropriate*?
List in *order of priority* the actions that the nurse takes.
The *most appropriate* response to the client is:
Which intervention is of *highest priority* in the preoperative teaching plan?
Select *all nursing interventions that apply* in the care of the client.
Which statement made by a nursing assistant indicates to the licensed practical nurse that the assistant *understands* how to perform the procedure?
Which statement made by the client indicates the *best understanding* of how to prevent transmission of the disease?
Which of the following outcomes indicates that the most important goal *has been achieved* for this client?
A nurse determines that the client is *adequately tolerating* the procedure if which of the following observations is made?

True Response Question: Multiple Choice

A client with suspected *active* tuberculosis is being scheduled for diagnostic tests. A nurse anticipates that which diagnostic test will *most likely* be prescribed to *confirm* the diagnosis?

1. Chest x-ray
2. Skin testing
3. White blood cell count
4. Sputum smear

Answer: 4

Test-Taking Strategy: This question identifies an example of a true response question. Note the key words "active," "most likely," and "confirm." Focus on the diagnosis presented in the question and the associated pathophysiology to assist in directing you to option 4. Remember, tuberculosis is an infectious disease caused by *Mycobacterium tuberculosis* and the demonstration of tubercle bacilli bacteriologically is essential for establishing a diagnosis. It is not possible to make a diagnosis solely on the basis of a chest x-ray. A positive reaction to a skin test indicates the presence of tuberculosis infection but does not show whether the infection is active or dormant. A white blood cell count may be increased but is not specifically related to the presence of tuberculosis. Focus on the key words!

True Response Question: Fill in the Blank

The nurse is preparing to administer digoxin (Lanoxin) 0.25 mg orally. The label on the medication bottle reads digoxin (Lanoxin) 0.125 mg per tablet. How many tablet(s) does the nurse *plan to administer* to the client?

Answer: 2

Test-Taking Strategy: Note the key words "plan to administer." Focus on the information in the question and note that a dose of 0.25 mg is prescribed. Use the computer's on-screen calculator and the formula for calculating a medication dose to answer the question. Focus on the key words!

True Response Question: Multiple Response

Select *all nursing interventions that apply* in the care of an infant following a cleft lip repair (cheiloplasty).

___ Position the child on the abdomen
___ Cleanse the suture line gently after feeding the infant
___ Keep elbow restraints on the infant at all times
___ Institute measures that will prevent vigorous and sustained crying
___ Observe for bleeding at the operative site
___ Assist the mother with breastfeeding if this is the feeding method of choice

Answer:

___ Position the child on the abdomen
_X_ Cleanse the suture line gently after feeding the infant
___ Keep elbow restraints on the infant at all times
_X_ Institute measures that will prevent vigorous and sustained crying
_X_ Observe for bleeding at the operative site
_X_ Assist the mother with breast-feeding if this is the feeding method of choice

Test-Taking Strategy: Note the key words "all nursing interventions that apply," and focus on the surgical procedure, a cleft lip repair. Visualize each intervention and think about its effect on the surgical repair to assist in selecting the correct interventions. Focus on the key words!

True Response Question: Using a Figure

The nurse is performing cardiopulmonary resuscitation on a *6-month-old infant.* Using the computer mouse, click on the anatomical area that the nurse would palpate to *assess circulation.*

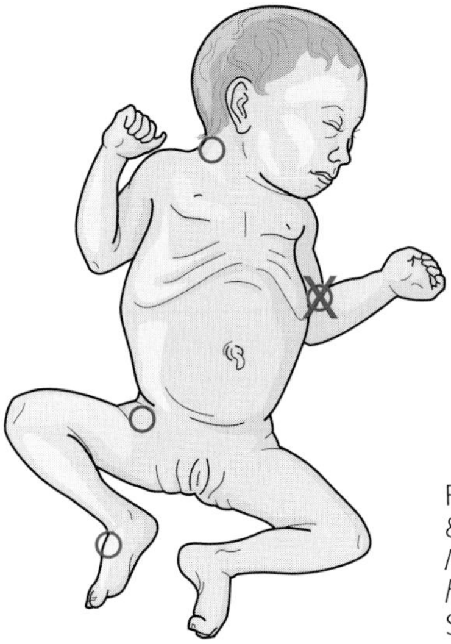

From Lowdermilk, D. & Perry, A. [2004]. *Maternity & women's health care* (8th ed.). St. Louis: Mosby.)

Answer: Answer is indicated by the circle containing the X

Test-Taking Strategy: Focus on the key words, "6-month-old infant" and "assess circulation." Visualize the body structure of a 6-month-old infant and recall that the very short and fat neck of the infant makes the carotid pulse difficult to palpate. In an infant less than 1 year of age, the brachial pulse is used to assess circulation. Focus on the key words!

True Response Question: Prioritizing (Ordered Response)

List in *order of priority* the interventions that the nurse would take in the care of a client who develops acute pulmonary edema. (Number 1 indicates the first action and number 4 indicates the last action.)

___ Place the client on a pulse oximetry
___ Place the client in high-Fowler's position
___ Prepare the client for endotracheal intubation and mechanical ventilation
___ Prepare for the administration of oxygen

Answer: 2, 1, 4, 3

Test-Taking Strategy: Focus on the key words, "order of priority." Think about the pathophysiology associated with acute pulmonary edema. This will assist in determining that positioning the client in high-Fowler's is the first action. Next select placing the client on a pulse oximetry because this action relates to data collection and does not require a physician's order. From the remaining interventions, recall that endotracheal intubation and mechanical ventilation is performed if oxygen administration via mask or nasal cannula is ineffective and therefore would be performed as a last intervention. Focus on the key words!

True Response Question: Chart/Exhibit

A nurse is reviewing the physician's preoperative orders for a client with appendicitis scheduled for an emergency appendectomy. Which order would a licensed practical nurse verify with a registered nurse before carrying it out?

1. Maintain an NPO status
2. Apply a heating pad on low setting to the abdomen
3. Position in a right side-lying or low to semi-Fowler's position
4. Monitor for changes in the level of pain

CLIENT'S CHART

ORDERS	LABS	MEDS
Maintain an NPO status Apply a heating pad on low setting to the abdomen Position in a right side-lying or low to semi-Fowler's position Monitor for changes in the level of pain		

Answer: 2

Test-Taking Strategy: Note the key words "verify with the registered nurse before carrying it out." Recalling that the primary concern for a client with appendicitis is rupture and recalling the effects of heat will direct you to option 2 as the order to verify. Focus on the key words!

FALSE RESPONSE QUESTIONS

What Is a False Response Question?

A false response question asks you to make a decision and select the option that is inaccurate or incorrect with regard to the data presented in the question. False response questions are used less frequently on the NCLEX-PN examination as compared with the true response questions, but you need to be alert in noting these types of questions. It is unlikely that false response questions will be presented in alternate test question formats. You will most likely note false response questions presented in a multiple-choice format. How will you know that the question is a false response one? Read carefully and focus on the stem of the question. The stem contains key words or phrases that indicate that the question is a false response question. Generally, false response questions are used in evaluation-type questions and evaluate the effectiveness of a treatment, procedure, medication, or teaching.

> False response question: Asks you to select the option that is inaccurate or incorrect with regard to the data presented in the case situation.

What Are the Key Words and Phrases Commonly Used in False Response Questions?

Remember to read the question carefully and focus on the stem of the question because it contains key words or phrases that indicate that the question is a false response question. Examples of question stems and sample questions that indicate that the question is a false response one are listed below.

FALSE RESPONSE QUESTIONS: KEY WORDS

- Least likely
- Least priority
- Least helpful
- Avoid
- Needs reinforcement of the discharge instructions
- Have not yet been fully met
- Ineffective
- Needs reinforcement of the medication administration instructions
- Has not met the outcome criteria

False Response Questions: Example Question Stems

Which of the following individuals is *least likely* to develop coronary artery disease?

Which nursing diagnosis is of *least priority?*

Which of the following approaches by the nurse would be *least helpful* in assisting this client?

A nurse would *avoid* which of the following actions?

A nurse determines that the family *needs reinforcement of the discharge instructions* if the nurse observes which of the following being done by the family?

Which of the following outcomes indicates to the nurse that the goals *have not yet been fully met?*

A nurse determines that the medication is *ineffective* if the client continues to experience which symptom?

A nurse determines that the client needs *reinforcement of the medication administration instructions* if the client makes which of the following statements?

A nurse determines that the client *has not met the outcome criteria* by discharge if the client:

False Response Question: Multiple Choice

A nurse is reviewing the nursing care plan of a client hospitalized with sickle cell crisis. Which nursing diagnosis written in the plan is of *least priority?*

1. Acute pain
2. Deficient fluid volume
3. Ineffective tissue perfusion
4. Ineffective coping

Answer: 4

Test-Taking Strategy: Focus on the key words "least priority." According to Maslow's Hierarchy of Needs theory, physiological needs are the priority, followed by safety needs and then psychosocial needs. Using Maslow's theory will direct you to option 4 because this is the only option that addresses a psychosocial need. Focus on the key words!

False Response Question: Multiple Choice

A nurse has collected data from four clients seen in the health care clinic. Which client is *least likely* to develop coronary artery disease?

1. A client with a blood cholesterol level of 289 mg/dL
2. A client with hypertension whose blood pressure has been maintained at 118/78 mm Hg
3. A client who has been smoking two packs of cigarettes daily for the past 20 years
4. A client who is obese, inactive, and has a stressful lifestyle

Answer: 2

Test-Taking Strategy: Focus on the key words, "least likely." Recalling the risk factors associated with coronary disease will direct you to option 2. Option 2 is the only option that identifies a risk factor that has been modified and controlled. Focus on the key words!

False Response Question: Multiple Choice

A nurse would *avoid* which of the following actions when communicating with a client with aphasia?

1. Increase environmental stimuli
2. Ask questions that can be answered with a "yes" or "no"
3. Speak with a normal volume or tone
4. Present one thought or idea at a time

Answer: 1

Test-Taking Strategy: Focus on the key word, "avoid." Recalling that the client with aphasia may need extra time to comprehend and respond to communication will direct you to option 1. Increased environmental stimuli may be distracting and disrupting to communication efforts. Focus on the key words!

False Response Question: Multiple Choice

A nurse is collecting data from a client who has been taking omeprazole (Prilosec) as prescribed. The nurse determines that the medication is *ineffective* if the client continues to experience which symptom?

1. Headaches
2. Muscle pains
3. Heartburn
4. Dizziness

Answer: 3

Test-Taking Strategy: Focus on the key word "ineffective." Recalling that omeprazole is a gastric acid pump inhibitor (most medication names that end with *-zole* are gastric acid pump inhibitors) will direct you to option 3. Focus on the key words!

False Response Question: Multiple Choice

A client treated for an episode of hyperthermia is being discharged to home from the emergency department. The nurse determines that the client *needs reinforcement of the discharge instructions* if the client states to:

1. stay in a cool environment when possible.
2. increase fluid intake for the next 24 hours.
3. monitor voiding for adequacy of urine output.
4. resume full activity level immediately.

Answer: 4

Test-Taking Strategy: Focus on the key words "needs reinforcement of the discharge instructions." Select the client statement that indicates that the nurse needs to provide further instructions. Resumption of full activity immediately is not helpful; rather rest periods are indicated. Focus on the key words!

False Response Question: Multiple Choice

An unconscious client has a nursing diagnosis of Imbalanced Nutrition: Less Than Body Requirements documented in the nursing care plan. Which outcome indicates to the nurse that the goals *have not yet been met?*

1. Stable weight
2. Intake equaling output
3. Blood urea nitrogen (BUN) 12 mg/dL
4. Total protein 4.5 g/dL

Answer: 4

Test-Taking Strategy: Focus on the key words "has not yet been met." Because stable weight and equal intake and output are satisfactory indicators and the BUN is normal, option 4 is the answer to the question. Focus on the key words!

REFERENCES

Chernecky, C. & Berger, B. (2004). *Laboratory tests and diagnostic procedures* (4th ed). Philadelphia: Saunders.

DeWit, S. (2005). *Fundamental concepts and skills for nursing* (2nd ed). Philadelphia: Saunders.

Gulanick, M., Myers, J., Klopp, A., Galanes, S., Gradishar, D., & Puzas, M. (2003). *Nursing care plans: nursing diagnosis and intervention* (5th ed). St. Louis: Mosby.

Hill, S. & Howlett, H. (2005). *Success in practical/vocational nursing: from student to leader* (5th ed). Philadelphia: Saunders.

Hodgson, B. & Kizior, R. (2005). *Saunders nursing drug handbook 2005.* Philadelphia: Saunders.

Ignatavicius, D. & Workman, M. (2006). *Medical-surgical nursing: critical thinking for collaborative care* (5th ed). Philadelphia: Saunders.

Linton, A. & Maebius, N. (2003). *Introduction to medical-surgical nursing* (3rd ed). Philadelphia: Saunders.

Lowdermilk, D. & Perry, A. (2004). *Maternity & women's health care* (8th ed). St. Louis: Mosby.

National Council of State Boards of Nursing, Inc. *Test Plan for the National Council Licensure Examination for Licensed Practical/Vocational Nurses* (effective date: April 2005), National Council of State Boards of Nursing, Chicago, 2004.

National Council of State Boards of Nursing, Inc. Online: available at www.ncsbn.org.

Potter, P. & Perry, A. (2005). *Fundamentals of nursing* (6th ed). St. Louis: Mosby.

Wong, D. & Hockenberry, M. (2003). *Wong's nursing care of infants and children* (7th ed). St. Louis: Mosby.

Chapter 9 Questions That Require Prioritizing

BE PREPARED!

Be prepared! Many of the test questions in the examination will require you to use the skill of prioritizing nursing actions. Most of the prioritizing questions will be presented in the multiple-choice format; however, you may be presented with a question in the prioritizing (ordered-response) format. Prioritizing questions address content in any nursing area. These types of questions can be difficult because when a question requires prioritization, all of the options may be correct but you need to determine the correct order of action. There are some test-taking strategies that you can use to assist in answering these questions correctly. These strategies include noting the key words or phrases that indicate the need to prioritize; the ABCs—airway, breathing, and circulation; Maslow's Hierarchy of Needs theory; and the steps of the nursing process (clinical problem-solving process). Let's review the definition of prioritizing and these test-taking strategies.

GUIDES FOR PRIORITIZING

- Key words or phrases
- The ABCs
- Maslow's Hierarchy of Needs theory
- The steps of the nursing process (clinical problem solving process)

PRIORITIZING

What Does Prioritizing Mean?

Prioritizing means that you need to rank the client's problems in order of importance. It is very important to read a question carefully and focus on the information in the question because the order of importance may vary depending on the issue of the question, the clinical setting, the client's condition, and the client's needs. It is also important to consider what the client deems as a priority, which may be quite different from what the nurse may feel is most important. Always consider what the client believes is the priority when planning care.

When you prioritize, you are deciding which needs or problems require immediate action and which ones could be delayed until later because they are not urgent. As you read a question and are trying to determine which option identifies the nurse's priority, use the priority classification system. The priority classification system ranks nursing actions as either a high priority, intermediate (middle) priority, or low priority. The description of these three types of classifications is listed below.

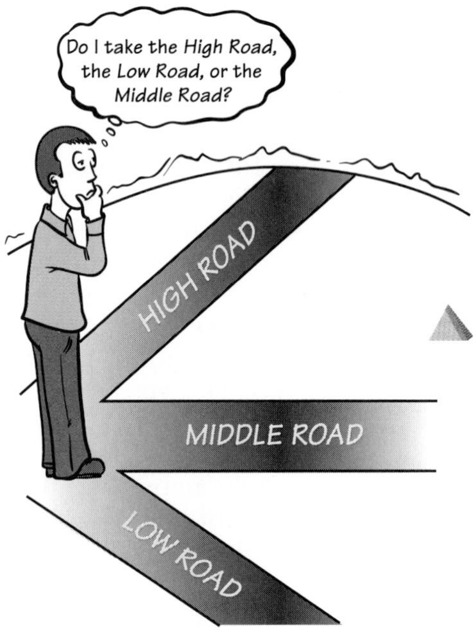
Do I take the High Road, the Low Road, or the Middle Road?
HIGH ROAD
MIDDLE ROAD
LOW ROAD

PRIORITY CLASSIFICATION SYSTEM

High Priority: A client need that is life-threatening or if untreated could result in harm to the client

Intermediate (Middle) Priority: A nonemergency and non–life-threatening client need that does not require immediate attention

Low Priority: A client need that is not directly related to the client's illness or prognosis, is not urgent, and does not require immediate attention

When Do You Select the Option, "Notify a Registered Nurse"?

An important point to remember is that the NCLEX examination is testing you on your competence and ability to care for a client and to implement measures that are necessary in a particular situation. It is critically important to read the question carefully, note the information in the question, and read all of the available options. If the question does not describe a life-threatening client situation or one that indicates a change in the client's condition, and there is an option that directly relates to a nursing action relevant to the situation, then it is best to select that option and not the option that reads *Notify a registered nurse.* If the question does describe a life-threatening client situation or one that indicates a change in the client's condition, then select the option that reads *Notify a registered nurse.*

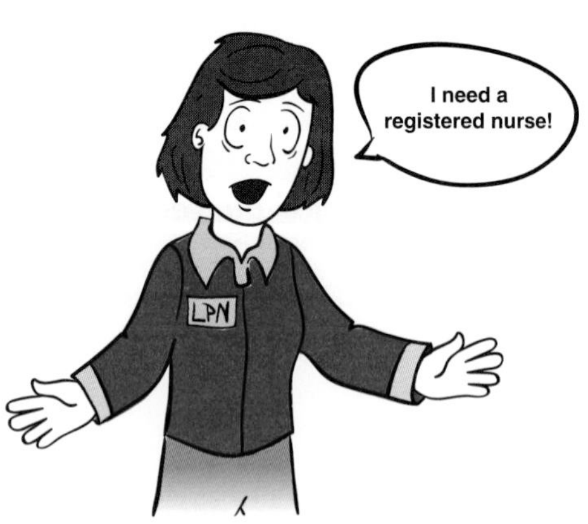
I need a registered nurse!
LPN

As a licensed practical/vocational nurse, you may be employed in an agency in which you will be in charge of the nursing unit and changes in a client's condition or life-threatening client situations may need to be reported directly to a physician. If you note an option that reads *Notify the physician,* use the same guidelines for deciding if it is necessary to *notify a registered nurse.* If there is a change in the client's condition or a life-threatening condition exists, *notify the physician.*

Remember, read the question and all of the options carefully. The data in the question will be a helpful guide in determining whether you should notify a registered nurse or physician.

Let's review some sample questions that illustrate client situations requiring and not requiring notification of a registered nurse.

When Not to Select the Option, "Notify a Registered Nurse"

A nurse is caring for a postoperative client who becomes restless. The nurse should take which *initial* action?

1. Check the client's vital signs.
2. Notify a registered nurse.
3. Medicate the client for pain.
4. Talk to the client in a calm voice.

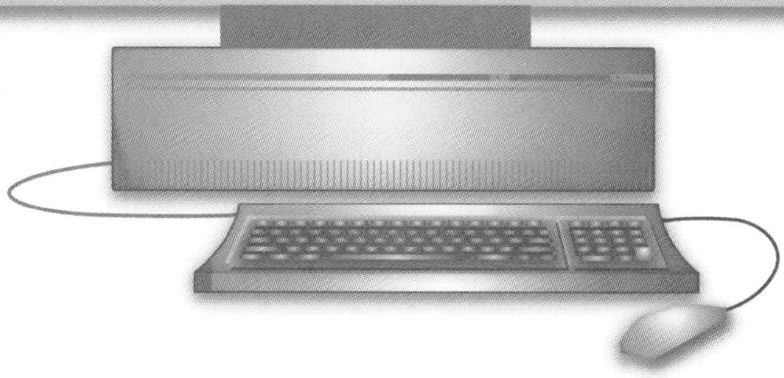

Answer: 1

Test-Taking Strategy: Read the question carefully, note the key word "initial," and focus on the issue, *a postoperative client who becomes restless.* There are no data in the question that indicate that the client has pain; therefore, eliminate option 3. Because option 4 is a psychosocial action rather than a physiological one (physiological needs are the priority), eliminate that option. Recall that restlessness indicates an early sign of shock. However, there are no data in the question that indicate a life-threatening condition. Therefore, the nurse would gather more data about the client's condition and *initially* check the client's vital signs.

When to Select the Option, "Notify a Registered Nurse"

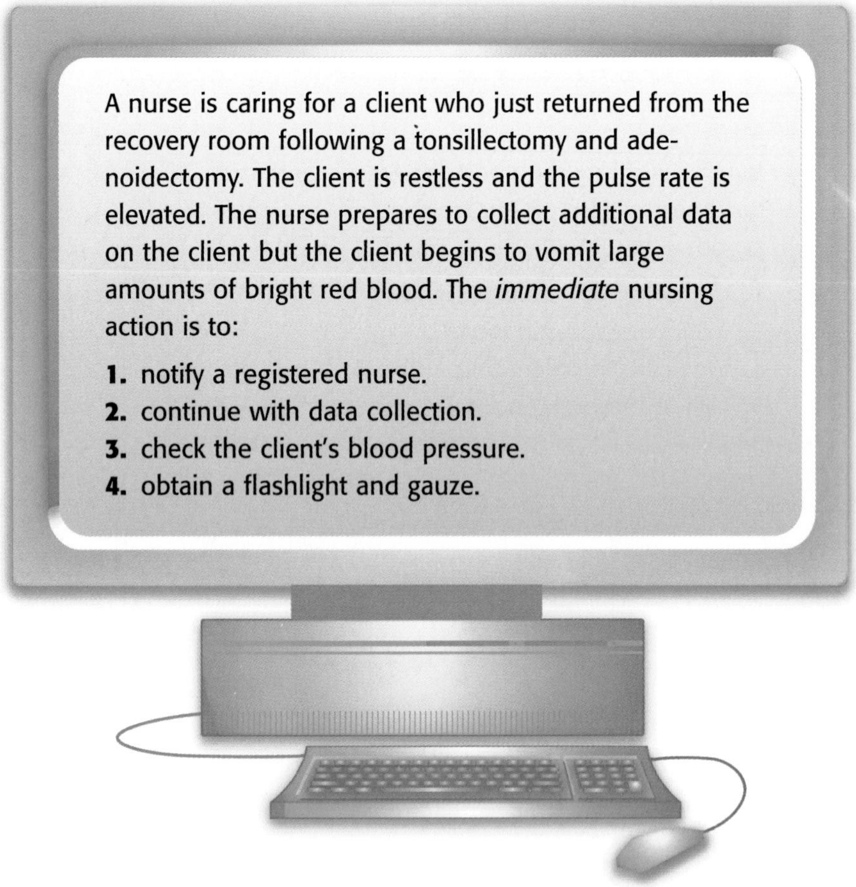

A nurse is caring for a client who just returned from the recovery room following a tonsillectomy and adenoidectomy. The client is restless and the pulse rate is elevated. The nurse prepares to collect additional data on the client but the client begins to vomit large amounts of bright red blood. The *immediate* nursing action is to:
1. notify a registered nurse.
2. continue with data collection.
3. check the client's blood pressure.
4. obtain a flashlight and gauze.

Answer: 1

Test-Taking Strategy: Read the question carefully and note the key words and the issue of the question. There are several key words in this question that you need to note. These include "restless," "pulse rate is elevated," "large amounts," "bright red blood," and "immediate." The issue of the question is that *the client is actively bleeding and is exhibiting signs of shock*. Remember to always read each option carefully. In this situation and from the options provided, the nurse would need to *notify a registered nurse*. Options 2, 3, and 4 would delay necessary interventions needed in this life-threatening situation.

KEY WORDS OR PHRASES

What Are the Key Words or Phrases That Indicate the Need to Prioritize Nursing Actions?

When a question requires prioritization, all options may be correct, and you need to determine the correct order of nursing action. Read the question carefully and look for the key words or phrases in the question that indicate the need to prioritize. Some of the common key words or phrases that indicate the need to prioritize are listed below and are followed by examples of how some of these words or phrases are used in a question.

> Note the key words that indicate the need to prioritize!

Common Key Words That Indicate the Need to Prioritize

Best
Essential
First
Highest priority
Immediately
Initial
Most appropriate
Most effective
Most important
Most likely
Next
Order of priority
Priority
Primary
Vital

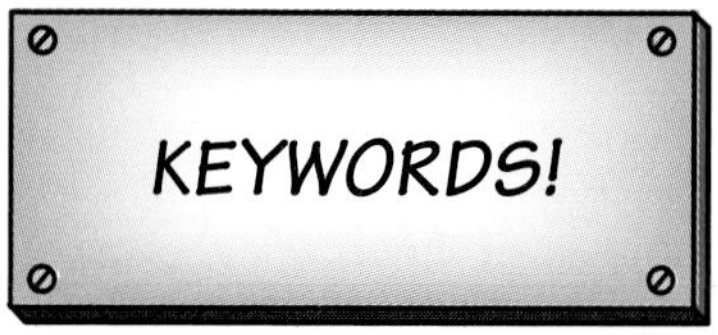

Sample Question: Key Words

A nurse is caring for a client with angina pectoris who begins to experience chest pain. The nurse administers a sublingual nitroglycerin (Nitrostat) tablet as prescribed, but the pain is unrelieved. Which action would the nurse take *next?*

1. Call a code blue.
2. Call the client's family.
3. Administer another nitroglycerin tablet.
4. Reposition the client.

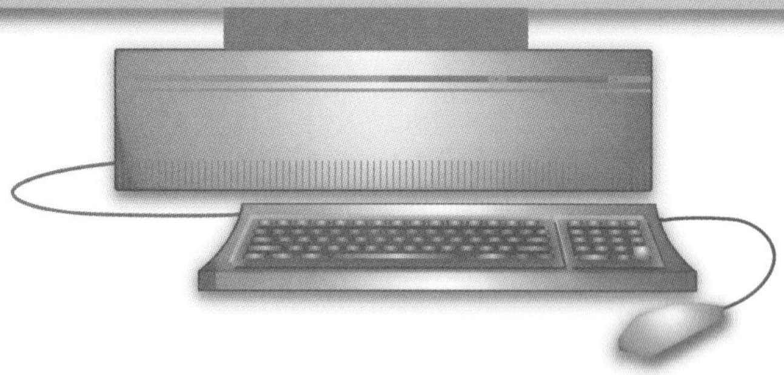

Answer: 3

Test-Taking Strategy: Note the key word "next" and focus on the issue, *that the client is experiencing chest pain.* Recalling that the nurse would administer three nitroglycerin tablets 5 minutes apart from each other to relieve chest pain will assist in directing you to option 3. Repositioning the client will not alleviate the pain associated with angina pectoris. There are no data in the question that indicate the need to call a code blue. A code blue is called if assistance with cardiopulmonary resuscitation measures is needed. There is no useful reason to call the client's family.

Sample Question: Key Words

An infant with tetralogy of Fallot experiences a hypercyanotic spell during a blood draw. List in *order of priority* the actions that the nurse would take (number 1 is the first priority and number 4 is the lowest priority).

___ Administer morphine subcutaneously as prescribed.
___ Administer 100% oxygen by face mask as prescribed.
___ Place the infant in a knee-chest position.
___ Administer intravenous fluids as prescribed.

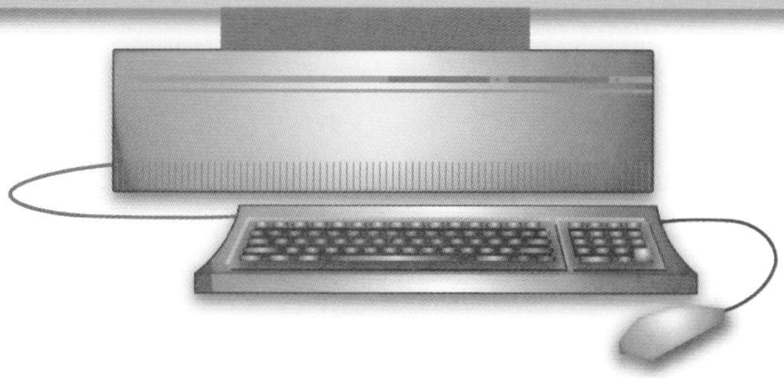

Answer: 3, 2 ,1, 4

Test-Taking Strategy: Note the key words "order of priority" and the issue of the question, *a hypercyanotic spell.* In questions that require you to determine the order of priority for nursing actions, if one of the options indicates client positioning, that option may be the first action. Positioning a client can relieve a symptom and is an intervention that takes only seconds to implement. Placing the infant in the knee-chest position reduces the venous return from the legs (which is desaturated) and increases systemic vascular resistance, which diverts more blood flow into the pulmonary artery. Note that the remaining options all require a physician's order. Recalling that airway is a priority, the next action is to administer oxygen to the infant. Knowing that morphine sulfate reduces spasm that occurs with these spells and that intravenous fluids are not always needed to treat these spells will assist in determining the order of priority for these remaining two interventions.

THE ABCs

What Are the ABCs and How Will They Help to Answer a Prioritizing Question?

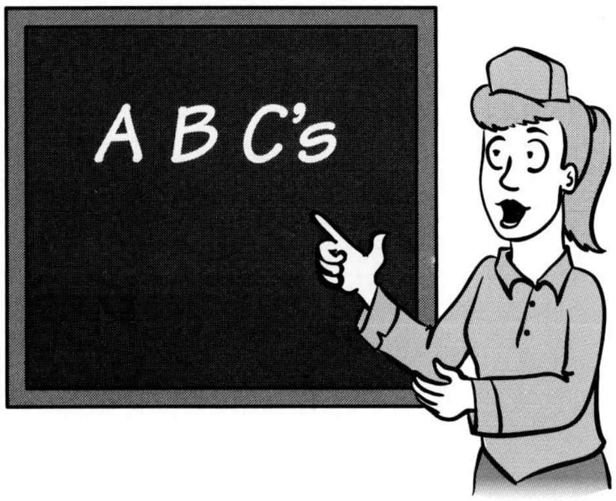

The ABCs indicate airway, breathing, and circulation and direct the order of priority of nursing actions. Airway is always the first priority in caring for any client. When you are asked a question that requires prioritization, use the ABCs to assist in determining the correct option. If an option addresses maintenance of a patent airway, that will be the correct option. If none of the options address airway, then move to B = breathing, followed by C = circulation. Some sample questions of how this strategy works are illustrated below.

> Use the ABCs to prioritize!

Sample Question: The ABCs

The client with a diagnosis of cancer is receiving morphine sulfate 10 mg subcutaneously every 3 to 4 hours for pain. When preparing a plan of care for the client, the nurse includes which *priority* action?

1. Monitor stools.
2. Monitor the urine output.
3. Encourage the client to cough and deep breathe.
4. Encourage fluid intake.

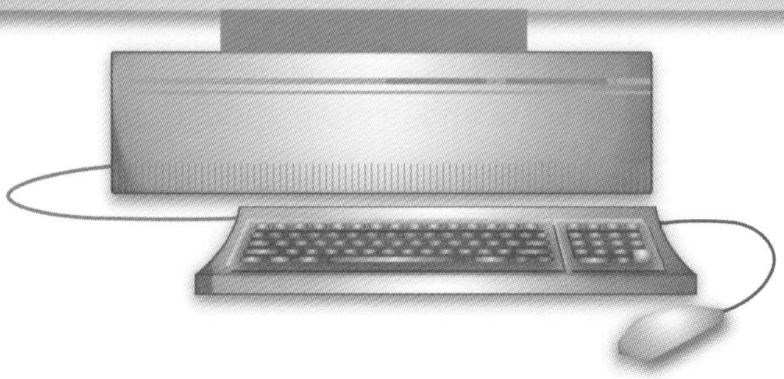

Answer: 3

Test-Taking Strategy: Note the key word "priority" and the issue, *morphine sulfate*. Use the ABCs—airway, breathing, and circulation—as a guide to direct you to the correct option. Recall that morphine sulfate suppresses the cough reflex and the respiratory reflex. Although options 1, 2, and 4 are components of the plan of care, the correct option addresses airway. Remember, use the ABCs—airway, breathing, and circulation—to prioritize.

Sample Question: The ABCs

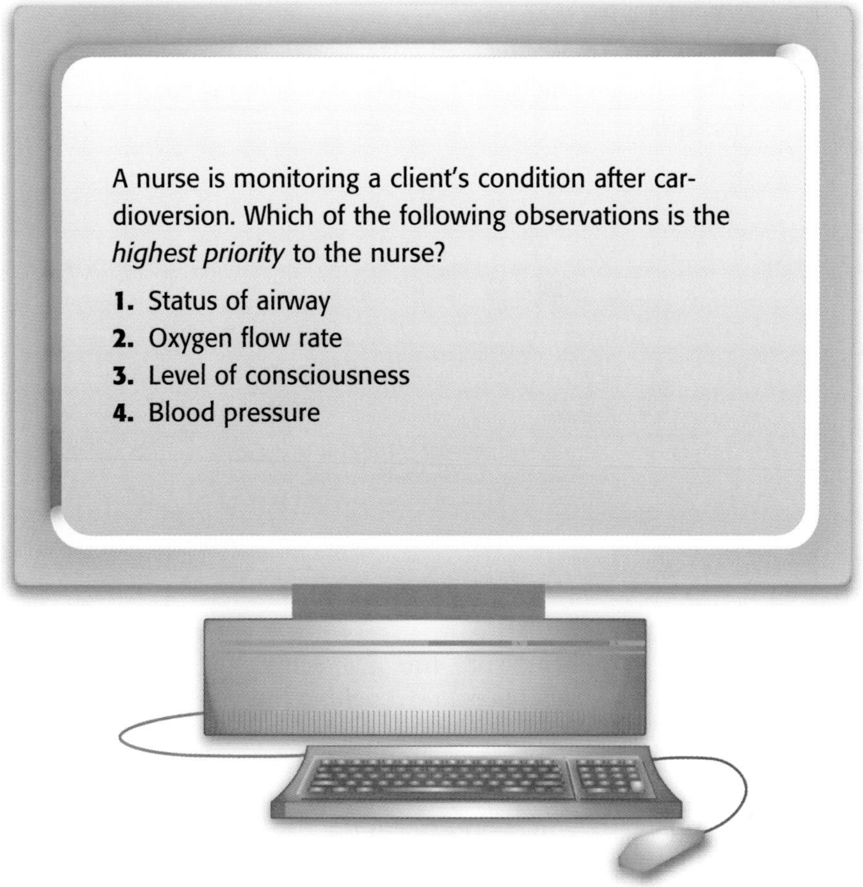

A nurse is monitoring a client's condition after cardioversion. Which of the following observations is the *highest priority* to the nurse?
1. Status of airway
2. Oxygen flow rate
3. Level of consciousness
4. Blood pressure

Answer: 1

Test-Taking Strategy: Note the key words, "highest priority" and the issue, *monitoring the client's condition after cardioversion*. Nursing responsibilities after cardioversion include maintaining a patent airway, administering oxygen, and monitoring vital signs and level of consciousness, and for cardiac irregularities. Airway however, is always the highest priority. Use the ABC's—airway, breathing, and circulation—to direct you to option 1.

Sample Question: The ABCs

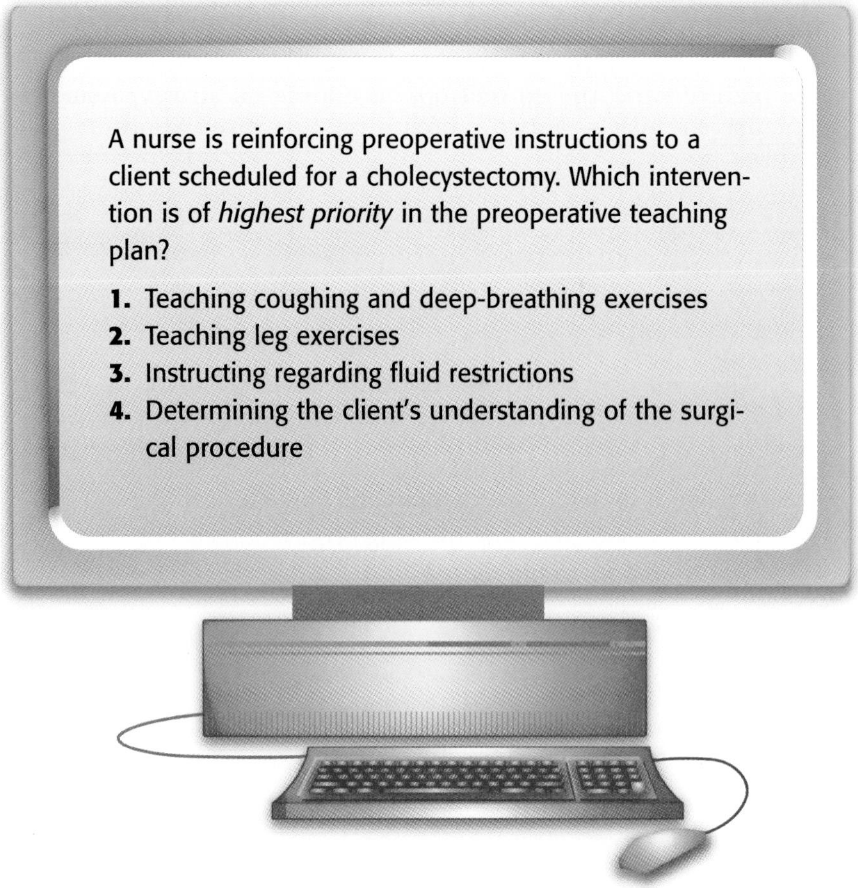

A nurse is reinforcing preoperative instructions to a client scheduled for a cholecystectomy. Which intervention is of *highest priority* in the preoperative teaching plan?

1. Teaching coughing and deep-breathing exercises
2. Teaching leg exercises
3. Instructing regarding fluid restrictions
4. Determining the client's understanding of the surgical procedure

Answer: 1

Test-Taking Strategy: Note the key words "highest priority" and note the issue, *preoperative teaching plan.* Use the ABCs—airway, breathing, and circulation—to answer the question. Option 1 relates to airway. After cholecystectomy, breathing tends to be shallow because deep breathing is painful as a result of the location of the incision. Teaching the importance of performing coughing and deep breathing exercises is the priority.

MASLOW'S HIERARCHY OF NEEDS THEORY

What Is Maslow's Hierarchy of Needs Theory and How Will It Help to Answer Prioritizing Questions?

Abraham Maslow theorized that human needs are satisfied in a particular order and arranged human needs in a pyramid or hierarchy. According to Maslow, basic physiological needs such as airway, breathing, circulation, water, food, and elimination are the priority. These basic physiological needs are then followed by safety and the psychosocial needs including security, love and belonging, self-esteem, and self-actualization, in that order.

Maslow's Hierarchy of Needs theory is a helpful guide to use to prioritize client needs. When you are answering a question that requires you to prioritize, select an option that relates to a physiological need, remembering that physiological needs are the priority.

If a physiological need is not addressed in the question or noted in one of the options, then continue to use Maslow's Hierarchy of Needs theory as a guide and look for the option that addresses safety. If neither physiological nor safety needs are addressed, then look for the option that addresses the client's psychosocial need. Figure 9-1 illustrates Maslow's Hierarchy of Needs theory. The sample questions below point out how Maslow's theory can be used as a guide to answer questions that require prioritizing.

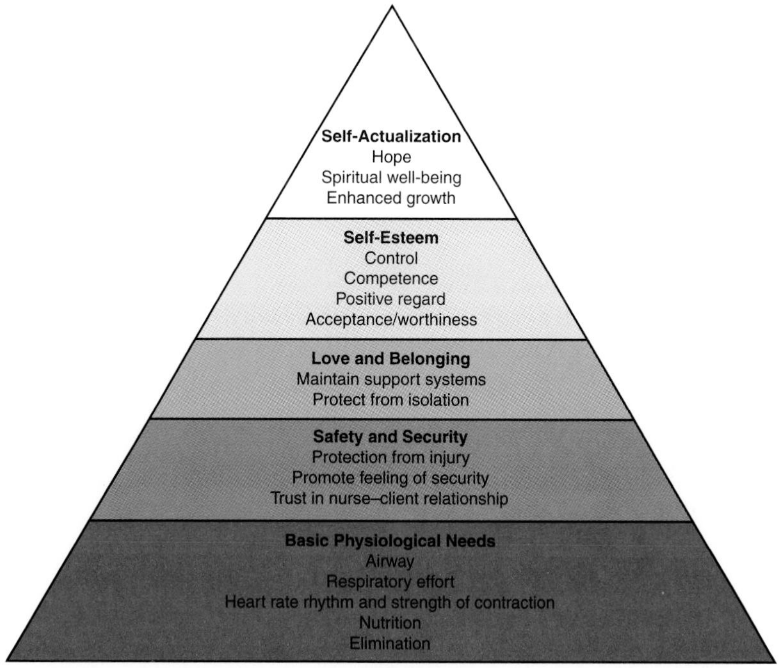

Figure 9-1 Nursing Priorities from Maslow's Hierarchy. From Harkreader, H. & Hogan, M.A. [2004]. *Fundamentals of nursing: caring and clinical judgment* (2nd ed.). Philadelphia: Saunders.

Use Maslow's Hierarchy of Needs theory to prioritize!

Sample Question: Maslow's Hierarchy of Needs Theory

A nurse is assisting with the admission of a client to the mental health unit with a diagnosis of post-traumatic stress disorder. The client is confused and disoriented. During data collection, the nurse's *primary* goal for this client is to:

1. stabilize the client's psychiatric needs.
2. orient the client to the unit.
3. explain the unit rules.
4. make the client feel safe.

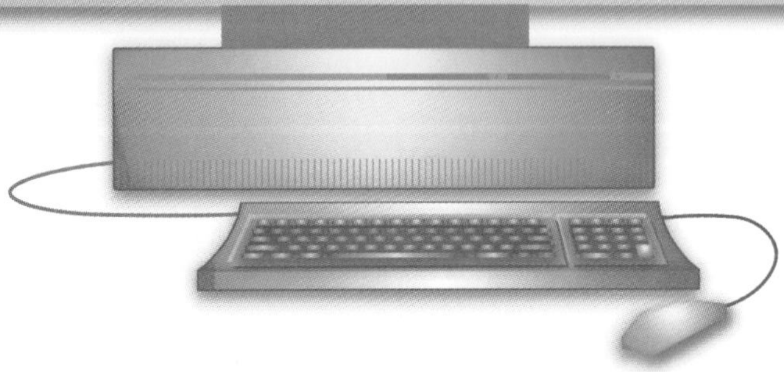

Answer: 4

Test-Taking Strategy: Note the key word "primary" and focus on the issue, *a client being admitted to the mental health unit.* Use Maslow's Hierarchy of Needs theory and remember that when a physiological need does not exist, then safety needs take precedence. It is important to make a confused and disoriented client feel safe. Stabilizing psychiatric needs is a long-term goal. Orientation and explaining the unit rules are part of any admission process.

Sample Question: Maslow's Hierarchy of Needs Theory

A nurse has helped develop a plan of care for a client diagnosed with anorexia nervosa. Which nursing diagnosis would the nurse select as the *priority* in the plan of care?

1. Disturbed Body Image
2. Defensive Coping
3. Deficient Knowledge
4. Imbalanced Nutrition: Less Than Body Requirements

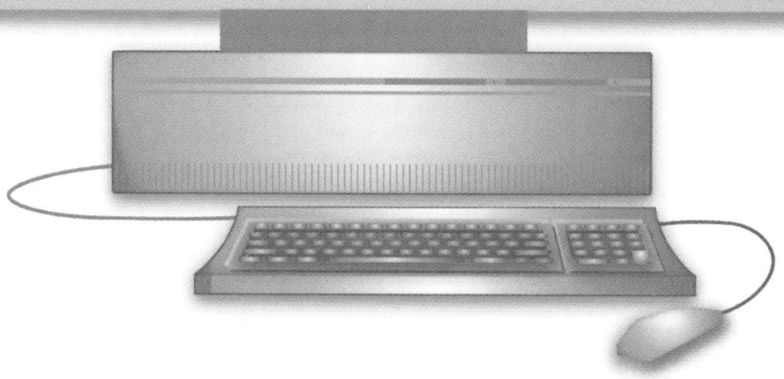

Answer: 4

Test-Taking Strategy: Note the key word "priority" and focus on the issue, *a nursing diagnosis.* Use Maslow's Hierarchy of Needs theory, recalling that physiological needs are the priority. This will assist in directing you to option 4. Options 1, 2, and 3 are psychosocial needs and are of a lesser priority.

Sample Question: Maslow's Hierarchy of Needs Theory

A nurse is preparing to reinforce instructions with a client about using crutches. Before reinforcing the instructions, the nurse collects which *priority* information from the client?

1. The client's fear related to the use of the crutches
2. The client's understanding of the need for increased mobility
3. The client's muscle strength and previous activity level
4. The client's feelings about the restricted mobility

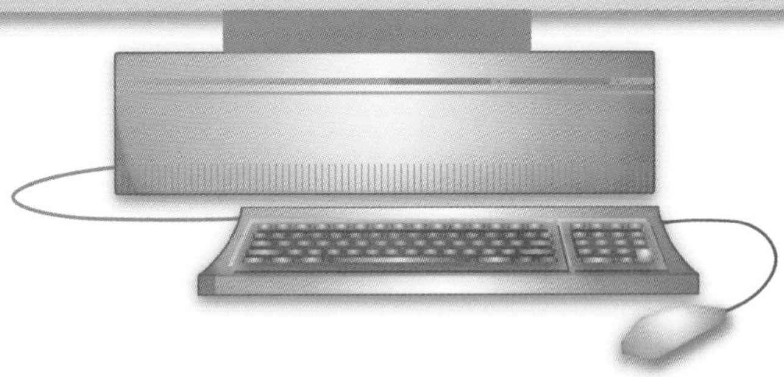

Answer: 3

Test-Taking Strategy: Note the key word "priority" and focus on the issue, *teaching a client how to use crutches*. Using Maslow's Hierarchy of Needs theory, remember that physiological needs take precedence over psychosocial needs. This should direct you to option 3. Information about muscle strength will help determine if the client has enough strength for crutch walking and if muscle-strengthening exercises are necessary. Previous activity level will provide information related to the tolerance of activity. Options 1, 2, and 4 are also important data but relate to psychosocial needs.

CLINICAL PROBLEM-SOLVING PROCESS (NURSING PROCESS)

How Will the Clinical Problem-Solving Process (Nursing Process) Help to Answer Prioritizing Questions?

The test plan for the NCLEX-PN examination identifies the clinical problem-solving process (nursing process) as an Integrated Process. The clinical problem-solving process (nursing process) provides a systematic method for providing care to a client. These steps include data collection, planning, implementation, and evaluation. These steps are usually followed in sequence, with data collection being the first step and evaluation being the last. However once the clinical problem-solving process (nursing process) begins, it becomes a cyclical process. The steps of the clinical problem-solving process (nursing process) can be used as a guide to help you to answer questions that require prioritization. Remember that it is always important to read the question carefully to determine what the question is asking. When a question asks for the first or initial nursing action, use these steps and look for a data collection action in one of the options. If a data collection action is not addressed in one of the options, then continue to use the clinical problem-solving process (nursing process) in a systematic order. Figure 9-2 illustrates the steps of the clinical problem-solving process (nursing process) and a description for each step is provided below.

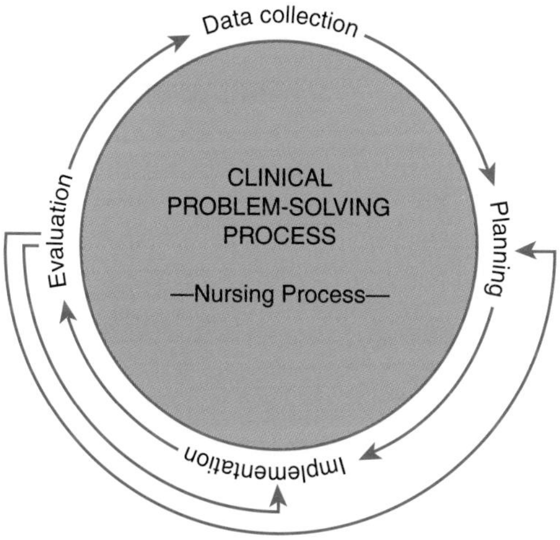

Figure 9-2 The Clinical Problem Solving Process (Nursing Process): A Systematic and Continuous Method for Providing Care to Clients.

> Use the steps of the clinical problem-solving process (nursing process) to prioritize!

Data Collection

Data collection questions address the process of gathering subjective and objective data relative to the client, confirming that data, and communicating and documenting the data.

Remember that data collection is the first step in the clinical problem-solving process (nursing process). When you are asked to select your first and initial nursing action, look for an option that addresses data collection. If an option contains the concept of the collection of client data, it is best to select that option. There are some key words to look for in the options that indicate a data collection action. Some of these key words, as well as a sample question, are listed below.

Key Words in Options That Indicate Data Collection

Check
Collect
Determine
Find out
Gather
Identify
Monitor
Observe
Obtain information
Recognize

If a data collection action is not noted in one of the options, follow the steps of the clinical problem-solving process (nursing process) as your guide to select your first action. There is a possible exception to using the process of data collection as a guide to prioritize. ***Possible exception to the guideline:*** If the question presents an emergency situation, read carefully; in an emergency situation, an intervention may be the priority!

Sample Question: Data Collection

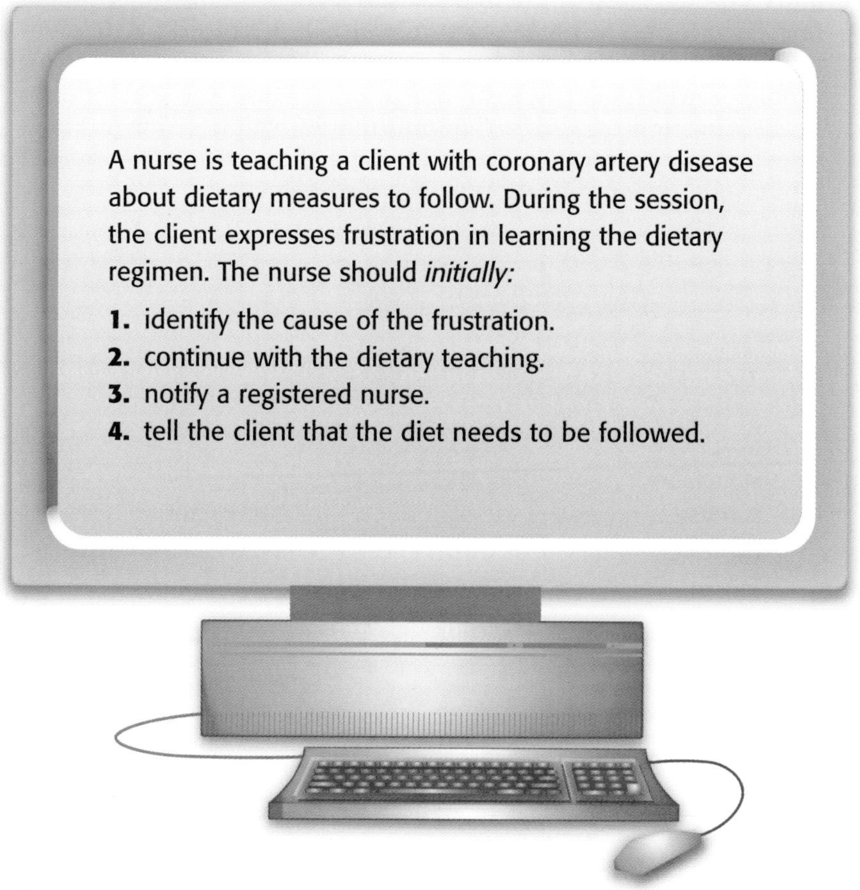

A nurse is teaching a client with coronary artery disease about dietary measures to follow. During the session, the client expresses frustration in learning the dietary regimen. The nurse should *initially:*

1. identify the cause of the frustration.
2. continue with the dietary teaching.
3. notify a registered nurse.
4. tell the client that the diet needs to be followed.

Answer: 1

Test-Taking Strategy: Note the key word "initially" and focus on the issue, *a nursing action.* Use the steps of the clinical problem-solving process (nursing process). Of the four options presented, the only data collection action is option 1. Options 2, 3, and 4 identify the implementation step of the clinical problem-solving process (nursing process). The initial action is to identify the cause of the frustration. Remember data collection in the first step of the clinical problem-solving process (nursing process).

Planning

Planning questions frequently address nursing diagnoses. These questions require prioritizing nursing diagnoses, assisting in determining goals and outcome criteria for goals of care, assisting in developing the plan of care, and communicating and documenting the plan of care. With regard to questions that address the planning step of the clinical problem-solving process (nursing process) there are two important points to keep in mind. The first point is to remember that this is a nursing examination and the answer to the question most likely involves something related to the nursing plan rather than the medical

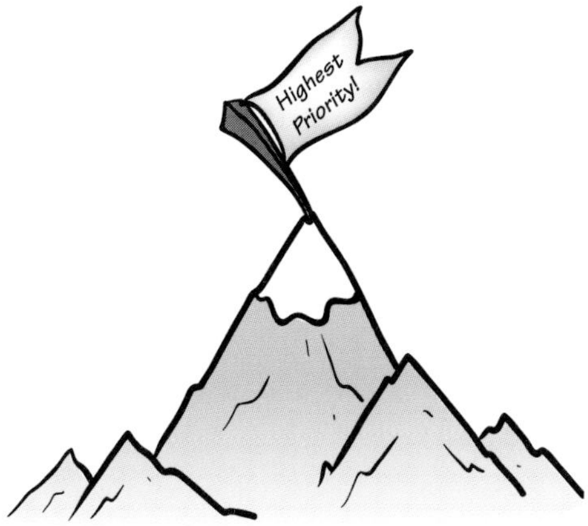

plan, unless the question asks what you anticipate the physician will prescribe. The second point to remember relates to questions that contain options listing nursing diagnoses and require you to prioritize them or to select the nursing diagnosis of highest priority. In these questions, it is important to remember that actual client problems rather than potential or at risk client problems will most likely be the priority. Read the information in the question carefully; this information will be your guide to selecting the correct option in this type of question. A sample of a planning type of question is provided below.

Sample Question: Planning

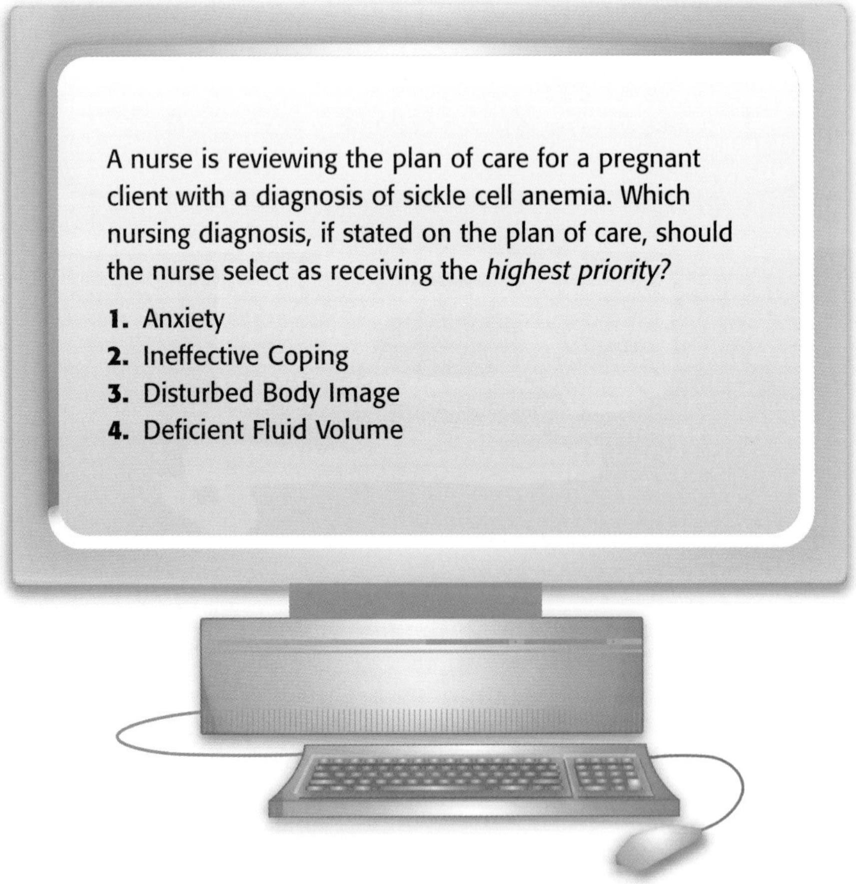

A nurse is reviewing the plan of care for a pregnant client with a diagnosis of sickle cell anemia. Which nursing diagnosis, if stated on the plan of care, should the nurse select as receiving the *highest priority?*
1. Anxiety
2. Ineffective Coping
3. Disturbed Body Image
4. Deficient Fluid Volume

Answer: 4

Test-Taking Strategy: Note the key words, "highest priority" and focus on the issue, *a nursing diagnosis in the plan of care.* To correctly answer this question, use Maslow's Hierarchy of Needs theory to prioritize, remembering that physiological needs come first. Using this guideline will direct you to option 4. Deficient fluid volume is a physiological need and is the priority nursing diagnosis. Options 1, 2, and 3 are psychosocial needs. Remember, physiological needs are the priority.

Implementation

Implementation questions address the process of assisting with organizing and managing care, providing care to achieve established goals, supervising unlicensed personnel and coordinating care, and communicating and documenting nursing interventions. Because the NCLEX examination tests your competence and ability to function as a nurse, many of the questions on the examination will be implementation-type questions.

When you are presented with a question that requires you to determine what the nurse will do, there are two important points to keep in mind. The first point is that the only client that you need to be concerned about is the client in the question; the client in the question is your only assigned client. This is an important point to bear in mind as you are trying to select the correct option.

You have only one client to be concerned about!

The second important point to keep in mind when you are answering NCLEX questions is that you need to answer the question from an ideal and textbook perspective not a reality perspective, and answer the question as if you had all the time available to care for the client and all the resources needed at the client's bedside.

Answer the question from an ideal and textbook perspective!

Answer the question as if you had all the time available to care for the client and all the resources needed at the client's bedside!

To illustrate these important points, let's look at the following questions.

Sample Question: Implementation

A nurse is caring for a preoperative male client who verbalizes a great deal of anxiety about the surgical procedure scheduled in 2 hours. Which action by the nurse would *best* alleviate the client's anxiety?

1. Tell the client that you will spend some time answering questions as soon as you get your other tasks completed.
2. Talk to the client for 15 minutes and return shortly thereafter to check on him.
3. Call the client's wife and ask her to visit the client before surgery.
4. Stay with the client until he is taken to the operating room.

Answer: 4

Test-Taking Strategy: Note the key word "best" and focus on the issue, *to alleviate the client's anxiety.* As you are reading the options, you may be hesitant to select option 4 and may say to yourself, "I could never stay with a client for 2 hours. I would never get any of my other clients taken care of." Stop right there and remember that on the NCLEX examination, the only client that you are caring for is the client in the question. Therefore the option that reads "Stay with the client until the client is taken to the operating room" is the *best* of the four options.

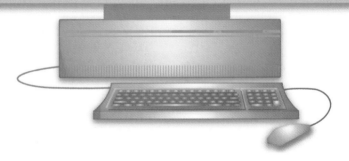

Sample Question: Implementation

A nurse is caring for a client following a cardiac catheterization. The client suddenly complains of a feeling of wetness in the groin at the catheter insertion site. The nurse checks the site, notes that the client is actively bleeding, and takes which *best* action?

1. Dons a clean glove and places pressure on the insertion site with the gloved hand
2. Dons a sterile glove and places pressure on the insertion site using a sterile gauze
3. Checks the client's blood pressure
4. Checks the client's peripheral pulse in the affected extremity

Answer: 2

Test-Taking Strategy: Note the key word "best" and focus on the issue, *a nursing action.* Active bleeding indicates the need for intervention and the application of pressure at the site of bleeding. This directs you to options 1 and 2 as the possible correct options. You may be hesitant to select option 2 because you may say to yourself, "I wouldn't use the sterile gloves or gauze because by the time I went to the treatment room, obtained these items, and returned to the room, the client would have lost a critically large amount of blood." Stop right there and remember that on the NCLEX examination, you have all of the supplies and resources needed and readily available at the client's bedside. Because the catheter insertion site is an open area, the *best* option is to don a sterile glove and place pressure on the insertion site using sterile gauze.

Evaluation

Evaluation questions focus on comparing the actual outcomes of care with the expected outcomes and focus on how the nurse should monitor or make a judgment concerning a client's response to therapy or to a nursing action. These questions also address evaluating the client's ability to implement self-care, unlicensed personnel ability to implement care, and the process of communicating and documenting evaluation findings.

In an evaluation question, it is important to note whether the question is a true response question or a false response question. Look for the words or phrases that indicate a false response question because they are frequently used in evaluation-type questions and ask for inaccurate information related to the issue of the question. (Key words or phrases used in both true response questions and false response questions can be located in Chapter 8.) Following is an example of an evaluation-type question.

Sample Question: Evaluation

A client recovering from an exacerbation of left-sided heart failure has a nursing diagnosis of Activity Intolerance. The nurse determines that the client *best* tolerates mild exercise if the client exhibits which of the following changes in vital signs during activity?

1. Pulse rate increased from 80 beats per minute to 104 beats per minute
2. Respiratory rate increased from 16 breaths per minute to 19 breaths per minute
3. Oxygen saturation decreased from 96% to 91%
4. Blood pressure decreased from 140/86 mm Hg to 112/72 mm Hg

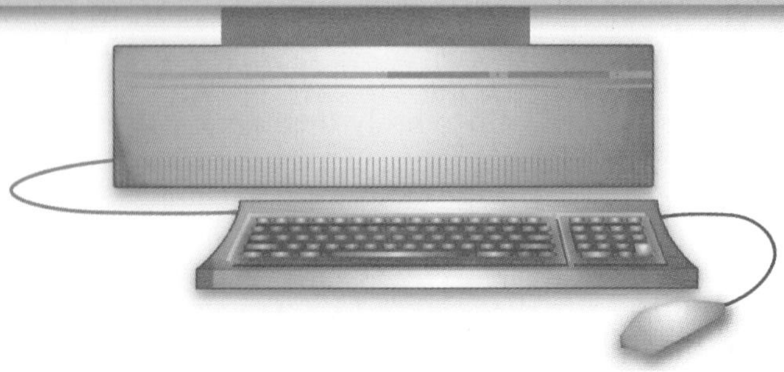

Answer: 2

Test-Taking Strategy: Note the key word "best" and focus on the issue, *the client's ability to tolerate exercise.* Use the process of elimination and nursing knowledge regarding normal vital sign values. Options 1 and 3 are incorrect because they represent changes from normal values to abnormal ones. Blood pressure decreases by more than 10 mm Hg is not a sign that indicates tolerance of activity. The only option that identifies values that remain within the normal range is option 2.

REFERENCES

Chernecky, C. & Berger, B. (2004). *Laboratory tests and diagnostic procedures* (4th ed). Philadelphia: Saunders.

DeWit, S. (2005). *Fundamental concepts and skills for nursing* (2nd ed). Philadelphia: Saunders.

Gulanick, M., Myers, J., Klopp, A., Galanes, S., Gradishar, D., & Puzas, M. (2003). *Nursing care plans: nursing diagnosis and intervention* (5th ed). St. Louis: Mosby.

Harkreader, H. & Hogan, M.A. (2004). *Fundamentals of nursing: caring and clinical judgment* (2nd ed). Philadelphia: Saunders.

Hill, S. & Howlett, H. (2005). *Success in practical/vocational nursing: from student to leader* (5th ed). Philadelphia: Saunders.

Hodgson, B. & Kizior, R. (2005). *Saunders nursing drug handbook 2005.* Philadelphia: Saunders.

Ignatavicius, D. & Workman, M. (2006). *Medical-surgical nursing: critical thinking for collaborative care* (5th ed). Philadelphia: Saunders.

Linton, A. & Maebius, N. (2003). *Introduction to medical-surgical nursing* (3rd ed). Philadelphia: Saunders.

Lowdermilk, D. & Perry, A. (2004). *Maternity & women's health care* (8th ed). St. Louis: Mosby.

National Council of State Boards of Nursing, Inc. *Test Plan for the National Council Licensure Examination for Licensed Practical/Vocational Nurses* (effective date: April 2005), National Council of State Boards of Nursing, Chicago, 2004.

National Council of State Boards of Nursing, Inc. online: Available at www.ncsbn.org.

Potter, P. & Perry, A. (2005). *Fundamentals of nursing* (6th ed). St. Louis: Mosby.

Varcarolis, E.M. (2002). *Foundations of psychiatric mental health nursing* (4th ed). Philadelphia: Saunders.

Wong, D. & Hockenberry, M. (2003). *Wong's nursing care of infants and children* (7th ed). St. Louis: Mosby.

Chapter 10

Managing and Delegating Care, and Client Care Assignment Questions

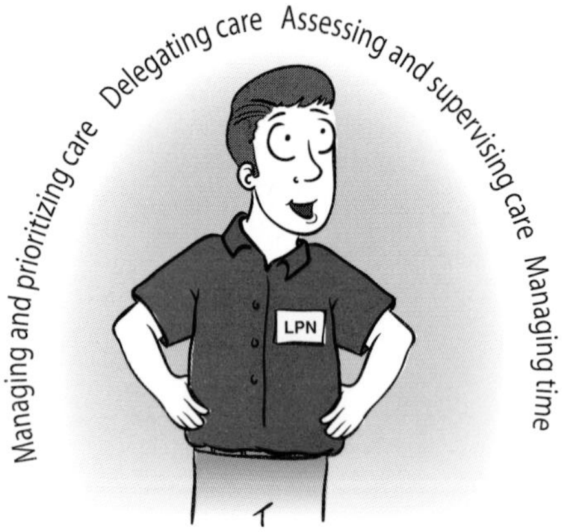

The licensed practical/vocational nurse manages, organizes, and prioritizes care; makes client care or related task assignments and delegates care; supervises care delivered by unlicensed personnel; and manages time efficiently. The NCLEX-PN® test plan, developed by the National Council of State Boards of Nursing, identifies the content related to these roles and responsibilities in the subcategory, Coordinated Care of the Safe, Effective Care Environment category of Client Needs. This subcategory, which entails 11% to 17% of the test plan, addresses content that tests the nurse's knowledge, skills, and abilities required to collaborate with health care team members to facilitate effective client care. Chapter 3, titled Client Needs, lists some of the content in the Coordinated Care subcategory that will be tested in this examination. It is important to review information related to this list of content to ensure that you are well prepared for questions regarding these role and responsibilities.

Some of the test questions in the subcategory of Coordinated Care relate to the nurse's responsibilities regarding delegating care and assignment-making and the supervisory role of these responsibilities. You may also be presented with questions that require you to determine the priority of care for a group of clients. The questions in the subcategory of Coordinated Care will most likely be in the multiple-choice format; however, you may be presented with questions that address these responsibilities in the multiple-response format or the prioritizing (ordered response) format. This chapter reviews the guidelines and principles related to delegating and assignment-making, two very important roles of the nurse. Guidelines for time management are also reviewed because managing time efficiently is a key factor for completing activities and tasks within a definite time period.

DELEGATION AND ASSIGNMENT-MAKING

What Is Delegation?

Delegation is the process of transferring a selected nursing task in a client situation to an individual who is competent to perform that specific task. It involves sharing activities and achieving outcomes with other individuals who have the competency to accomplish the task. The nurse practice acts and any other practice limitations, such as agency policies and procedures define the aspects of care that can be delegated and the tasks and activities that need to be performed by licensed and unlicensed personnel, such as a nursing assistant. When the nurse delegates an activity, the nurse needs to determine the degree of supervision that the delegatee may require and provide supervision as appropriate.

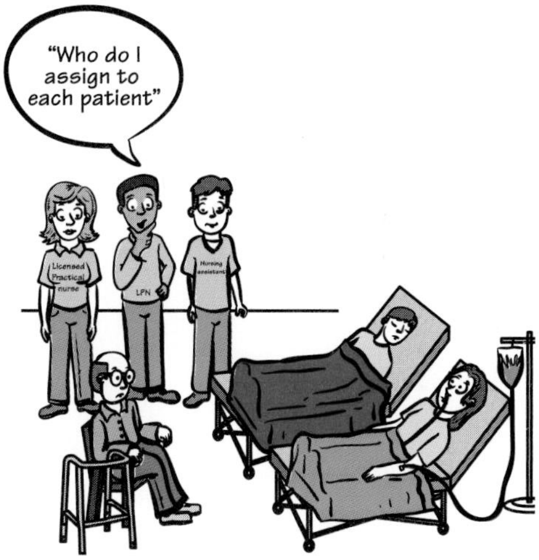

Delegation: Transferring a nursing task to an individual who is competent to perform the task.

What Is Assignment-Making?

Assignment-making is a specific activity that involves planning care activities for a client or a group of clients and determining specifically who will provide the care or perform certain activities. As with delegating, the nurse practice acts and any other practice limitations such as agency policies and procedures that define the aspects of care need to be used as a guide when planning assignments for activities and client care. Supervision of performance of the activity as appropriate is also important.

Assignment-making: Planning care activities for a client or a group of clients and determining who will provide the care or perform certain activities.

What Are the Important Points to Keep in Mind When Delegating or Making Assignments?

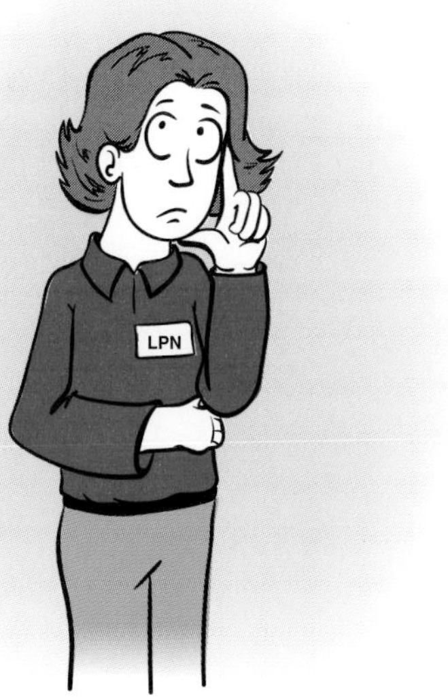

When you are answering questions related to either delegating or assignment-making there are two important points to keep in mind. The first is that even though a task or activity may be delegated to someone, the nurse who delegates the task or activity maintains accountability for the overall nursing care of the client. Remember, only the task, not the ultimate accountability, may be delegated to another.

The second point to keep in mind is that this examination is a national examination. Therefore, use general guidelines, such as the nurse practice acts, regarding what a health care provider can competently and legally perform to answer the question correctly. Avoid using agency policies and procedures and agency position descriptions to answer the question, unless the question provides information to do so, because they are specific to the agency.

Let's review two sample questions: one that illustrates the use of general guidelines related to delegating and assignment-making, and one that relates to specific agency policies and procedures.

Sample Question: General Guidelines

A licensed practical nurse is planning client assignments for the day and has another licensed practical nurse and a nursing assistant on the nursing team. The nurse *most appropriately* assigns which client to the licensed practical nurse?

1. An older client recovering from pneumonia who requires ambulation every 3 hours
2. A client with a tracheostomy who requires frequent suctioning
3. An older client who requires turning and repositioning every 2 hours and range of motion exercises every 4 hours
4. A client who requires the collection of urine for a 24-hour period

Answer: 2

Test-Taking Strategy: This question requires that you determine which client should *most appropriately* be assigned to the licensed practical nurse. There is no information in the question that indicates the need to use agency policies, procedures, or position descriptions to determine the most appropriate assignment; therefore, use general guidelines such as the nurse practice acts. As you read each option, think about and visualize the client's needs. The client described in option 2 has needs that cannot be met by the nursing assistant. Remember that the health care provider needs to competent and skilled to perform the assigned task or client activity.

Sample Question: Specific Agency Policies and Procedures

A licensed practical nurse employed in a long-term care facility is assigning client care activities to a nursing assistant. The nursing assistant is a first-semester senior nursing student and works at the facility as a nursing assistant part-time on weekends. The facility position description for a nursing student who is employed as a nursing assistant indicates that he or she may perform procedures learned in nursing school if supervised by a licensed nurse. Based on the facility's position description, the licensed practical nurse assigns which *most appropriate* activity to the nursing assistant?

1. Hang an intravenous solution of 0.9% normal saline
2. Insert an intravenous catheter
3. Change a sterile abdominal dressing
4. Administer digoxin (Lanoxin)

Answer: 3

Test-Taking Strategy: In this question, information is provided that directs you to use the facility's position description to determine the most appropriate activity to assign to the nursing assistant. The key words in the question are "most appropriate." Based on the data provided in the question and in the options, it is best to select the least invasive activity. Also, recall that intravenous and medication administration must be performed by a licensed health care provider.

Inserting an intravenous catheter is an invasive procedure that needs to be performed by a health care provider specially trained to perform it. Remember that the health care provider needs to be competent and skilled to perform the assigned task or client activity.

What Principles and Guidelines Can Be Used to Delegate and Make Assignments?

If you are presented with a question on the examination that requires you to delegate or plan assignments for a group of clients, there are principles and guidelines to use to assist in answering the question correctly. As you are using the process of elimination to determine the correct option, keep these principles and guidelines in mind. Also, read each option carefully. Think about and visualize the client's needs to determine which health care provider could best meet the client's needs. Following is a review of the principles and guidelines for delegating and assignment-making:

Always ensure client safety—never select an option that could potentially cause harm to the client.

Focus on the issue of the question and what the question is asking; for example, is the question asking you to delegate to another licensed practical or vocational nurse, or a nursing assistant?

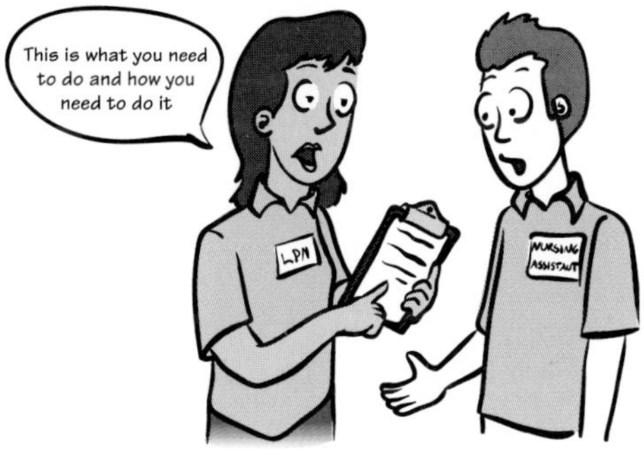
This is what you need to do and how you need to do it
LPN
NURSING ASSISTANT

Determine which tasks or client care activities can be delegated and to whom, and match the task to the delegatee on the basis of the nurse practice act or agency policies and procedures or position descriptions as appropriate; in other words, think about the activities that the delegatee can safely and legally perform.

Think about individual variations in work abilities and determine the degree of supervision that may be required; for example, if the question asks to delegate or assign a client care activity to a new nursing graduate, then you need to think about the need for providing adequate supervision and the need to teach the new graduate about the assigned activity.

Always provide directions to the delegatee that are clear, concise, accurate, and complete and validate the person's understanding of the directions and expectations; in other words, ask the delegatee to verbalize the procedure for performing the task and activity that was delegated.

Communicate a feeling of confidence to the delegatee, and provide feedback promptly after the task or activity is performed regarding his or her performance; in other words, ensure that the delegatee completed the task, and evaluate the outcome of the care provided.

Provide the delegatee with a timeline for completion of the task or activity; for example, if a client is scheduled for a diagnostic test and an activity or task needs to be completed before the test, it is important to identify this timeline to the delegatee.

Maintain continuity of care as much as possible when assigning client care; for example, it is best for the client to be cared for by a nurse with whom a therapeutic relationship has developed. However, it is also important to remember that there are some client situations in which maintaining continuity of care would be unfavorable with regard to ensuring a safe environment for a health care provider, such as with the client who has an infectious disease or the client with a radiation implant.

Sample Question: Assignment-Making

A nurse is planning the client assignments for the day and is reviewing client data and the needs of the clients on the nursing team. To maintain continuity of care, the nurse would ensure that which client is cared for by the nurse who cared for the client on the previous day?

1. A client with a cervical radiation implant
2. A client with active tuberculosis
3. A client with herpes zoster (chickenpox)
4. A client recently diagnosed with inoperable cancer

Answer: 4

Test-Taking Strategy: Focus on the issue of the question, *to maintain continuity of care.* Read each option carefully, keeping two points in mind: the client's needs and ensuring a safe environment for the health care provider. The clients described in options 1, 2, and 3 can potentially present a risk to the health care provider. The client in option 4 will likely have psychosocial needs that can best be met if the client is cared for by a health care provider with which the client has developed a therapeutic relationship.

Who Can Do What?

There are some general guidelines to follow when answering a question that requires determining what tasks and client care activities would be assigned to which health care provider. Remember these are general guidelines and the general guidelines are the ones that you need to follow when taking a national examination. These guidelines are followed by sample questions in both multiple choice and multiple response formats.

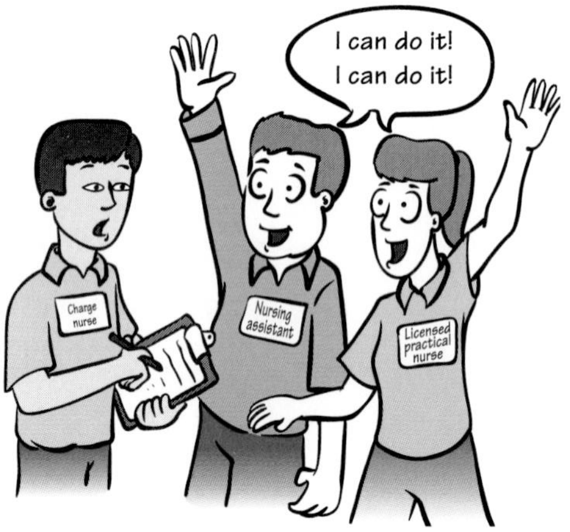

Unlicensed Personnel, such as a Nursing Assistant

Generally, noninvasive tasks and client care activities can be assigned to an unlicensed individual. Some of these tasks and activities include the following:

Ambulation
Bathing

Grooming
Hygiene measures
Positioning
Range-of-motion exercises
Skin care
Some specimen collections, such as a urine or stool
Transporting a client

Licensed Practical or Vocational Nurse

A licensed practical or vocational nurse can perform the tasks that the unlicensed personnel can perform as well as certain invasive tasks and client care activities. Some of these additional tasks include the following:

Administering oral medications
Administering intramuscular injections
Administering subcutaneous injections
Changing dressings
Irrigating wounds
Monitoring an intravenous flow rate
Performing urinary catheterization
Suctioning
Teaching about basic hygienic and nutritional measures
Using the clinical problem-solving process (nursing process): data collection, planning, implementing, and evaluating
Wound irrigations

Registered Nurse

A registered nurse is competent to perform many tasks and client care activities. In addition to the tasks and client care activities that a licensed practical or vocational nurse can perform, there are numerous procedures that the registered nurse can perform. To assist you in differentiating the role of the registered nurse and the licensed practical or vocational nurse, some of the tasks and client care activities that only the registered nurse can perform are listed below.

Administering intravenous medications
Leading others and managing the client care environment
Teaching
Using the nursing process: assessment, analyzing data, planning client care, implementing care, and evaluating care

Sample Question: Multiple Response

Select all clients that could be safely assigned to a nursing assistant.

___ A client with an open abdominal wound that requires wound irrigations every 3 hours
___ A client requiring a bed bath
___ A client with a spinal cord injury who requires intermittent urinary catheterization every 4 hours

___ A client who needs to be transported to the x-ray department via wheelchair
___ A client newly diagnosed with diabetes mellitus who requires reinforced teaching about insulin administration
___ A client who requires frequent ambulation with a walker

Answer:

___ A client with an open abdominal wound that requires wound irrigations every 3 hours
_X_ A client requiring a bed bath
___ A client with a spinal cord injury who requires intermittent urinary catheterization every 4 hours
_X_ A client who need to be transported to the x-ray department via wheelchair
___ A client newly diagnosed with diabetes mellitus who requires reinforced teaching about insulin administration
_X_ A client who requires frequent ambulation with a walker

Test-Taking Strategy: Focus on the issue of the question, *safe client assignments for a nursing assistant.* Use general principles and guidelines to assist in answering the question correctly. Think about and visualize the client's needs and determine if the nursing assistant can competently, safely, and legally perform activities to meet these needs. A client who requires wound irrigations, a client who requires intermittent urinary catheterization every 4 hours, and a client who requires reinforced teaching about insulin administration have needs that require the skills of a licensed nurse. Remember, the health care provider needs to be competent and skilled to perform the assigned task or client activity.

Sample Question: Multiple Choice

A nurse is planning client assignments for the day and needs to assign four clients. There is a licensed practical nurse and two nursing assistants on the nursing team. Which client would the nurse *most appropriately* assign to the licensed practical nurse?

1. A client with a right leg amputation who requires a dressing change
2. A client requiring a bed bath
3. A client who requires frequent ambulation
4. A client who requires a 24-hour urine collection

Answer: 1

Test-Taking Strategy: Note the key words "most appropriately." Focus on the issue of the question, *a client assignment to a licensed practical nurse.* Use general principles and guidelines to assist in answering the question correctly. Think about and visualize the client's needs. The needs of the client with a right leg amputation who requires a dressing change can best be met by the licensed practical nurse because the licensed practical nurse can perform dressing changes. The nursing assistant can most appropriately give a bed bath, ambulate a client, and collect urine specimens. Remember, the health care provider needs to be competent and skilled to perform the assigned task or client activity.

Sample Question: Multiple Choice

A nurse is planning the client assignments for the day. Which of the following is the *most appropriate* assignment for the nursing assistant?

1. A client with difficulty swallowing food and fluids
2. A client who requires stool specimen collections
3. A client requiring colostomy irrigation
4. A client receiving continuous tube feedings

Answer: 2

Test-Taking Strategy: Focus on the issue of the question, *a client assignment to a nursing assistant.* Use general principles and guidelines to assist in answering the question correctly. Think about and visualize the client's needs and determine if the nursing assistant can competently, safely, and legally perform activities to meet these needs. In this situation, the most appropriate assignment for a nursing assistant would be to care for the client who requires stool specimen collections. The client with difficulty swallowing food and fluids is at risk for aspiration. Colostomy irrigations and tube feedings are not performed by unlicensed personnel. Remember, the health care provider needs to be competent and skilled to perform the assigned task or client activity.

TIME MANAGEMENT

What Is Time Management and Why Is It Important?

Time management is a technique used by a nurse to assist in completing tasks within a definite time. It involves learning how, when, and where to use one's time and involves establishing personal goals and time frames. Time management requires an ability to anticipate the day's activities, to combine activities when possible, and to not be interrupted by nonessential activities. It also involves efficiency in completing tasks as quickly as possible, and effectiveness in deciding on the most important task to do, and doing it correctly. The ability to manage time efficiently is important in order to complete tasks and client care activities within a reasonable time frame. In many client care situations, time management requires prioritizing. The nurse needs to be skilled in planning time resourcefully and needs to assist other health care providers with time management. Some of the principles and guidelines to use to assist in managing time efficiently are listed below.

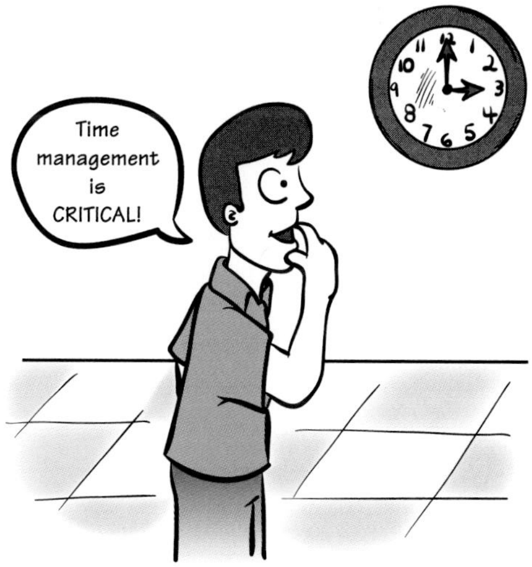
Time management is CRITICAL!

Time management: The ability to manage time effciently in order to complete tasks and client care activities within a reasonable time frame.

Principles and Guidelines of Time Management

Identify tasks, obligations, and client care activities, and write them down.

Organize the workday; identify which tasks and client care activities must be completed in specified time frames.

Prioritize client needs.

Anticipate the needs of the day, and provide time for unexpected and unplanned tasks or client care activities that may arise.

Focus on beginning the daily tasks, working on the most important first, while keeping goals in mind; look at the final goal for the day, which will help to break down tasks into manageable parts.

Begin client rounds at the beginning of the shift, collecting data on each assigned client.

Delegate tasks to others as appropriate.

Keep a daily hour-by-hour log to assist in providing structure to the tasks that must be accomplished, and cross tasks off the list as they are accomplished.

Use hospital and agency resources intelligently, anticipating resource needs, and gathering the necessary supplies before beginning the task.

Organize paperwork, and continuously document task completion and necessary client data throughout the day.

At the end of the day, evaluate the effectiveness of time management.

TIME MANAGEMENT

Think! Plan!
Organize! Prioritize!

Sample Question: Prioritizing (Ordered Response)

A nurse on the day shift is assigned to care for four clients. Following report from the night shift, the nurse plans to perform client rounds and collect data from each client. Number in order of priority how the nurse will plan the client rounds. (Number 1 is the first client that the nurse will check and collect data from and number 4 is the last client that the nurse will check and collect data from.)

___ Client scheduled for a cardiac catheterization at 11:00 AM
___ Client diagnosed with diabetes mellitus who is scheduled for discharge to home at 12:00 noon
___ Client with emphysema who is receiving oxygen therapy
___ Client scheduled to have an electrocardiogram (ECG) at 2:00 PM

Answer: 2, 3, 1, 4

Test-Taking Strategy: This question describes a situation in which the nurse needs to prioritize assigned clients. Use the ABCs—airway, breathing, and circulation—to determine which client the nurse will check and collect data from first. Airway is always a high priority and the nurse would *first* collect data from the client with emphysema who is receiving oxygen therapy. The nurse would next collect data from the client scheduled for the cardiac catheterization because this client will require preprocedure preparation and is scheduled at 11:00 AM. The client scheduled for discharge would be checked next. Although the client may have discharge needs that require attention, the client is not scheduled to be discharged until 12:00 noon. The client scheduled for an ECG at 2:00 PM can be checked last.

REFERENCES

DeWit, S. (2005). *Fundamental concepts and skills for nursing* (2nd ed). Philadelphia: Saunders.

Harkreader, H. & Hogan, M.A. (2004). *Fundamentals of nursing: caring and clinical judgment* (2nd ed). Philadelphia: Saunders.

Hill, S. & Howlett, H. (2005). *Success in practical/vocational nursing: from student to leader* (5th ed). Philadelphia: Saunders.

Linton, A. & Maebius, N. (2003). *Introduction to medical-surgical nursing* (3rd ed). Philadelphia: Saunders.

National Council of State Boards of Nursing, Inc. *Test Plan for the National Council Licensure Examination for Licensed Practical/Vocational Nurses* (effective date: April 2005), National Council of State Boards of Nursing, Chicago, 2004.

National Council of State Boards of Nursing, Inc. Online: available at www.ncsbn.org.

Potter, P. & Perry, A. (2005). *Fundamentals of nursing* (6th ed). St. Louis: Mosby.

Yoder-Wise, P. (2003). *Leading and managing in nursing* (3rd ed). St. Louis: Mosby.

Chapter 11

Communication Questions

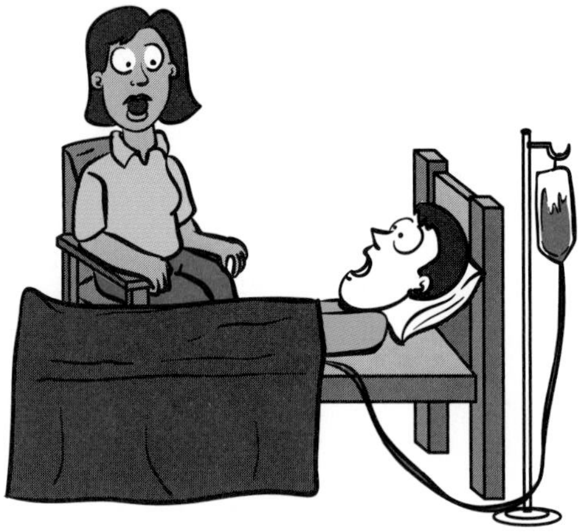

Communication is a process in which information is exchanged, either verbally or nonverbally, between two or more individuals. According to the National Council of State Boards of Nursing (NCSBN), an Integrated Process of the test plan is a process that is fundamental to the practice of nursing and is incorporated through the Client Needs categories of the test plan. In the NCLEX-PN® test plan, the NCSBN identifies the concept of communication as a component of one of the Integrated Processes. Additionally, in the Psychosocial Integrity category of Client Needs (8%-14% of test items), Therapeutic Communication is listed as content that is tested on the NCLEX-PN examination. Therefore, it is likely that you will be presented with questions that relate to the communication process. This chapter reviews the guidelines to use when answering communication questions. Several sample questions are included that illustrate how these guidelines are used.

HOW ARE COMMUNICATION CONCEPTS TESTED IN A QUESTION?

Communication is an important characteristic of the nurse-client relationship. Therefore, test questions that refer to the concept of communication may address a client situation in any clinical setting and any nursing care area. In other words, communication questions may address client situations in the adult health area, the maternity area, the pediatric area, or the mental health area in settings such as the hospital, clinic, physician's office, or other health care setting.

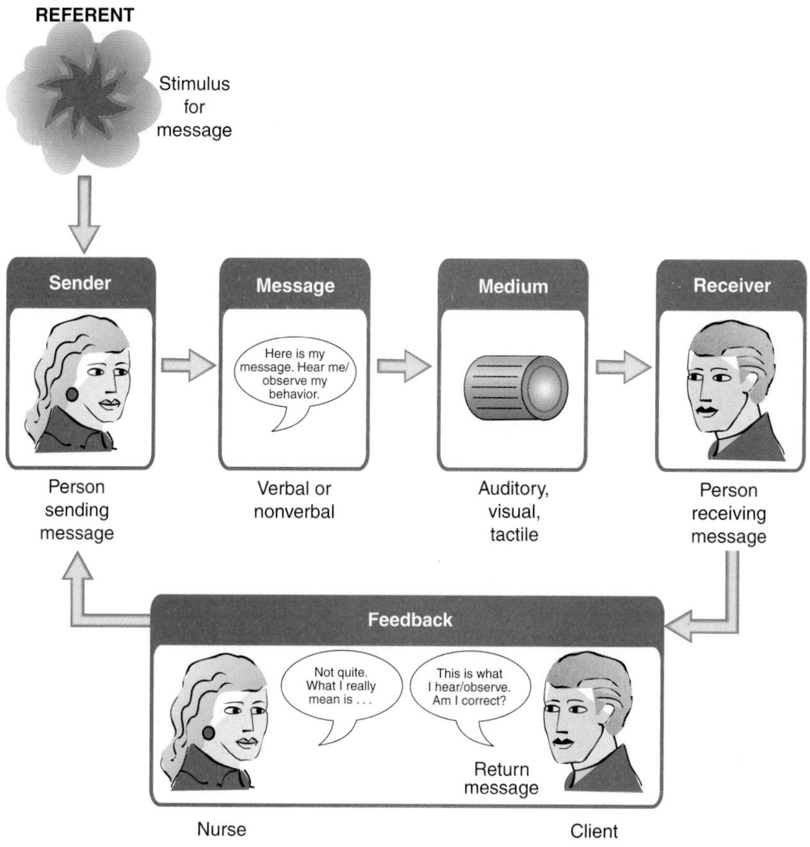

Communication Model. From Varcarolis, Elizabeth M. [2002]. *Foundations of psychiatric mental health nursing* (4th ed.) Philadelphia: Saunders.

Communication questions may address a client situation in any clinical setting and any nursing care area!

When we think about communication concepts and the nurse-client relationship, we usually visualize an interaction between the nurse and the client. Although this is an accurate visualization, it is important to broaden our thinking with regard to the communication process and the concepts that will be tested on the examination. Test questions address not only the communication process between the nurse and the client but also address this process between the nurse and a client's family member or significant other, or the nurse and another member of the health care team, such as another nurse, a nursing assistant, or a physician. For example, you may be asked about how you would respond to a nursing assistant who makes an inappropriate statement or how you would respond to a physician who is demanding. Most of the questions that test the concept of communication are in the multiple-choice format and relate to how the nurse would respond to the person that he or she is communicating with.

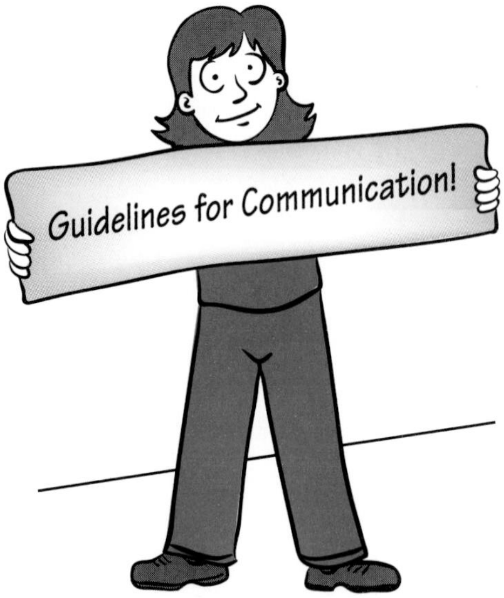

WHAT GUIDELINES CAN BE USED TO ANSWER COMMUNICATION QUESTIONS?

There are four primary guidelines to use when answering communication questions. These guidelines are as follows.

1. Use therapeutic communication techniques to answer communication questions because of their effectiveness in the communication process. As you read the question and each option, look for the option that indicates the use of a therapeutic communication technique.
2. Nontherapeutic communication techniques are ineffective and are avoided when responding to a client, a client's family member or significant other, or another member of the health care team. As you read the question and each option, eliminate the options that indicate the use of a nontherapeutic communication technique.
3. Focus on feelings, concerns, anxieties, or fears. As you read the question and each option, look for the option that indicates the use of a therapeutic communication technique and focuses on the client's, client's family member or significant other's, or health care team member's feelings, concerns, anxieties, or fears.
4. Consider cultural differences as you answer the question. If you note that a question contains information that identifies a specific cultural group, you need to think about specific cultural characteristics to answer the question correctly. Remember each culture is unique with regard to the characteristics related to the process of communication.

GUIDELINES FOR COMMUNICATION

Use therapeutic communication techniques.
Avoid nontherapeutic communication techniques.
Focus on the client's feelings, concerns, anxieties, or fears.
Consider cultural differences

COMMUNICATION TECHNIQUES

What Are the Therapeutic Communication Techniques?

Using therapeutic communication techniques encourages the client, or other individual that the nurse is communicating with, to express his or her thoughts and feelings. There are many therapeutic communication techniques that can be used to promote verbalization. You have probably learned these techniques in your first nursing course in nursing school; however, the following section provides a brief review.

Therapeutic Communication Techniques

Technique	Description
Active listening	Noting carefully what the client is saying and observing the client's nonverbal behavior
Broad openings	Encouraging the client to select topics for discussion
Clarifying	Providing a means for making the message clearer, to correct any misunderstandings, and to promote mutual understanding
Focusing	Directing the conversation on the topic being discussed
Informing	Giving information to the client
Offering self to help	Can include staying with the client or talking to the client
Open-ended questions	Encouraging conversation because these questions require more than one-word answers
Paraphrasing	Restating in different words what the client said
Reflecting	Directing the client's question or statement back to the client for consideration
Restating	Repeating what the client has said and directing the statement back to the client to provide the client the opportunity to agree or disagree or to clarify the message further
Silence	Allowing time for formulating thoughts
Summarizing	Stating briefly what was discussed during the conversation
Validating	Verifying that both the nurse and the client are interpreting the topic or message in the same way

What Are the Nontherapeutic Communication Techniques?

Nontherapeutic communication techniques impair or block the flow of a conversation. These techniques are also known as the barriers to an effective communication process. There are many nontherapeutic communication techniques and you are probably quite familiar with them and have learned that these techniques need to be avoided when communicating because of their ineffectiveness. The following section briefly reviews some of the nontherapeutic communication techniques.

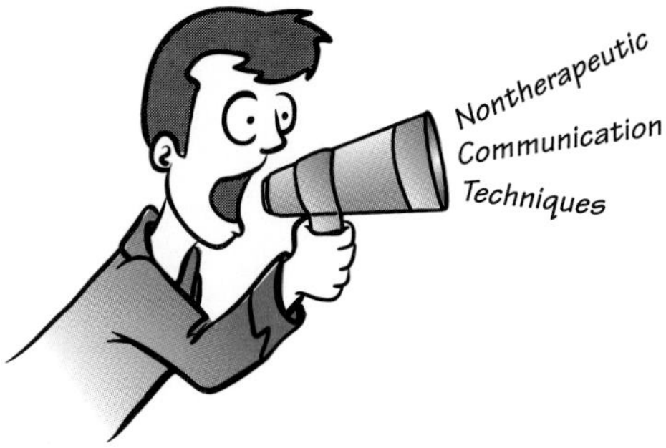

Nontherapeutic Communication Techniques

Technique	Description
Approval	Implying that the client is thinking or doing the right thing and is not thinking or doing what is wrong; this may direct the client to focus on thinking or behavior that pleases the nurse
Asking excessive questions	Demanding information from the client without respect for the client's willingness or readiness to respond
Changing the subject	Avoiding addressing the client's thoughts, feelings or concerns; implies that the client's statement is not important
Closed-ended questions	Questions that ask for specific information such as a yes or no answer and therefore inhibit communication
Disagreeing	Opposing the client's thinking or opinions, implying that the client is wrong
Disapproving	Indicating a negative value judgment about the client's behavior or thoughts
False reassurance	Statement implying that the client has no reason to be worried or concerned; belittling a client's concerns
Giving advice	Assuming that the client can't think for him- or herself, which inhibits problem solving and fosters independence
Minimizing the client's feelings	Statement implying that the client's feelings are not important
Parroting	Repeating the client's words before determining what the client has said
Placing client's feelings on hold	Avoiding addressing the client's thoughts, feelings, or concerns; making a statement that places the responsibility of addressing the client's thoughts, feelings, or concerns elsewhere or on another person
Value judgments	Making a comment that addresses the client's morals; this can make the client feel angry or guilty, or make the client feel as though he or she is unsupported
"Why?" questions	Questions that cause the client to feel defensive; these types of questions often imply criticism

WHY ARE CULTURAL CONSIDERATIONS IMPORTANT?

A nurse needs to be aware of certain cultural characteristics that relate to the communication process that may be different from one's own cultural uniqueness. Questions on the NCLEX-PN examination may address the concept of communication with a client from a specific cultural group. If you note that a question contains information that identifies a specific cultural group, you need to think about specific cultural characteristics to answer the question correctly.

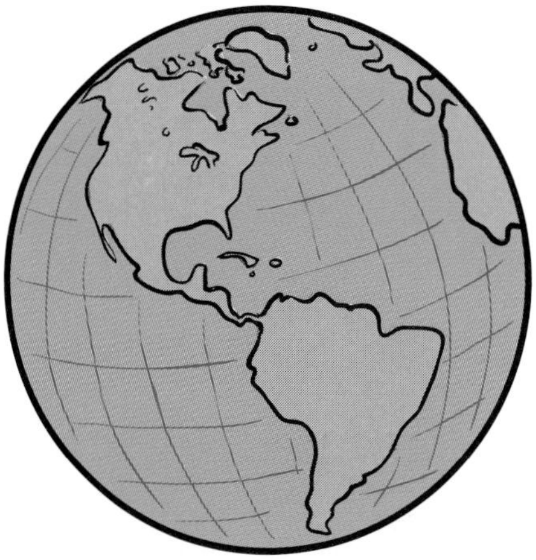

With regard to communication, there are three cultural characteristics to consider: communication style, use of eye contact, and the meaning of touch. It is important to review the characteristics associated with a specific culture and to become familiar with them before taking the NCLEX-PN examination. Identified below are some of the characteristics of specific cultural groups that you need to consider. If you are unfamiliar with content related to the characteristics of various cultures then refer to the *Saunders Comprehensive Review for the NCLEX-PN® Examination*. This product contains information about cultural characteristics and a specific chapter titled Cultural Diversity that describes many features related to cultural differences for various cultural groups.

CULTURAL COMMUNICATION POINTS TO CONSIDER!

Communication style
Use of eye contact
Meaning of touch

Communication Style

The following sections provide some background information to consider when developing your communication style with specific cultural groups.

African Americans

Personal questions asked on initial contact with the client may be viewed as intrusive.

Head nodding by the client does not necessarily mean agreement.

Asian Cultures

Asian cultures may believe that feelings and emotions are private and an open expression of emotions is regarded as a weakness.

Silence is valued by the client.

Criticism or disagreement is not expressed verbally by the client.
Head nodding by the client does not necessarily mean agreement.
The client may interpret the word "no" as disrespect for others.
The client does not use hand gestures.

European (White) Americans

Silence can be used by the client to show respect or disrespect for another, depending on the situation.

French and Italian Americans

The client may use expressive hand gestures and animated facial expression during conversation.

German and British Americans

The client may show little facial emotion because these clients highly value the concept of self-control.

Hispanic Americans

The client may use dramatic body language such as gestures or facial expressions to express emotion or pain.
The client may tend to be verbally expressive, yet confidentiality is important.
Hispanic Americans may believe that direct confrontation is disrespectful, and the expression of negative feelings is impolite.

Native Americans

To Native Americans, silence indicates respect for the speaker.
Many of these clients speak in a low tone of voice and expect others to be attentive.
Body language is important.
Obtaining input from members of the extended family is important.

Use of Eye Contact

The following sections provide information regarding how the use of eye contact is viewed by clients of specific cultural groups.

African Americans

Direct eye contact may be interpreted as rudeness or aggressive behavior.

Asian Cultures

Eye contact is limited and may be considered inappropriate or disrespectful.

European (White) Americans

Eye contact is viewed as indicating trustworthiness.

Native Americans

Eye contact is viewed as a sign of disrespect.
The nurse needs to understand that the client may be attentive even when eye contact is absent.

Hispanic Americans

Some Hispanic Americans believe that avoiding eye contact with a person in authority indicates respect and attentiveness.

Meaning of Touch

The following sections discuss how touch is viewed in specific cultural groups.

African Americans

African Americans may be comfortable with close personal space when interacting with family and friends.

Asian Cultures

These clients prefer a formal personal space except with family and close friends.
They usually do not touch others during conversation.
Touching is unacceptable with members of the opposite sex; if possible, a female client prefers a female health care provider.
The head is considered to be sacred; therefore, touching someone on the head is disrespectful.
The nurse should avoid physical closeness and excessive touching and touch a client's head only when necessary, informing the client before doing so.

European (White) Americans

European Americans tend to avoid physical contact.
The nurse needs to respect the client's personal space.

Native Americans

Personal space is very important for these clients.
Native American clients may lightly touch another person's hand during greetings.
In this culture, massage is used for the newborn infant to promote bonding between the infant and mother.
Touching a dead body may be prohibited in some tribes.

Hispanic Americans

Hispanic Americans are comfortable with close proximity with family, friends, and acquaintances and value the physical presence of others.
The nurse needs to protect the client's privacy.
Hispanic Americans are very tactile and use embraces and handshakes.
The nurse needs to ask if it would be okay to touch a child before examining him or her.

SAMPLE COMMUNICATION QUESTIONS

Following are sample communication questions that illustrate the use of therapeutic and nontherapeutic communication techniques. Remember to use the following communication guidelines:

Use therapeutic communication techniques.
Avoid the use of nontherapeutic communication techniques.
Focus on the client's feelings, concerns, anxieties, or fears.
Consider cultural differences.

Sample Question: Communication

A mother says to a nurse in the physician's office, "I am afraid that my child might have another seizure." Which response by the nurse is *therapeutic?*

1. "Why worry about something that you cannot control?"
2. "Most children will never experience a second seizure."
3. "Tell me what frightens you the most about seizures."
4. "Phenytoin [Dilantin] can prevent another seizure from occurring."

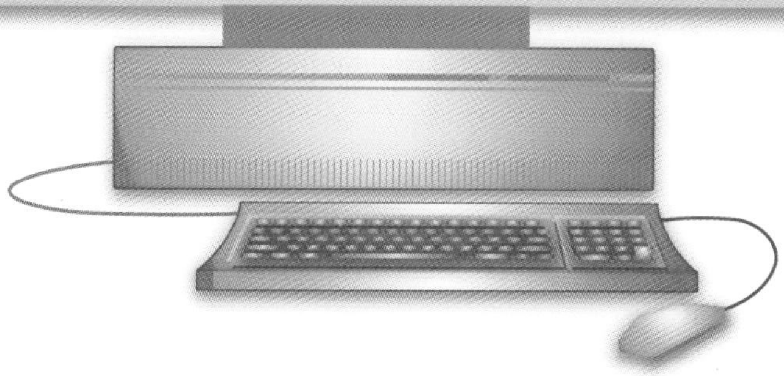

Answer: 3

Test Taking Strategy: Note the key word "therapeutic." Option 3 is the only option that addresses the client's fears. Option 1 is a nontherapeutic response because it states that the mother should not worry. Options 2 and 4 are incorrect because the nurse is giving false assurance to the mother that a seizure will not recur, or can be prevented in this child. Use therapeutic communication techniques and focus on the client's feelings, concerns, anxieties, or fears!

Sample Question: Communication

A client seen in the health care clinic has been diagnosed with hypertension and has been taking a prescribed antihypertensive medication. On a follow-up visit the client says to the nurse, "I don't understand why I have to take this medication. It makes me feel awful." The *appropriate* nursing response is which of the following?

1. "You will need to ask your doctor about that."
2. "Everyone that takes that medication says the same thing."
3. "You have to take this medication if you want to prevent a stroke."
4. "Describe what you mean when you say that the medication makes you feel awful."

Answer: 4

Test-Taking Strategy: Note the key word "appropriate." Option 1 avoids the client's concern and places the client's feelings on hold. Option 2 minimizes the client's feelings and implies that the client's complaint is not important. In option 3 the nurse gives advice and provides false reassurance that the medication will prevent a stroke. In this option the nurse also avoids the client's complaint and is threatening in a sense and induces fear in the client. In option 4 the nurse uses the therapeutic communication technique of restating. In this technique the nurse explores by repeating what the client has said and directing the statement back to the client to provide the client the opportunity to clarify the message further. Be sure to use therapeutic communication techniques and focus on the client's feelings, concerns, anxieties, or fears!

Sample Question: Communication

A client with a history of cardiac disease is brought to the emergency department because of experiencing an episode of chest pain while mowing the lawn. During data collection, the client tells the nurse that he stopped taking his cardiac medication. The *appropriate* response by the nurse is which of the following?

1. "Tell me some of the reasons that led you to stop taking your medication."
2. "Why did you stop taking your medication?"
3. "Everything is going to be just fine. We'll get you started on those medications right away."
4. "You stopped the medication! You know that you are never supposed to do that with cardiac medications?"

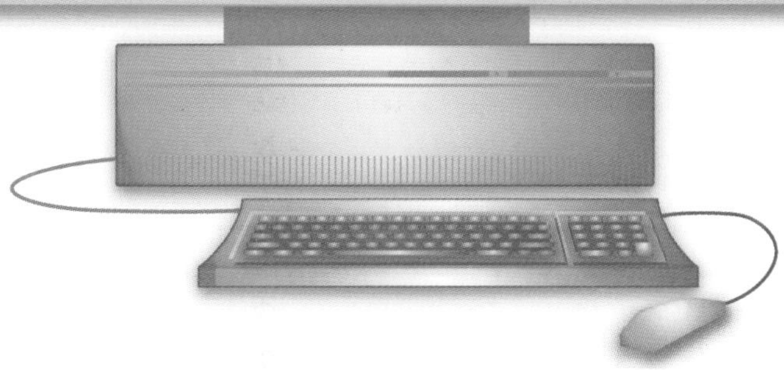

Answer: 1

Test-Taking Strategy: Note the key word "appropriate." Option 1 is an open-ended and a broad opening question that will promote and encourage the client to communicate. The statement in option 2 uses the word "why," which implies criticism and often makes the client feel defensive. In option 3 the nurse provides false reassurance by telling the client that everything is going to be fine. Additionally, the nurse avoids exploring the reason(s) that led the client to stopping the medication. In option 4 the nurse demoralizes and belittles the client and lectures the client, which is nontherapeutic. Remember, use therapeutic communication techniques and focus on the client's feelings, concerns, anxieties, or fears!

Sample Question: Communication

A client recently diagnosed with ovarian cancer says to the nurse, "I can't believe this has happened to me. I wish that I were dead!" Which nursing response is *therapeutic?*

1. "I know what you mean but there are a lot of treatments available for ovarian cancer."
2. "Every client diagnosed with this type of cancer says the same thing."
3. "You must be feeling very upset. Are you thinking of hurting yourself?"
4. "Why are you talking that way? Your children wouldn't want to hear you say that, would they?"

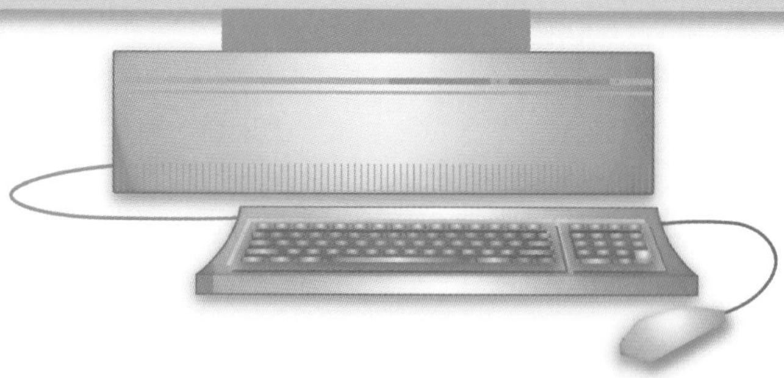

Answer: 3

Test-Taking Strategy: Note the key word "therapeutic." In option 3 the nurse focuses on the client's statement and addresses the client's feeling in the response. In options 1 and 2, the nurse minimizes the client's feelings. Additionally, option 1 provides false reassurances. In option 4, the nurse uses the word "why," which implies criticism and often makes the client feel defensive. Additionally, option 4 focuses on the client's children and their feelings rather than the client's feelings. Use therapeutic communication techniques and focus on the client's feelings, concerns, anxieties, or fears!

Sample Question: Communication

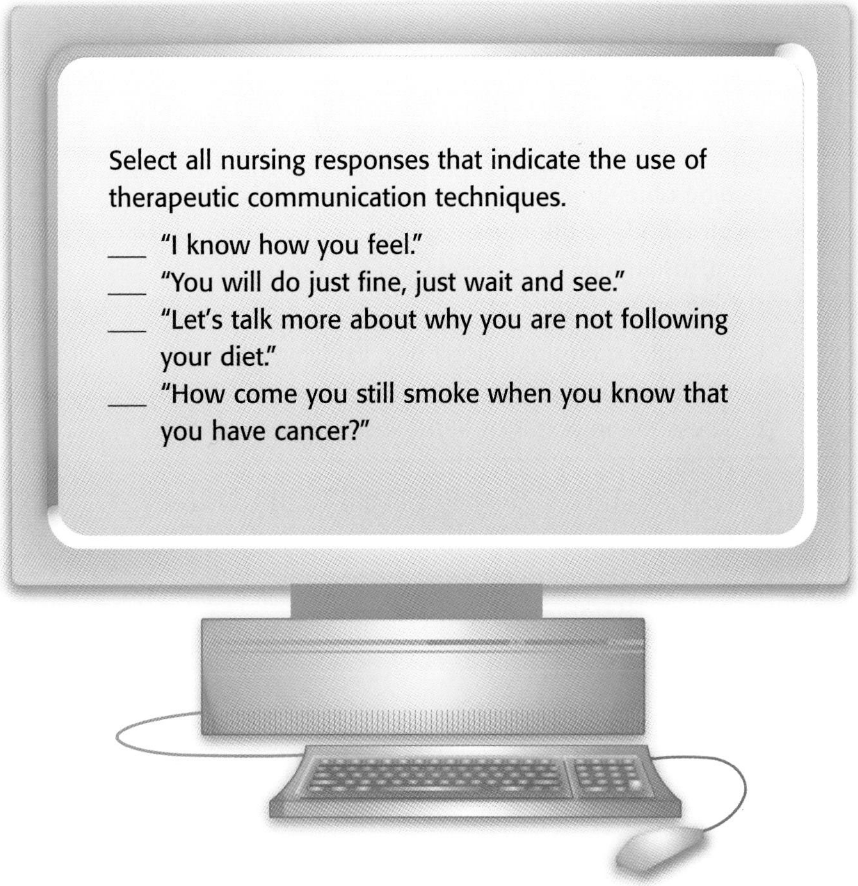
Select all nursing responses that indicate the use of therapeutic communication techniques.
___ "I know how you feel."
___ "You will do just fine, just wait and see."
___ "Let's talk more about why you are not following your diet."
___ "How come you still smoke when you know that you have cancer?"

Answer:

___ "I know how you feel."
___ "You will do just fine, just wait and see."
_X_ "Let's talk more about why you are not following your diet."
___ "How come you still smoke when you know that you have cancer?"

Test-Taking Strategy: Focus on the issue, *therapeutic communication techniques.* Review the following nursing responses.

"I know how you feel."—Nontherapeutic and minimizes the client's feelings.

"You will do just fine, just wait and see."—Nontherapeutic and minimizes and avoids the client's feelings.

"Let's talk more about why you are not following your diet."—Therapeutic and uses the technique of focusing.

"How come you still smoke when you know that you have cancer?"—Nontherapeutic and demoralizes the client and can make the client feel guilty, angry, anxious, or unsupported.

Remember to use therapeutic communication techniques and focus on the client's feelings, concerns, anxieties, or fears when answering communication questions!

Sample Question: Communication

A nurse is providing instructions to an Asian client regarding obtaining a stool specimen for testing for occult blood. As the nurse explains the instructions, the client continually turns away from the nurse. Which nursing action is *appropriate?*

1. Continue with the instructions, verifying client understanding.
2. Stress the importance of the instructions with the client.
3. Walk around the client so that the nurse constantly faces the client.
4. Give the client the list of instructions and return later to continue with the instructions.

Answer: 1

Test-Taking Strategy: In this question you need to consider the characteristics of the Asian culture. Many Asian clients maintain a formal distance with others, which is a form of respect. Many Asian clients are uncomfortable with face-to-face communications, especially when there is direct eye contact. If the client turns away from the nurse during a conversation, the appropriate nursing action is to continue with the conversation. Walking around to the client so that the nurse faces the client is in direct conflict with the cultural practice. Telling the client about the importance of the instructions may be viewed as degrading. The client may view returning later to continue with the explanation as a rude gesture. If the question identifies a specific cultural group, you need to consider the characteristics of the culture to answer the question!

Sample Question: Communication Concepts

A nurse in an ambulatory care clinic is collecting admission data from an African American client scheduled for a laparoscopic cholecystectomy. Which of the following questions would be *inappropriate* for the nurse to ask on an *initial data collection?*

1. "Do you have any difficulty breathing?"
2. "Do you have a close family relationship?"
3. "Do you ever experience chest pain?"
4. "Do you frequently have episodes of abdominal pain?"

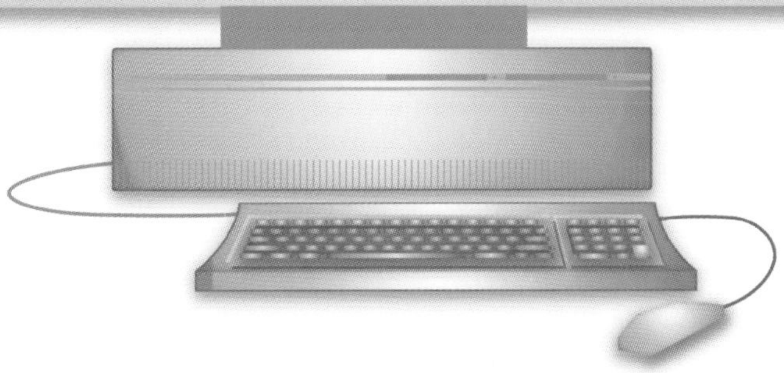

Answer: 2

Test-Taking Strategy: In this question you need to consider the characteristics of the African American culture. Note the key words "inappropriate" and "initial data collection." In the African American culture, it is considered to be intrusive to ask personal questions on the initial contact or meeting. African Americans are highly verbal and express feelings openly to family or friends, but what transpires within the family is viewed as private. Respiratory, cardiovascular, and gastrointestinal assessments are physiological assessments that are the priority. You can also use Maslow's Hierarchy of Needs theory to answer the question. Note that options 1, 3, and 4 address physiological needs. Option 2 addresses the psychosocial need. Remember, if the question identifies a specific cultural group, you need to consider the characteristics of the culture to answer the question!

REFERENCES

Chernecky, C. & Berger, B. (2004). *Laboratory tests and diagnostic procedures* (4th ed). Philadelphia: Saunders.

DeWit, S. (2005). *Fundamental concepts and skills for nursing* (2nd ed). Philadelphia: Saunders.

Gulanick, M., Myers, J., Klopp, A., Galanes, S., Gradishar, D., & Puzas, M. (2003). *Nursing care plans: nursing diagnosis and intervention* (5th ed). St. Louis: Mosby.

Hill, S. & Howlett, H. (2005). *Success in practical/vocational nursing: from student to leader* (5th ed). Philadelphia: Saunders.

Hodgson, B. & Kizior, R. (2005). *Saunders nursing drug handbook 2005.* Philadelphia: Saunders.

Ignatavicius, D. & Workman, M. (2006). *Medical-surgical nursing: critical thinking for collaborative care* (5th ed). Philadelphia: Saunders.

Linton, A. & Maebius, N. (2003). *Introduction to medical-surgical nursing* (3rd ed). Philadelphia: Saunders.

Lowdermilk, D. & Perry, A. (2004). *Maternity & women's health care* (8th ed). St. Louis: Mosby.

National Council of State Boards of Nursing, Inc. *Test Plan for the National Council Licensure Examination for Licensed Practical/Vocational Nurses* (effective date: April 2005), National Council of State Boards of Nursing, Chicago, 2004.

National Council of State Boards of Nursing, Inc. Online: available at www.ncsbn.org.

Potter, P. & Perry, A. (2005). *Fundamentals of nursing* (6th ed). St. Louis: Mosby.

Varcarolis, E.M. (2002). *Foundations of psychiatric mental health nursing* (4th ed). Philadelphia: Saunders.

Wong, D. & Hockenberry, M. (2003). *Wong's nursing care of infants and children* (7th ed). St. Louis: Mosby.

Chapter 12

Pharmacology Questions

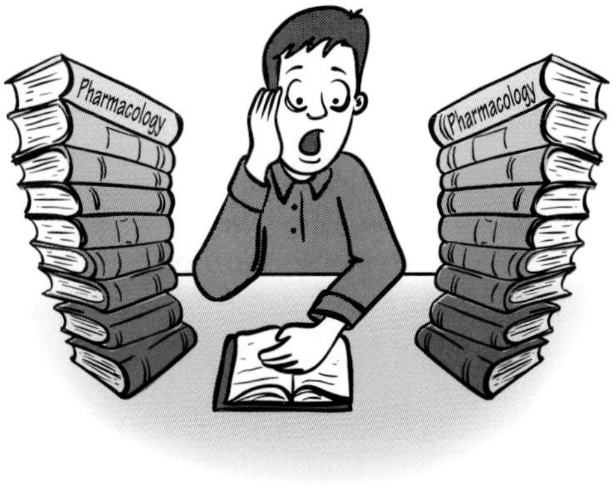

Pharmacology is one of the most difficult nursing content areas to master and feel comfortable with. One reason why it is so difficult is because of the enormous number of medications available. Another reason is because there is a vast amount of information to know about each medication. The NCLEX-PN® test plan addresses pharmacological therapies in the Physiological Integrity category and identifies 9% to 15% as the percentage of test questions that will possibly appear on your examination. What this means is, if you took a 100-question examination, 9 to 15 of the questions would be pharmacology questions. Therefore, it is important for you to spend ample time reviewing pharmacology in preparation for this examination, and it is best to do your review from a question-and-answer perspective.

Pharmacological and parenteral therapies = 9% to 15%

This chapter provides you with strategies for preparing to answer pharmacology questions and the guidelines and strategies to use to answer the question correctly.

Remember to read the question carefully, noting the key words and the issue of the question, and always use the process of elimination to select the correct option. As with any type of question, it is best to use your nursing knowledge to answer the question. However, a question may appear on your examination that contains a medication that you are unfamiliar with. When this occurs, the guidelines and the strategies to answer a pharmacology question correctly will be valuable. After you read this chapter, practice as many pharmacology questions as you can. There are several resources available that contain hundreds of pharmacology practice questions. Some of these include the *Saunders Comprehensive Review for the NCLEX-PN® Examination*, the *Saunders Q&A Review for the NCLEX-PN® Examination*, and the *Saunders Review Cards for the NCLEX-PN® Examination*.

These products can be obtained at the Elsevier Health website at *www.elsevierhealth.com.*

GUIDELINES AND STRATEGIES

Read the question carefully
Note the key words
Note the issue
Use the process of elimination
Use nursing knowledge
Use pharmacology guidelines
Use test-taking strategies

PHARMACOLOGY GUIDELINES

How Will the Pharmacology Guidelines Be Helpful in Answering a Pharmacology Question and What Are These Guidelines?

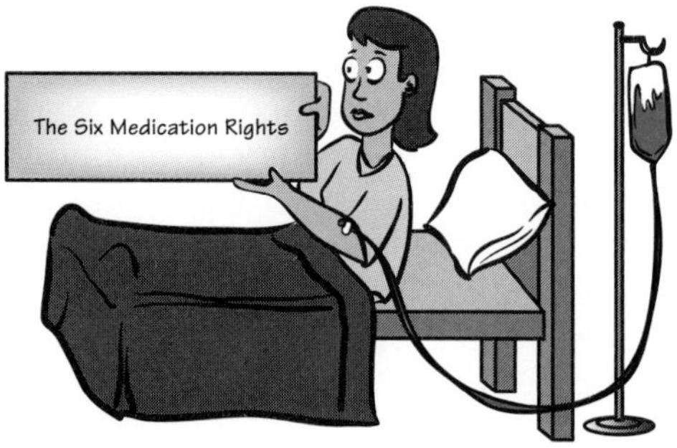

There are some specific guidelines to follow when you administer a medication to a client. In addition to the six rights for medication administration, these guidelines include data collection from the client and data collection of other factors related to the medication, such as certain laboratory values or vital signs; checking for potential interactions or contraindications related to the medication; client teaching, monitoring for intended effects, side effects, adverse effects, or toxic effects; and evaluating the client's response to the medication therapy. When you are presented with a pharmacology question and are trying to select the correct option, using the guidelines will assist you in eliminating incorrect options. Some of these guidelines are listed below.

SIX MEDICATION RIGHTS

Right Client
Right Medication
Right Dose
Right Time and frequency
Right Route
Right Documentation

Pharmacology: Data Collection Guidelines to Follow

Always check for client allergies or hypersensitivity to a medication.

Always ask the client about existing medical disorders that are contraindicated with the administration of a prescribed medication.

Always check for potential interactions related to the medication.

Always check pertinent laboratory results.
Always check the client's vital signs, particularly if antihypertensives or cardiac medications are being administered.
Always monitor the client for intended effects, side effects, adverse effects, or toxic effects of the medication.
Always monitor the client's response to the medication.

These guidelines will be particularly helpful if the question asks for the priority nursing action when administering a medication. Below is a sample pharmacology question that illustrates how these guidelines may be helpful.

Sample Question: Pharmacology

The nurse notes that a physician has prescribed co-trimoxazole (Bactrim) for a client with a urinary tract infection. Which *priority* action will the nurse take before administering this medication?

1. Call the pharmacy to order the medication.
2. Ask the client about an allergy to sulfonamides.
3. Check the medication supply room to find out if the medication needs to be ordered.
4. Inform the client about the need to increase fluid intake.

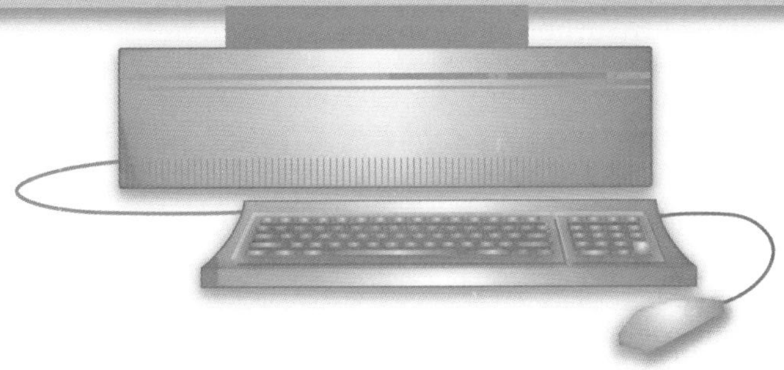

Answer: 2

Test-Taking Strategy: Remember to read the question carefully, noting the issue of the question and the key words. In this question, the key word is "priority" and the issue is *the action that the nurse will take.* Using the pharmacology guidelines will direct you to option 2. Also, using the steps of the clinical problem-solving process (nursing process) will direct you to the correct option because option 2 is the only option that addresses data collection.

What Other Guidelines Will Be Helpful?

There are some very general guidelines to keep in mind as you are trying to select the correct option.

Pharmacology: General Guidelines to Follow

Medication absorption, distribution, metabolism, and excretion are affected by age and physiological processes; the older client and the neonate and infant are at greater risk for toxicity than an adult.

Many medications are contraindicated in pregnancy and during breastfeeding.

Antacids are not usually administered with medication because the antacid will affect the absorption of the medication.

Grapefruit juice is not usually administered with medication because it contains a substance that will interact with the absorption of the medication.

Enteric-coated and sustained-release tablets should not be crushed; additionally, capsules should not be opened.

Nursing interventions always include monitoring for intended effects, side effects, adverse effects, or toxic effects of the medication.

Nursing interventions always include client teaching.

A nurse or client should never adjust or change a medication dose, abruptly stop taking a medication, or discontinue a medication.

A nurse may withhold a medication if the nurse suspects that the client is experiencing an adverse effect or a toxic effect of the medication; the nurse must immediately notify a registered nurse, who will then contact the physician if either of these effects occurs.

A client needs to avoid taking any over-the-counter medications or any other medications such as herbal preparations unless they are approved for use by the health care provider.

A client needs to know how to correctly administer the medication.

A client needs to be aware of the side effects of medications and how to check his or her own temperature, pulse, and blood pressure.

A client needs to take the prescribed dose for the prescribed length of therapy and understand the necessity of compliance.

A client needs to avoid consuming alcohol and smoking.

A client needs to avoid driving and using heavy machinery if taking a central nervous system depressant, until the effects of the medication are known.

A client should wear a Medic-Alert bracelet if he or she is taking medications, such as but not limited to anticoagulants, oral hypoglycemics or insulin, certain cardiac medications, corticosteroids and glucocorticoids, antimyasthenic medications, anticonvulsants, and monoamine oxidase inhibitors.

A client needs to follow-up with a health care provider as prescribed.

Below is a sample pharmacology question that illustrates how these general pharmacology guidelines may be helpful.

Sample Question: Pharmacology

A client taking amitriptyline hydrochloride (Elavil) calls the nurse at the physician's office and reports that he develops an upset stomach whenever he takes the medication. The nurse *appropriately* tells the client to:

1. take the medication with an antacid.
2. stop the medication for 2 days and then resume the prescribed medication schedule.
3. take the medication on an empty stomach.
4. take the medication with food.

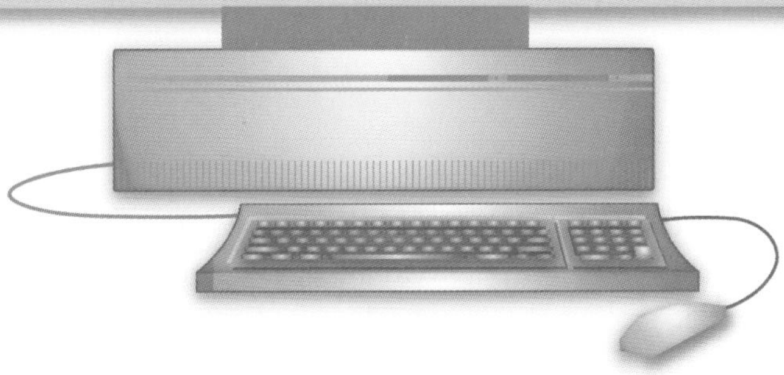

Answer: 4

Test-Taking Strategy: Remember to read the question carefully, noting the issue of the question and the key words. In this question, the key word is "appropriately" and the issue is *the client's complaint of an upset stomach.* Recalling that antacids are not usually administered with medication and that a nurse would not tell a client to discontinue a medication will assist in eliminating options 1 and 2. From the remaining options, focusing on the issue will assist in eliminating option 3.

MEDICATION EFFECTS

What Is the Difference Between an Intended Effect, a Side Effect, an Adverse Effect, and a Toxic Effect of a Medication?

It is important to understand the difference between an intended effect, a side effect, an adverse effect, and a toxic effect. Understanding these differences will assist in eliminating the incorrect options in a pharmacology question that asks about one of these effects. When you are presented with a question on the examination that asks about an effect of a medication, note the specific issue: is the issue of the question an intended effect, a side effect, an adverse effect, or a toxic effect? The differences are described in the following sections, and include a sample question related to the specific effect discussed in that section.

Intended Effect

An intended effect is a desirable effect and is the effect that you would expect to occur from a medication. For example, the intended effect of morphine sulfate is pain relief. Below is a sample of a question that asks about an intended effect.

INTENDED EFFECT
A desirable effect

Sample Question: Intended Effect

Acetylsalicylic acid (aspirin) is prescribed for a client with rheumatoid arthritis. On a follow-up visit to the physician's office the nurse asks the client if the medication has *provided relief from* which of the following?

1. Joint pain
2. Dyspepsia
3. Diarrhea
4. Flatulence

Answer: 1

Test-Taking Strategy: Remember to read the question carefully, noting the issue of the question and the key words. In this question, the key words are "provided relief from" and the issue is *an intended effect of the medication.* Note that the question provides the client's diagnosis. Recalling the pathophysiology related to rheumatoid arthritis will assist in directing you to option 1. Also note that options 2, 3, and 4 are similar in that they all address gastrointestinal symptoms. When options are similar, it is best to eliminate those options because they are unlikely to be correct.

Side Effect

A side effect is a physiological effect of a medication that is unrelated to the desired medication effects. For example, a side effect of an antihistamine medication is drowsiness. A side effect of a medication is not usually life-threatening and normally there are measures that will either eliminate the side effect or alleviate the discomfort associated with it. Below is a sample of a question that asks about a side effect.

SIDE EFFECT

Not a desired effect

Not usually life-threatening

Can usually be alleviated with specific measures

Sample Question: Side Effect

Erythromycin (E-Mycin) has been prescribed for a client with a respiratory infection. The nurse tells the client that which frequent *side effect* can occur from this medication?

1. Yellow discoloration to the white part of the eye
2. Abdominal cramping
3. Severe diarrhea
4. Yellow skin

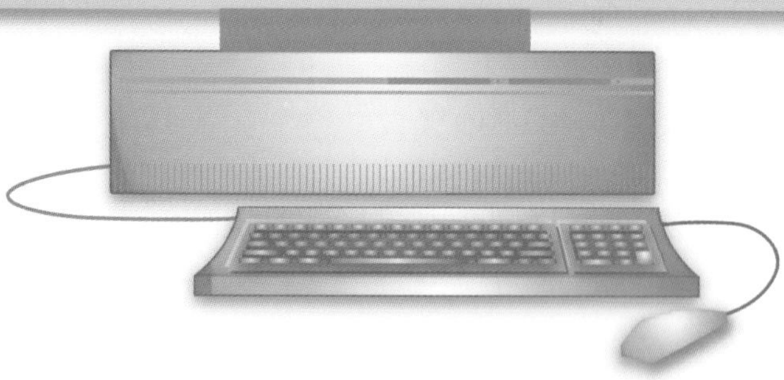

Answer: 2

Test-Taking Strategy: Remember to read the question carefully, noting the issue of the question and the key words. In this question, the key words and the issue are *a "side effect" of the medication.* Eliminate options 1 and 4 first because they are similar and both indicate the presence of hepatitis, an adverse effect of the medication. From the remaining options, eliminate option 3 because of the word "severe." Remember, the question asks about a side effect, not an adverse effect.

Adverse Effect

An adverse effect is more severe than a side effect and is always an undesirable effect. For example, an adverse effect of a sulfonamide is hypersensitivity that may be evidenced by a rash, fever, and shortness of breath. An adverse effect can range from a mild effect to a severe effect such as anaphylaxis. Adverse effects are always reported to a registered nurse, who in turn will notify the physician. Below is a sample of a question that asks about an adverse effect.

ADVERSE EFFECT

More severe than a side effect
Always an undesirable effect
Always reported to a registered nurse and physician

Sample Question: Adverse Effect

A client with congestive heart failure is receiving furosemide (Lasix). The nurse monitors the client for which *adverse effect* of the medication?

1. Nausea
2. Increase in urinary output
3. Gastric upset
4. Muscle weakness

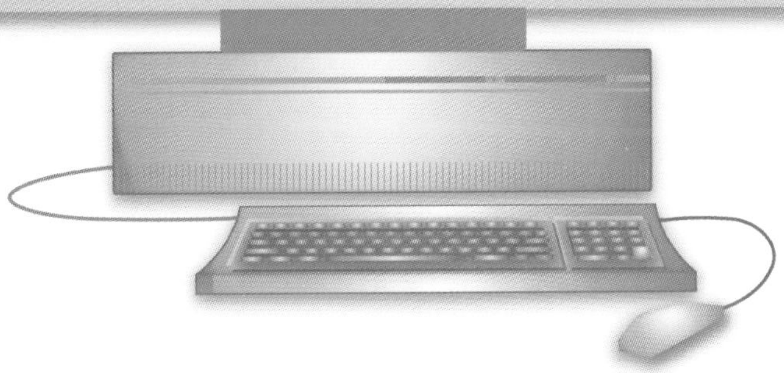

Answer: 4

Test-Taking Strategy: Remember to read the question carefully, noting the issue of the question and the key words. In this question, the key words and the issue are *an "adverse effect" of the medication.* Eliminate options 1 and 3 first because they are similar and both relate to the gastrointestinal system. From the remaining options, eliminate option 2 because it is an intended effect of the medication. Also, recall that furosemide is a diuretic and can cause electrolyte imbalances, and that muscle weakness is an indication of hypokalemia. Remember, the question asks about an adverse effect.

Toxic Effect

A toxic effect (toxicity) of a medication occurs when the medication level in the body exceeds the therapeutic level either from overdosing or medication accumulation. Toxic effects are always reported to a registered nurse, who will then notify the physician. Toxic effects are most often identified by monitoring the plasma (serum) therapeutic range of the medication. For example, the therapeutic blood level of digoxin (Lanoxin) is 0.5 to 2 ng/mL; if the blood level is greater than 2 ng/mL, the client experiences toxicity. The client will normally exhibit certain signs and symptoms (depending on the medication) that indicate toxicity, and the nurse needs to monitor for these signs and symptoms. For example, in digoxin toxicity the client may experience gastrointestinal disturbances such as anorexia, nausea, and vomiting, or ocular disturbances such as photophobia, light flashes, or halos around bright objects. Below is a list of medications commonly used in the clinical setting and their therapeutic blood level; a sample question about a toxic effect follows.

TOXIC EFFECT

Medication level in the body exceeds the therapeutic level.

Therapeutic Blood Medication Levels

Medication	Therapeutic Range
Acetaminophen (Tylenol)	10-20 mcg/mL
Carbamazepine (Tegretol)	5-12 mcg/mL
Digoxin (Lanoxin)	0.5-2 ng/mL
Gentamicin (Garamycin)	5-10 mcg/mL
Lithium (Lithobid)	0.5-1.3 mEq/L
Magnesium sulfate	4-7 mg/dL
Phenytoin (Dilantin)	10-20 mcg/mL
Salicylate	100-250 mcg/mL
Theophylline (Aminophylline, Theo-Dur)	10-20 mcg/mL

Sample Question: Toxic Effect

A nurse reviews the results of a therapeutic blood level that was drawn from a client taking theophylline (Theo-Dur) and notes that the level is 21 mcg/mL. The nurse would *appropriately:*

1. administer the next scheduled dose of theophylline.
2. place the results of the blood test in the client's medical record.
3. report the result to a registered nurse.
4. ask the laboratory to draw another blood specimen to verify the result.

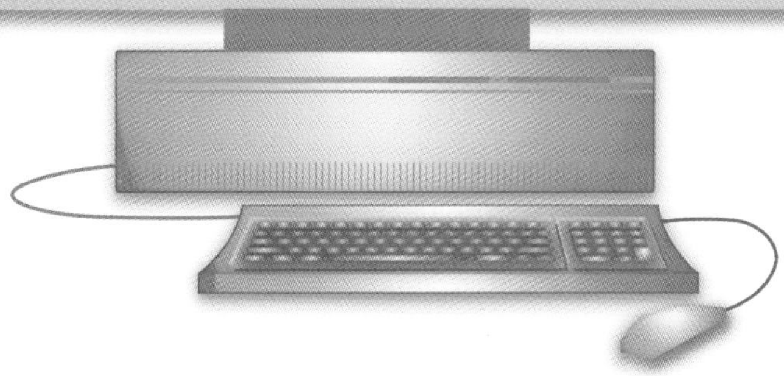

Answer: 3

Test-Taking Strategy: Read the question carefully, noting the issue of the question and the key words. In this question, the key word is "appropriately" and the issue is *a toxic effect of the medication.* Recalling that the therapeutic blood level of theophylline is 10 to 20 mcg/mL will assist in determining that the client is experiencing toxicity. Remember, toxic effects are always reported to a registered nurse, who will then notify the physician.

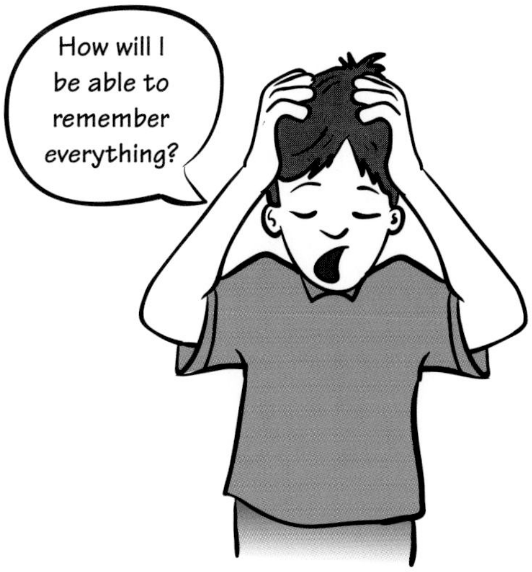
How will I be able to remember everything?

MEDICATION NAMES

Do You Need to Memorize Both the Generic Name and the Trade Name of a Medication?

No memorizing is necessary! When a pharmacology question appears on the computer screen, both the generic name and the trade name will appear. This will be very helpful to assist you in answering the question correctly. One medication name, perhaps the generic name, may be unfamiliar to you but you may recognize the trade name. For example, a question may ask about a medication named furosemide (Lasix). You may not be familiar with the medication name, furosemide, but it is very likely that you will be familiar with the medication name Lasix because it is a commonly administered medication.

How Will Medical Terminology Skills Help to Answer a Pharmacology Question?

BREAK THE WORD DOWN!

If a pharmacology question appears on your examination that contains the name of a medication that you are unfamiliar with, try to break the generic or trade name of the medication into parts and use medical terminology to assist in determining the medication action. Following is a pharmacology question and an example of how this strategy works.

Sample Question: Medical Terminology Skills

Metoprolol (Lopressor) has been prescribed for a client. The nurse takes which most important action before administering the medication to the client?

1. Checks the client's lung sounds
2. Checks the client for peripheral edema
3. Takes the client's blood pressure
4. Takes the client's temperature

Answer: 3

Test-Taking Strategy: Read the question carefully, noting the issue of the question and the key words. In this question, the key words are "most important" and the issue is *the most important action.* Focus on the name of the medication; if you are unfamiliar with the medication try to break the name of the medication into parts and use medical terminology to assist in determining the medication's action. *Lopressor* lowers *(lo)* the blood pressure *(pressor).*

MEDICATION CLASSIFICATIONS

How Will It Help to Identify a Medication by the Classification to Which It Belongs?

Medications that belong to a particular classification have similar actions and usually have commonalities in their side effects and nursing interventions related to administration. It is very difficult and nearly impossible to learn every feature about every medication. Learning medications by a "classification system method" groups several medications with similar properties and makes the amount of information that needs to be learned condensed and manageable.

With regard to side effects and nursing interventions, do not try to memorize every side effect and every nursing intervention for every medication. It is best if you associate side effects with nursing interventions. Learn to recognize the common side effects associated with each medication classification, and then relate the appropriate nursing interventions to each side effect. For example, if a side effect is hypertension, then the associated nursing intervention would be to monitor the blood pressure; if a side effect is hypokalemia, then the associated nursing interventions are to monitor the client for signs of hypokalemia and to monitor the client's potassium blood level. Again, this makes the vast amount of information that you need to remember manageable.

> Relate nursing interventions to the side effects of a medication!

How Can You Determine the Medication Classification if You Are Unfamiliar with the Medication?

If you are presented with a pharmacology question that contains the name of a medication that you are unfamiliar with, some of the strategies to use include the following:

1. Note if the question identifies the client's diagnosis. For example, if the question states: "Cyclophosphamide [Cytoxan] has been prescribed for a client with metastatic breast cancer," focusing on the client's diagnosis will help you to determine that cyclophosphamide is an antineoplastic medication.
2. Break the name of the medication (either the generic or trade name) down into parts. For example, if the question states: "Terbutaline sulfate [Brethine] has been prescribed for a client." Think about "breath" when you look at the medication name *Breth*ine to help you determine that this medication is a respiratory medication.
3. Note the letters in the medication name and look for those letters that identify a particular medication classification. Several examples of commonalities in medication names that belong to a particular classification are listed below. These examples are followed by sample questions.

COMMONALITIES IN MEDICATION NAMES

Following is a list of commonalities in medication names.

Androgens: Most medication names end with *-terone* such as testosterone (Androderm, Testoderm)

Angiotensin-converting enzyme (ACE) inhibitors: Most medication names end with *-pril* such as enalapril (Vasotec)

Antidiuretic hormones: Most medication names end with *-pressin* such as desmopressin (DDAVP)

Antilipemic medications: Most medication names end with *-statin* such as atorvastatin (Lipitor)

Antiviral medications: Most antiviral medications contain *vir* in their names such as ritonavir (Norvir)

Benzodiazepines: Includes some medications such as alprazolam (Xanax), chlordiazepoxide (Librium), clorazepate (Tranxene), estazolam (ProSom), and triazolam (Halcion); most other benzodiazepines names end with *-pam* such as diazepam (Valium)

Beta-adrenergic blockers: Most medication names end with *-lol* such as atenolol (Tenormin)

Calcium channel blockers: Most medication names end with *-pine* such as amlodipine (Norvasc); some exceptions include diltiazem (Cardizem, Cardizem SR) and verapamil (Calan, Isoptin)

Carbonic anhydrase inhibitors: Most medication names end with *-mide* such as acetazolamide (Diamox)

Estrogens: Most estrogen medication contain *est* in their names such as conjugated estrogen (Premarin)

Glucocorticoids and corticosteroids: Most medication names end with *-sone* such as prednisone (Deltasone)

Histamine H_2 receptor antagonists: Most medication names end with *-dine* such as cimetidine (Tagamet)

Nitrates: Most medications contain *nitr* in their names such as nitroglycerin (Nitrostat)

Pancreatic enzyme replacements: Most medications contain *pancre* in their names such as pancrelipase (Pancrease)

Phenothiazines: Most phenothiazine medication names end with *-zine* such as chlorpromazine (Thorazine)

Proton pump inhibitors: Most medication names end with *-zole* such as lansoprazole (Prevacid)

Sulfonamides: Most medications include *sulf* in their names such as sulfasalazine (Azulfidine)

Sulfonylureas: Most medication names end with *-mide* such as chlorpropamide (Diabinese)

Thiazide diuretics: Most medication names end with *-zide* such as hydrochlorothiazide (Hydrodiuril)

Thrombolytic medications: Most medication names end in *-ase* such as alteplase (Activase)

Thyroid hormones: Most medications contain *thy* in their names such as levothyroxine (Synthroid)

Xanthine bronchodilators: Most medication names end with *-line* such as aminophylline (Tryphylline)

Sample Question: Commonalities in Medication Names

A nurse is collecting data from a client who is taking pantoprazole (Protonix). The nurse determines that the medication is effective if the client states relief of:

1. a nighttime cough.
2. heartburn.
3. constipation.
4. migraine headaches.

Answer: 2

Test-Taking Strategy: Read the question carefully, noting the issue of the question and the key words. In this question, the key words are "is effective" and "relief of" and the issue is *an intended effect*. Remembering that most proton pump inhibitor medication names end with the suffix *-zole*, will direct you to option 2.

Sample Question: Commonalities in Medication Names

A nurse is taking a health history on a client. When the nurse asks the client about current prescribed medications, the client tells the nurse that amprenavir (Agenerase) is taken twice daily. Based on this finding, the nurse suspects the presence of which condition?

1. Peptic ulcer disease
2. Inflammatory bowel disease
3. Human immunodeficiency virus (HIV)
4. Diverticulitis

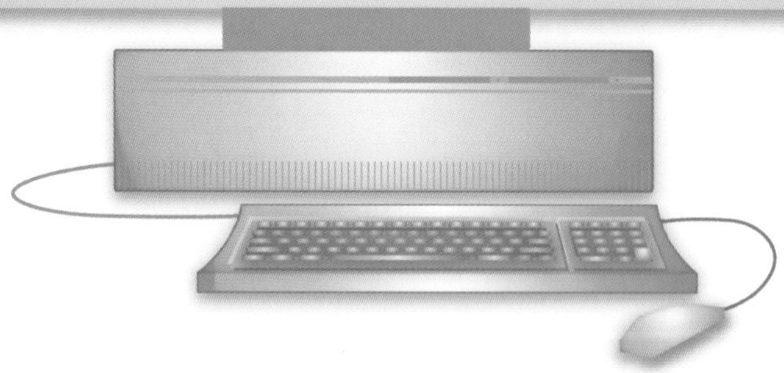

Answer: 3

Test-Taking Strategy: Read the question carefully, noting the issue of the question and the key words. In this question, the key words are "suspects the presence" and the issue is *the nurse's finding*. Remembering that many antiviral medication names contain the letters *vir* will direct you to option 3. Also note the similarity in options 1, 2, and 4. These options all relate to a gastrointestinal disorder.

Sample Question: Commonalities in Medication Names

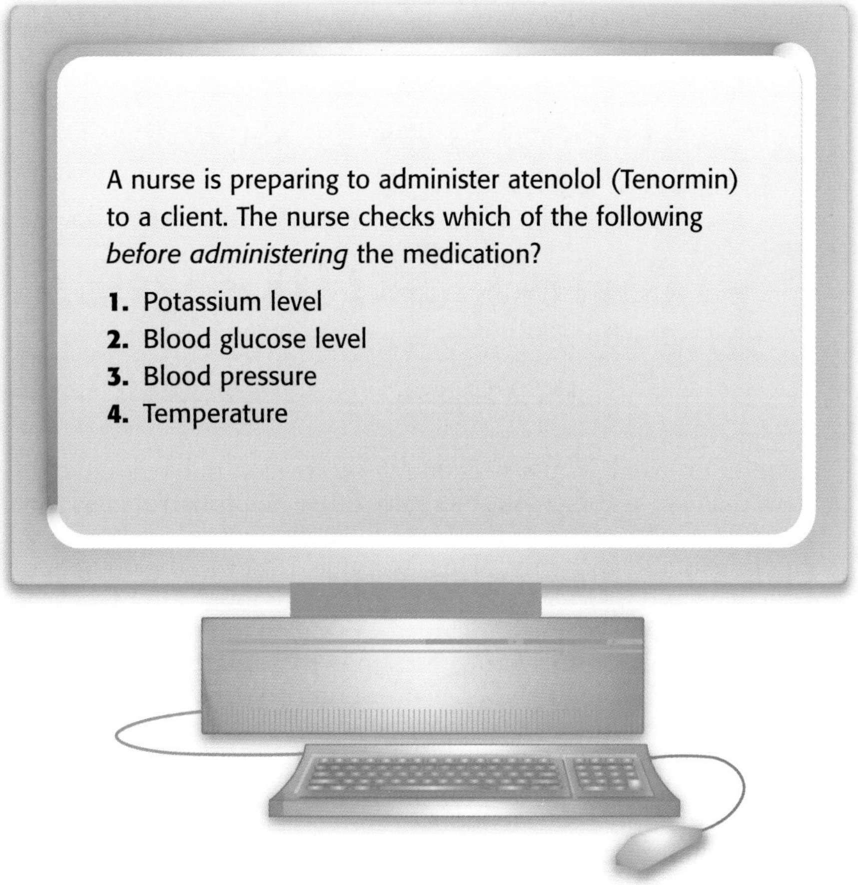

A nurse is preparing to administer atenolol (Tenormin) to a client. The nurse checks which of the following *before administering* the medication?

1. Potassium level
2. Blood glucose level
3. Blood pressure
4. Temperature

Answer: 3

Test-Taking Strategy: Read the question carefully, noting the issue of the question and the key words. In this question, the key words are "before administering" and the issue is *the item that the nurse checks*. Note the name of the medication *atenolol*. Recalling that most beta adrenergic blockers medication names end with *-lol* and that these medications are used to control blood pressure will direct you to option 3.

REFERENCES

Hodgson, B. & Kizior, R. (2005). *Saunders nursing drug handbook 2005.* Philadelphia: Saunders.

Kee, J. & Hayes, E. (2003). *Pharmacology: a nursing process approach* (4th ed). Philadelphia: Saunders.

Lehne, R. (2004). *Pharmacology for nursing care* (5th ed). Philadelphia: Saunders.

National Council of State Boards of Nursing, Inc. *Test Plan for the National Council Licensure Examination for Licensed Practical/Vocational Nurses* (effective date: April 2005), National Council of State Boards of Nursing, Chicago, 2004.

National Council of State Boards of Nursing, Inc. Online: available at www.ncsbn.org.

Chapter 13 Additional Pyramid Strategies

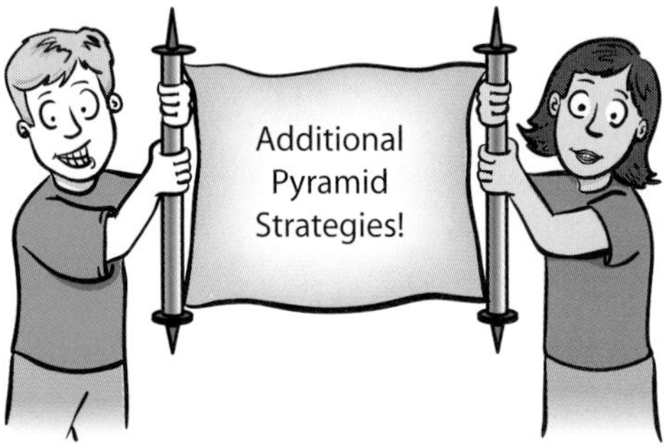

In addition to all of the test-taking strategies that you have reviewed so far in this book, there are other helpful strategies that you can use to assist in the process of elimination and answering questions correctly. This chapter reviews these helpful strategies and provides sample questions to illustrate how these strategies are used. Also included in this chapter are strategies that are useful for answering questions that relate to medication and intravenous calculations, questions that relate to laboratory values, and questions that relate to client positioning. The additional pyramid strategies include the following:

1. Eliminating options that contain absolute words and selecting options that contain not-so-absolute words
2. Eliminating options that contain medical rather than nursing interventions
3. Eliminating similar options
4. Ensuring that all components of an option are correct
5. Selecting the umbrella option
6. Visualizing the information in the case situation and in the options
7. Looking for similar concepts in the question and in one of the options

ELIMINATING OPTIONS THAT CONTAIN ABSOLUTE WORDS AND SELECTING OPTIONS THAT CONTAIN NOT-SO-ABSOLUTE WORDS—HOW WILL THIS HELP?

In most situations, if an option contains an absolute word, then it is incorrect. As you read each option, if you note a word that is absolute, eliminate the option. Conversely, as you read an option and note a not-so-absolute word, then that may be the correct option. Below is a list of absolute words and those words that are not so absolute.

Absolute Words	***Not-So-Absolute Words***
All	Generally
Always	May
Can't	Possibly
Every	Usually
Must	
Never	
None	
Not	
Only	
Won't	

> Absolute words may indicate an incorrect option!
> Not-so-absolute words may indicate a correct option!

Following are sample questions that illustrate the strategy of absolute versus not-so-absolute words.

Sample Question: Eliminating Options That Contain Absolute Words

A nurse is providing dietary instructions to a client about a low-fat diet. The nurse tells the client to:

1. never use butter for cooking.
2. read the labels on food items to determine their fat content.
3. eat only foods that have less than 1% fat content.
4. drink fluids only if they are fat-free.

Answer: 2

Test-Taking Strategy: Read every word in each option carefully. Note the absolute word "never" in option 1 and "only" in options 3 and 4. These options should be eliminated because they are incorrect. Remember, the use of an absolute word in an option will most likely make the option incorrect!

Sample Question: Selecting Options That Contain Not-So-Absolute Words

A client scheduled for a computed tomography (CT) scan of the abdomen asks the nurse when the results of the test will be available. The nurse makes which *appropriate* response to the client?

1. "The results won't be available for at least 1 week."
2. "You must ask the CT technician for that information."
3. "Your physician may have the results in about 3 days."
4. "Every scan is read by a radiologist and this process always takes 1 week,"

Answer: 3

Test-Taking Strategy: Read every word in each option carefully and note the key word "appropriate." If you were unable to answer this question using nursing knowledge, note the use of the not-so-absolute word "may" in option 3. Also, note the absolute word "won't" in option 1, "must" in option 2 and "every" and "always" in option 4. These options should be eliminated because they are incorrect. Remember, the use of an absolute word in an option will most likely make the option incorrect and the use of a not-so-absolute word in an option tends to make the option correct.

ELIMINATING OPTIONS THAT CONTAIN MEDICAL RATHER THAN NURSING INTERVENTIONS—HOW WILL THIS HELP?

An important point to remember is that the NCLEX-PN examination is a nursing examination, not a medical one. Therefore, focus on nursing and select the option that relates to a nursing intervention rather than a medical one. The only situation in which you may need to select a medical intervention is if the question indicates to do so. For example, if the question stem states, "Which intervention does the nurse anticipate the physician to prescribe?" then you may need to select the option that contains a medical action or prescription. Following is a review of sample questions that illustrate this strategy.

Focus on nursing rather than medical interventions!

Sample Question: Eliminating Options That Contain Medical Rather Than Nursing Interventions

A nurse is caring for a client with a diagnosis of congestive heart failure who suddenly experiences severe dyspnea, and the nurse suspects that the client developed pulmonary edema. The nurse *immediately:*

1. obtains a vial of furosemide (Lasix) and a syringe.
2. places the client in high-Fowler's position.
3. obtains a dose of morphine sulfate from the narcotic medication drawer.
4. inserts a Foley catheter.

Answer: 2

Test-Taking Strategy: Note the key word "immediately" and note the issue of the question, *a nursing action.* Although options 1, 3, and 4 are interventions that would be done in this situation, they all require a medical order from a physician. Option 2 is a nursing action that does not require a medical order. Remember, this is a nursing examination, not a medical examination!

Sample Question: Selecting an Option That Indicates a Medical Intervention

A nurse is assisting in admitting an infant to the pediatric unit with a diagnosis of respiratory syncytial virus (RSV). The nurse expects a physician's order for which of the following?

1. Ribavirin (Virazole)
2. Contact precautions
3. A private room
4. Strict handwashing procedures

Answer: 1

Test-Taking Strategy: Note the issue of the question, *the intervention that the physician will prescribe.* Although the physician may document options 2, 3, and 4 on the medical order sheet, these are interventions that the nurse can implement for an infant with RSV. In other words, a physician's order is not required for these interventions. On the other hand, option 1 requires a physician's order. Remember, this is a nursing examination, not a medical examination and the only situation in which you may need to select a medical intervention is if the question indicates to do so!

ELIMINATING SIMILAR OPTIONS—HOW WILL THIS HELP?

An important point for you to remember is that in multiple choice questions, there is only one correct option. As you read the options, if you note options that are similar with regard to their context, eliminate these options. The correct answer to the question will be the option that is different. Following is a sample question that illustrates this strategy of eliminating similar options.

> Eliminate similar options!

Sample Question: Eliminating Similar Options

A nurse is assisting in preparing a plan of care for an older client with a history of heart failure who will be receiving a blood transfusion. The nurse suggests writing which intervention in the plan that relates to monitoring for a transfusion reaction?

1. Monitor the client's intake and output during the transfusion.
2. Weigh the client before and after the transfusion.
3. Monitor the client's temperature during the transfusion.
4. Check the client's lung sounds hourly for crackles.

Answer: 3

Test-Taking Strategy: Note the issue of the question, *a transfusion reaction.* If you know the signs of a transfusion reaction, then you can answer this question easily. If you do not know these signs, then read the options carefully. Note that options 1, 2, and 4 are similar in that they all relate to the complication of fluid overload. Because they are all similar they are incorrect and need to be eliminated. Remember, the correct answer to the question will be the option that is different!

ENSURING THAT ALL PARTS OF AN OPTION ARE CORRECT—HOW WILL THIS HELP?

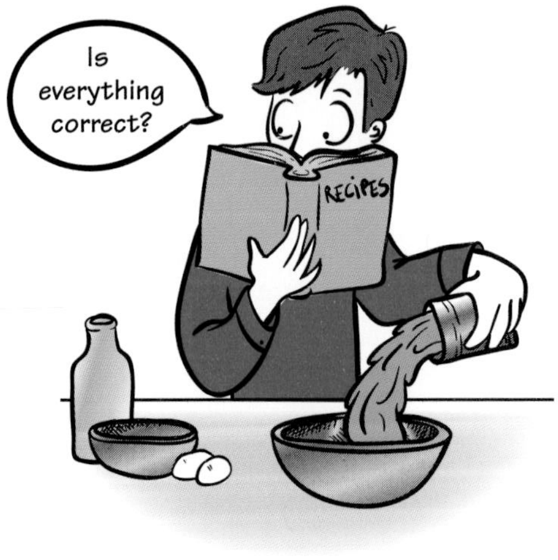
Is everything correct?
RECIPES

There may be some questions that contain options that include two parts and each part of the option will be separated by the word "and." Read the question carefully, note the key words, and focus on the issue. As you read the options, read both parts. If you note that one part of the option is incorrect, then the entire option is incorrect; therefore, eliminate the option. In these types of questions it is important to ensure that both parts of the option are correct. Following is a sample question that illustrates this strategy of ensuring that all parts of an option are correct.

Ensure that all parts of an option are correct!

Sample Question: Ensuring That All Parts of an Option Are Correct

A nurse is collecting data from a client diagnosed with a cataract of the right eye. The nurse should *expect to obtain* which data?

1. Complaints of blurred vision and excessive tearing of the eye
2. A cloudy white pupil and complaints of eye pain

3. Complaints of a gradual loss of vision and photophobia
4. Complaints of a frontal headache and photophobia

Answer: 3

Test-Taking Strategy: The options in this question contain two parts, each of which is separated by the word "and." Read the question carefully, note the key words, and focus on the issue. The key words are "expect to obtain" and the issue of the question is *data noted in a client with a cataract.* In this question knowledge regarding the differences of the signs and symptoms of a cataract and glaucoma will assist in answering correctly. Although a cloudy white pupil and photophobia occur in a client with a cataract, eye pain, and frontal headaches do not. Therefore, these options (options 2 and 4) are not entirely correct and can be eliminated. Eye pain and frontal headaches occur in the client with glaucoma. From the remaining two options, recalling that excessive tearing occurs in the client with glaucoma not the client with a cataract, will assist in eliminating option 1. Remember, all parts of the option needs to be correct for the option to be correct!

SELECTING THE UMBRELLA OPTION—HOW WILL THIS HELP?

The umbrella option is the option that is a general statement and may incorporate the content of the other options within it. The umbrella option may also be termed as a global option or a comprehensive option. When you are answering a question and note that more than one option appears to be correct, look for the umbrella option. The umbrella option will be the correct answer. Following is a sample question that illustrates this strategy.

> Look for the umbrella option!

Sample Question: Selecting the Umbrella Option

A nurse in the emergency department receives a telephone call from emergency medical services and is told that several victims who survived a plane crash and are suffering from cold exposure will be transported to the hospital. The *initial* nursing action is which of the following?

1. Supply the trauma rooms with bottles of sterile water and normal saline
2. Call the laundry department and ask the department to send as many warm blankets as possible to the emergency department
3. Call the nursing supervisor to activate the agency disaster plan
4. Call the intensive care unit to request that nurses be sent to the emergency department

Answer: 3

Test-Taking Strategy: Note the key word "initial" and focus on the issue, *the nursing action in the event of a disaster.* As you read each option you will note that all of the options are correct. In this type of question, look for the umbrella option, which is option 3. Activating the agency disaster plan will ensure that the interventions in options 1, 2, and 4 will occur. Remember, the umbrella option incorporates the ideas of the other options within it.

VISUALIZING THE INFORMATION IN THE CASE SITUATION AND IN THE OPTIONS—HOW WILL THIS HELP?

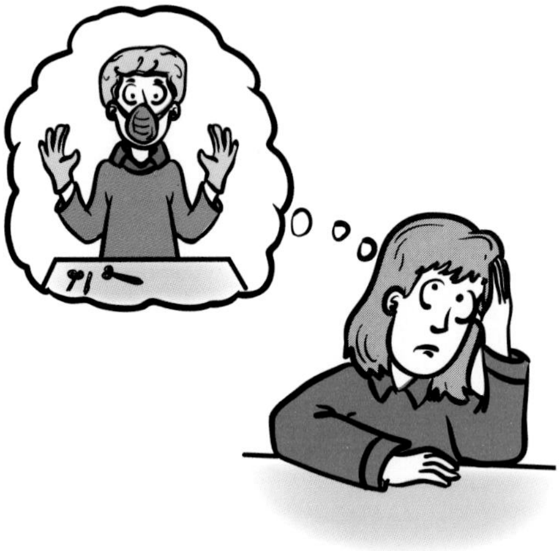

As you read the question, it is helpful to visualize the case situation. Forming a mental image of the situation places you as the nurse into the scenario. This may be useful because as you create the mental image, you may recall a similar situation that you experienced in the actual clinical area and recall what you as the nurse did in the situation. Additionally, visualize each option as you read it. This process will assist in determining the correct option. Visualizing and relating the case situation to a similar clinical experience can be a valuable strategy as you attempt to eliminate incorrect options. Following is a sample question that illustrates this strategy of visualizing the information.

> Visualize the information!

Sample Question: Visualizing the Information in the Case Situation and in the Options

A nurse prepares to perform a sterile dressing change on an abdominal incision. The nurse explains the procedure to the client, washes her hands, and sets up the sterile field. The nurse takes which action *next?*

1. Dons sterile gloves
2. Dons clean gloves and removes the old dressing
3. Cleans the wound with povidone-iodine (Betadine) solution as prescribed
4. Inspects the integrity of the abdominal incision

Answer: 2

Test-Taking Strategy: Note the key word "next." Form a mental image of this procedure and visualize the steps that you would take. You cannot clean the wound or inspect the wound unless you remove the old dressing; therefore, eliminate options 3 and 4. From the remaining options, recall that sterile gloves are necessary for cleaning and dressing the incision once the old dressing is removed. This will direct you to option 2. Visualizing and relating the case situation to a similar clinical experience can be a valuable strategy as you attempt to eliminate incorrect options!

LOOKING FOR SIMILAR CONCEPTS IN THE QUESTION AND IN ONE OF THE OPTIONS—HOW WILL THIS HELP?

Read the question carefully, noting the key words and the issue of the question. As you read each option, look for the option that contains similar concepts or has a relationship to those identified in the question. This strategy may be helpful as you are eliminating the incorrect options. Following is a sample question that illustrates this strategy.

> Look for similar concepts in the question and in one of the options!

Sample Question: Looking for Similar Concepts in the Question and in One of the Options

A client is admitted to the hospital with a diagnosis of pericarditis. A nurse monitors the client for which manifestation that differentiates pericarditis from other cardiopulmonary problems?

1. Chest pain that worsens on inspiration
2. Pericardial friction rub
3. Anterior chest pain
4. Weakness and irritability

Answer: 2

Test-Taking Strategy: Note the key word "differentiates," and focus on the issue, *a manifestation that differentiates pericarditis from other cardiopulmonary problems.* This tells you that the correct option is one that is unique to this health problem. Note the relationship between the word "pericarditis" in the question and the word "pericardial" in the correct option. Also recall that a pericardial friction rub is heard when there is inflammation of the pericardial sac, during the inflammatory phase of pericarditis. Remember, look for the option that contains a similar concept or has a relationship to the information in the question!

WHAT STRATEGIES WILL BE HELPFUL WHEN ANSWERING MEDICATION AND INTRAVENOUS CALCULATION QUESTIONS?

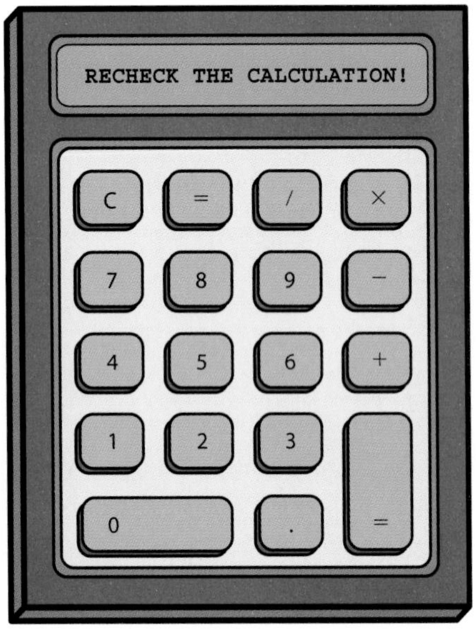

When a medication or intravenous calculation question is presented, you should always use the appropriate formula to solve the problem. Shortcuts should not be used in making these calculations. The problem and the answer should be expressed in the correct units of measure. Always be careful with decimal points. It is important to place the decimal points in the correct places, or the answer will be incorrect. Remember if you need to record the answer to the question such as in a fill-in-the-blank question, place a zero before a decimal point if the value lacks a numeral before the decimal point (example, 0.5 *not* .5) and avoid placing a decimal point and zero after a whole number (example 2.0 is *incorrect* and needs to written as 2). When solving a medication calculation problem, always determine whether the answer is within reason and makes sense.

On the NCLEX-PN examination, medication and intravenous calculation questions will most likely be in the multiple-choice or the fill-in-the blank format. You will be provided with an on-screen calculator for these medication and intravenous problems. Even if you use the calculator to calculate dosages and flow rates, it is important to recheck the calculation before selecting an option or typing the answer. Follow the formula, place the decimal points in the correct places, and check the accuracy of the calculation. Following are two sample questions that relate to medication and intravenous calculations.

MEDICATION AND INTRAVENOUS CALCULATIONS

- Use the on-screen calculator.
- Convert the unit of measure if necessary.
- Follow the formula.
- Place the decimal points in the correct places.
- Place a zero before a decimal point if the value lacks a numeric before the decimal point.
- Avoid placing a decimal point and zero after a whole number.
- Recheck the accuracy of the calculation!

Sample Question: Medication Calculation

A physician's order reads phenytoin (Dilantin) 0.2 g orally twice daily. The medication label states 100-mg capsules. A nurse prepares how many capsule(s) to administer one dose?

1. 1 capsule
2. 2 capsules
3. 3 capsules
4. 4 capsules

Answer: 2

Test-Taking Strategy: In this medication calculation problem, it is necessary to first convert grams to milligrams. Once you have done the conversion and reread the medication calculation problem, you will know that 2 capsules is the correct answer. Follow the formula for the calculation of the correct dose. Use the onscreen calculator and then recheck your work and make sure that the answer makes sense.

In the metric system, to convert larger to smaller, multiply by 1000 or move the decimal three places to the right. Therefore, 0.2 g = 200 mg. The formula and the calculation using the formula are provided below. Remember, follow the formula, recheck your answer, and make sure that the answer makes sense before selecting an option or typing the answer!

Formula:

$$\frac{\text{Desired}}{\text{Available}} \times \text{capsules} = \text{Capsules per dose}$$

Calculation:

$$\frac{200 \text{ mg}}{100 \text{ mg}} \times 1 \text{ capsule} = 2 \text{ capsules}$$

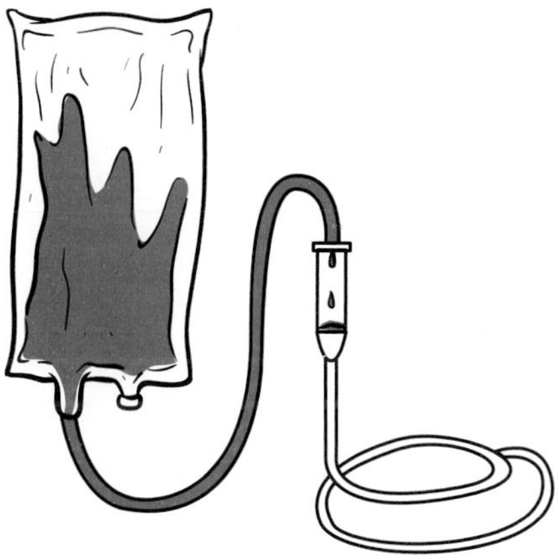

Sample Question: Intravenous (IV) Calculation

A physician orders 1000 mL of one-half normal saline to infuse over 8 hours. The drop factor is 15 drops (gtt) per 1 mL. The nurse sets the flow rate at how many drops per minute? (Round the answer to the nearest whole number)

Answer:__________

Answer: 31

Test-Taking Strategy: This question is in the fill-in-the-blank format. Use the formula for calculating IV flow rates when answering the question. Use the onscreen calculator and then recheck your work and make sure that the answer makes sense. Be careful with the multiplication and division. The formula and the calculation using the formula are provided below. Remember, follow the formula, recheck your answer, and make sure that the answer makes sense before typing the answer. Also remember to round the answer to the nearest whole number!

Formula:

$$\frac{\text{Total volume} \times \text{gtt factor}}{\text{Time in minutes}} = \text{gtt per minute}$$

$$\frac{1000 \text{ mL} \times 15 \text{ gtt}}{480 \text{ minutes}} = \frac{15{,}000}{480} = 31.2, \text{ or } 31 \text{ drops per minute}$$

WHAT STRATEGIES WILL BE HELPFUL WHEN ANSWERING QUESTIONS THAT RELATE TO LABORATORY VALUES?

LEARN NORMAL LABORATORY VALUES!

The questions on NCLEX-PN related to laboratory values will require you to identify whether the laboratory value is normal or abnormal, and then you will be required to think about the effects of the laboratory value in terms of the client. If you are familiar with the normal values, you will be able to determine if an abnormality exists when a laboratory value is presented in a question. Pyramid points to review are the normal values for the most common laboratory tests, therapeutic serum medication levels of commonly prescribed medications, and determination of the need to implement specific actions based on the findings. Remember that most blood samples should not be drawn during hemodialysis.

When a question is presented on the NCLEX-PN examination regarding a specific laboratory value, note the disorder presented in the question and the associated body organ that is affected as a result of the disorder. This process will assist you in determining the correct option. For example, if the question is asking you about the immune status of a client receiving chemotherapy, laboratory results of the white blood cell count and the neutrophils will be most important. You will need to determine that the results are probably going to be low, and then determine the specific client need, which in this case would be the risk for infection. In the client receiving chemotherapy who has a low white blood cell count, your plan centers on the immune system and protecting that client from infection. Interventions focus on preventive interventions related to infection, perhaps protective isolation measures. Evaluation may focus on maintenance of a normal temperature in the client. Following is a review of a sample question that relates to a laboratory test.

LABORATORY VALUES

Identify whether the laboratory value is normal or abnormal.
Note the disorder presented in the question.
Identify the associated body organ that is affected as a result of the disorder.

Sample Question: Laboratory Values

A client with a diagnosis of sepsis is receiving antibiotics by the intravenous route. The nurse monitors for nephrotoxicity by checking the results of which laboratory value *most closely?*

1. Blood urea nitrogen
2. White blood cell count
3. Platelet count
4. Lipase level

Answer: 1

Test-Taking Strategy: Note the key words "most closely." Focus on the information in the question and note that the issue is *nephrotoxicity.* Read each option carefully and note that option 1 is the only option that relates to kidney function. Option 2 relates to the immune system. Option 3 relates to the hematological system. Option 4 relates to pancreatic function. Remember, note the disorder or issue presented in the question and the associated body organ that is affected as a result!

WHAT STRATEGIES WILL BE HELPFUL WHEN ANSWERING QUESTIONS THAT RELATE TO CLIENT POSITIONING?

Nursing responsibility includes positioning clients in a safe and appropriate manner to provide safety and comfort. Knowledge regarding the client position required for a certain procedure or condition is expected. It is the nurse's responsibility to reduce the likelihood and prevent the development of complications related to an existing condition, prescribed treatment, or medical or surgical procedure. It is imperative that the nurse review the physician's orders after treatments or procedures and take note of instructions regarding positioning and mobility.

When you are presented with a question that relates to positioning a client, focus on the information in the question, the client's diagnosis, and the anatomical location of the client's diagnosis, and consider the pathophysiology of the disorder and the goals of care. In other words, think about what complications you want to prevent. There are also some guidelines to remember when answering questions that relate to positioning. These guidelines are listed below.

CLIENT POSITIONING

- Always review physician's orders!
- Focus on the client's diagnosis.
- Identify the anatomical location of the client's diagnosis.
- Consider the pathophysiology of the disorder and the goals of care.
- Think about what complications you want to prevent.

Guidelines Related to Positioning

Following is a list of guidelines related to positioning:

- Elevation of an affected body part reduces edema.
- Clients who have had neck or head surgery are placed in a semi-Fowler's or Fowler's position.
- Following a liver biopsy, the client is placed in a right lateral (side-lying) position to provide pressure to the site and prevent bleeding.
- Clients receiving irrigations or feeding through a nasogastric, gastrostomy, or jejunostomy tube are placed in a semi-Fowler's or Fowler's position to prevent aspiration.
- The left Sims' position is used to administer a rectal enema or irrigation to allow the solution to flow by gravity in the natural direction of the colon.
- A client with a respiratory disorder or cardiovascular disorder is placed in a semi-Fowler's or Fowler's position.
- Clients with peripheral arterial disease may be advised to elevate their feet and legs at rest, because swelling can prevent arterial blood flow, but they should not raise their legs above the level of the heart because extreme elevation slows arterial blood flow; some clients may be advised to maintain a slightly dependent position to promote perfusion.
- Clients with peripheral venous disease are usually advised to elevate their feet and legs.
- Clients with a head injury are placed in a semi-Fowler's or Fowler's position.
- If a client develops autonomic dysreflexia, the head of the bed is elevated.
- In clients with hemorrhagic strokes, the head of the bed is usually elevated to 30 degrees to reduce intracranial pressure and facilitate venous drainage.
- For clients with ischemic strokes, the head of the bed is usually kept flat.

Following craniotomy, the client should NOT be positioned on the site that was operated on, especially if the bone flap has been removed, because the brain has no bony covering on the affected site; a semi-Fowler's to Fowler's position is maintained with the head in a midline, neutral position to facilitate venous drainage from the head, and extreme hip and neck flexion is avoided.

With increased intracranial pressure, the client is placed in a semi-Fowler's to Fowler's position; the head is maintained in a midline, neutral position to facilitate venous drainage from the head, and extreme hip and neck flexion is avoided.

In a spinal cord injury, the client is immobilized on a spinal backboard, with the head in a neutral position, to prevent incomplete injury from becoming complete; head flexion, rotation, or extension is avoided and the client is logrolled.

In the client who underwent a total hip replacement, positioning will depend on the surgical techniques used, the method of implantation, the prosthesis, and physician's preference; extreme internal and external rotation and adduction is avoided and side-lying on the operative side is usually not allowed (unless specifically prescribed by the physician).

The following question relates to positioning a client.

Sample Question: Client Positioning

A nurse assists a physician in performing a liver biopsy. After the biopsy, the nurse plans to place the client in which of the following positions?

1. Supine
2. Prone
3. A left side-lying position with a small pillow or folded towel under the puncture site
4. A right side-lying position with a small pillow or folded towel under the puncture site

Answer: 4

Test-Taking Strategy: Focus on the information in the question, the anatomical location of the procedure, and think about what complication that you want to prevent; in this situation you want to prevent bleeding. Remember that the liver is on the right side of the body, and that the application of pressure on the right side will minimize the escape of blood or bile through the puncture site because this position compresses the liver against the chest wall at the biopsy site. Remember to focus on the information in the question, the client's diagnosis, and the anatomical location of the client's diagnosis, and consider the pathophysiology of the disorder and the goals of care!

REFERENCES

Chernecky, C. & Berger, B. (2004). *Laboratory tests and diagnostic procedures* (4th ed). Philadelphia: Saunders, p. 158.

DeWit, S. (2005). *Fundamental concepts and skills for nursing* (2nd ed). Philadelphia: Saunders.

Kee, J. & Marshall, S. (2004). *Clinical calculations: with applications to general and specialty areas* (5th ed). Philadelphia: Saunders.

Lewis, S., Heitkemper, M., & Dirksen, S. (2004). *Medical-surgical nursing: assessment and management of clinical problems* (6th ed). St. Louis: Mosby.

Peckenpaugh, N. (2003). *Nutrition essentials and diet therapy* (9th ed). Philadelphia: Saunders.

Potter, P. & Perry, A. (2005). *Fundamentals of nursing* (6th ed). St. Louis: Mosby.

Wong, D., Perry, S. & Hockenberry, M. (2002). *Maternal-child nursing care* (2nd ed). St. Louis: Mosby.

"A study method that I used to help me pass NCLEX exam involved three easy steps. First, I did several practice questions from my review books and CD-ROMs and made a list of every disease process or drug with which I was not familiar. Next, I took the list and made flash cards with all of the pertinent details of the content area in which I was unfamiliar. I then studied each flash card and attempted to learn the "hows" and "whys" of the material instead of just memorizing it. In the third and final step, I decided to "teach" the information to another person, which dramatically helped reinforce my own understanding of each concept.

—Robert, Clayton College and State University, Morrow, Georgia

"Answer questions every day for at least half an hour to an hour! I did Linda Silvestri's CD questions, and I also purchased a strategies book and read over that. Also when you answer the questions make sure you read over the strategies to explain why an answer was right or wrong. Often you learn a lot just from the responses. Don't study, just answer questions! It really helps and it's important to use the critical thinking strategies that are discussed in the first chapter. I highly recommend all of the products in Saunders Pyramid to Success for the NCLEX examination."

—Mindy, Salve Regina University, Newport, RI

Part 3 Additional Tips for Test-Takers

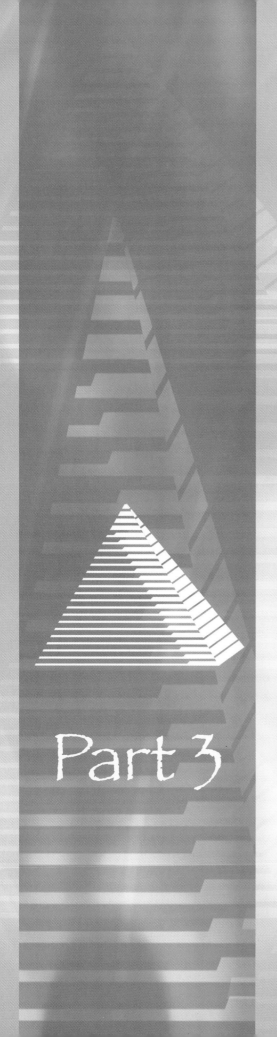

Chapter 14 Tips for Repeat Test-Takers

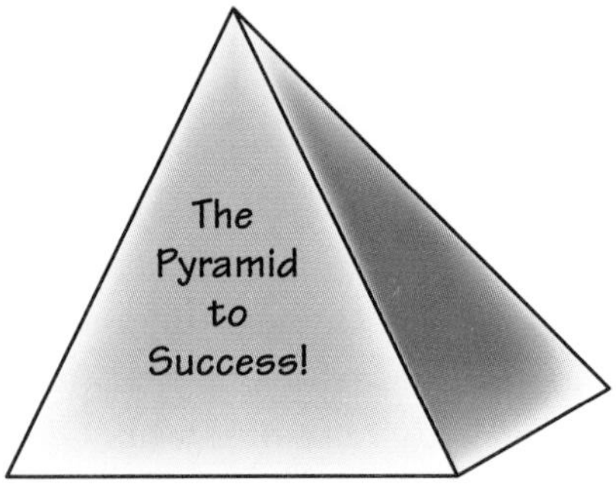

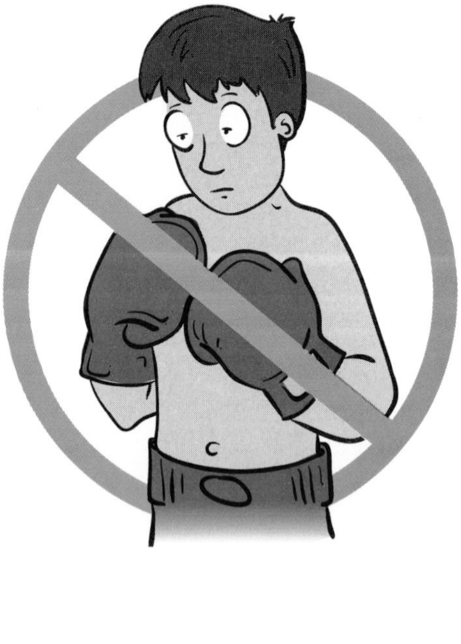

If you need to read this chapter because you have to retake the NCLEX-PN® examination, don't be discouraged or lose hope. You *will* be successful when you retake the examination. If you believe in yourself and believe that you can be successful you *will* pass this examination. Don't beat yourself up about the fact that you were unsuccessful!

You did the very best that you could! Never think that you are a failure because you did not pass this examination. Yes, you were unsuccessful but you are not a failure. And never feel as if you are all alone. There are other nursing graduates who were unsuccessful when taking this examination the first time.

Part of the preparation for retaking the examination involves maintaining a positive attitude and confidence in yourself that you can be successful. Think about all of the achievements that you have made and all of your life goals that you have met. You have been successful in receiving your diploma from the nursing program that you have attended, and that is one major achievement.

Everyone faces obstacles during their lifetime that they need to overcome. Now you are faced with an obstacle. Can you overcome it? Yes, of course you can! You need to remember that success is like climbing a mountain. You will have challenging obstacles to deal with as you climb, but the only way to reach the top of the mountain is to face these challenges in a positive way.

Let's be realistic. Receiving the large envelope in the mail that contained retake information was a devastating experience and you probably experienced a number of different feelings about the fact that you were unsuccessful. You probably needed to inform your family and perhaps children, friends, and your employer that you need to retake the examination. Sharing the news can be distressing and embarrassing. The fact that you need to retake this examination may have also created a financial burden because you are unable to start your career as a licensed practical/vocational nurse as you planned. So now what do you do? Stand tall, think about all of the accomplishments that you have achieved, stay positive, maintain your self-confidence, face those challenging obstacles, retake the examination, and think success!

Stand tall.
Think about your accomplishments.
Stay positive.
Maintain your self-confidence.
Face the challenges.
Retake the examination.
Think success!

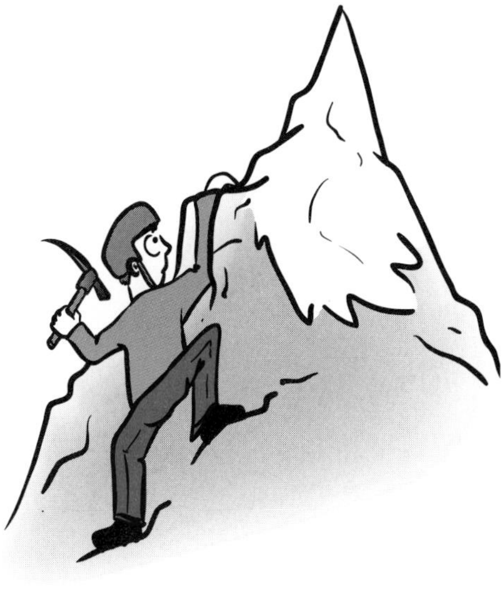

This chapter provides you with the tips and strategies that will help you to prepare to retake this examination. Specific tips and strategies address the procedure for self-assessment, developing a remediation plan, the steps in a remediation plan, and planning a retake date.

POSITIVES? ARE THERE ANY?

Believe it or not there are some positive points that you can think about and focus on to help you remain optimistic. Think about it, you have been through the entire experience and know what the examination process is all about. Let's review some of these positives.

The Positives

You have seen the test and know what the test is all about.
You are familiar with the computer.
You are familiar with the test center.
You are familiar with the testing procedures.
You have reviewed nursing content once.
You know what content areas need some fine-tuning.

WHEN DO YOU SCHEDULE A DATE TO RETAKE THE EXAMINATION?

Retake policies vary from state to state; therefore, it is important to carefully review the materials that were sent to you for registering to retake the examination. Depending on the state board of nursing, you will need to wait a minimum of 45 to 91 days before you can retake the examination. Readiness to retake this examination is highly individual and your readiness may be very different from someone else's. What you need to do is to develop your remediation plan and determine how much time it will take you to implement your plan. It is best to retake this examination as soon as you can as long as you have prepared by following your remediation plan. The longer you wait the more risk you run of forgetting critical nursing content that was learned in nursing school. So don't delay. Develop your remediation plan, get started with your review, and stick to your plan!

WHERE DO YOU START TO PREPARE FOR THE RETAKE EXAMINATION?

Your first task is self-assessment.

The first task that you have is to perform a self-assessment. Think about your testing experience and identify the factors or obstacles that you believe contributed to being unsuccessful. Write these factors down on a piece of paper so you can be sure that you pay attention to them as you prepare. Some self-assessment questions that you may want to consider include the following.

Self-Assessment Questions

Following is a list of self-assessment questions:

Did you adequately prepare?
Did you stick to your plan for review?
Did you review nursing content and practice test questions?
Do you understand how to use test-taking strategies?
Did you prepare for this examination holistically? In other words, did you include exercise, fun, and relaxation and did you eat a balanced diet?
Did you eat properly on the day of the examination? In other words, did you eliminate caffeine and high-fat foods from your diet?
Did you have test anxiety on the day of the examination? Were you able to control your test anxiety?
Did you face any obstacles on the way to the testing center that caused a delay such as traffic or road construction?
Did you encounter any distractions as you were taking the examination, and if so, what were they?
Were you able to focus and concentrate during the examination?
Were your self-expectations too high?
Did you expect the test to end after 85 questions, and when it didn't end did you begin to lose your stamina, ability to concentrate, and self-confidence?

WHAT IS THE NCLEX-PN® CANDIDATE PERFORMANCE REPORT AND HOW WILL IT HELP WITH DEVELOPING A REMEDIATION PLAN?

> Use the NCLEX-PN® Candidate Performance Report as a guide in developing a remediation plan.

The NCLEX-PN® Candidate Performance Report is prepared by the National Council of State Boards of Nursing (NCSBN) and is provided only to the nursing graduate who needs to retake the examination. This report provides extremely valuable information about your areas of strengths and the areas that you need to particularly focus on as you prepare to retake the examination.

The NCLEX-PN® Candidate Performance Report provides you with information about the number of questions that you answered and about your performance on specific content areas of the examination.

Specific Content Areas

Following is a list of some of the specific content areas:

Basic Care and Comfort
Coordinated Care
Health Promotion and Maintenance
Pharmacological Therapies
Psychosocial Integrity
Physiological Adaptation
Reduction of Risk Potential
Safety and Infection Control

In addition to the specific content area, the report provides you with the percentage of test questions in the content area, a description of the content area and a list of subject matter related to it, and a report of your performance. Your performance is stated as Above the Passing Standard, Near the Passing Standard, or Below the Passing Standard. This report is your guide to develop a remediation plan because it identifies your specific strengths and areas that need to be improved.

HOW DO YOU DEVELOP AN ACADEMIC REMEDIATION PLAN?

It is important to use the NCLEX-PN® Candidate Performance Report as your guide in developing a remediation plan. There are some steps to follow in developing the plan. Let's review the

Pyramid to Success 10-step remediation plan and how these steps can be implemented.

Steps of a Remediation Plan

1. Include nonacademic preparation strategies in the remediation plan.
2. Review the performance report.
3. Prioritize the content areas.
4. Start the review with content areas Below the Passing Standard with the highest percentage of test questions.
5. Review nursing content using NCLEX-PN review resources.
6. Practice test questions using the Study Mode on a CD-ROM.
7. Take a test using the Quiz Mode on a CD-ROM.
8. Take a test using the Exam Mode on a CD-ROM.
9. Review any content areas that still need some fine-tuning.
10. Retake the NCLEX-PN examination.

Step 1: Include Nonacademic Preparation Strategies in the Remediation Plan

Nonacademic preparation strategies are an important component of preparing for this examination. Review your self-assessment and identify the areas related to nonacademic preparation that were obstacles in your path to success. It is critical that you address these obstacles as part of your remediation plan because you don't want to have to face these barriers to success again when you retake the examination. Chapter 6 of this book, Nonacademic Preparation: Your Path to Success, describes the ways to prepare yourself for this examination from a nonacademic perspective and identifies the methods that can be used to deal with any obstacles that you have faced when you took your examination the first time.

Step 2: Review the Performance Report

Start by reviewing your performance report sent to you by the NCSBN and identify the content areas that were most difficult for you. It is very important to read the description of the subject matter tested in each reported content area because this provides you with information regarding what you need to review.

Step 3: Prioritize the Content Areas

Prioritize the content areas noted on your performance report that require review, and write these content areas in order of priority in your remediation plan. Remember, all content areas of the test need to be reviewed even those that were reported as Above the Passing Standard. But what you need to do is to prioritize the content areas with those areas Below the Passing

Standard as the priority, followed by those content areas Near the Passing Standard, and lastly those areas Above the Passing Standard.

Step 4: Start the Review with Content Areas Below the Passing Standard with the Highest Percentage of Test Questions

You need to start your review with the content areas that were most difficult for you. These content areas will be those that were identified as Below the Passing Standard. If you have more than one content area Below the Passing Standard, then look at the percentage of test questions in those areas and begin your review with the area that identifies the highest percentage of test questions. Once you have completed your review in the content areas identified as Below the Passing Standard then proceed to review content areas identified as Near the Passing Standard followed by content areas identified as Above the Passing Standard.

Step 5: Review Nursing Content Using NCLEX-PN® Review Resources

Use NCLEX-PN® review resources to prepare.

In the Pyramid to Success, there are several NCLEX-PN® review resources available to help you prepare for retaking this examination. It is extremely beneficial to use NCLEX-PN review resources because the content and practice test questions that they contain focus on the subject matter identified in the NCLEX-PN test plan. Do not attempt to prepare to retake this examination by studying all of your class notes that you have from nursing school because they are much too detailed and you will become overwhelmed. And do not prepare to retake this examination by planning to read all of your nursing textbooks. You have already read them and now you need to focus specifically on the subject matter that will be tested on the NCLEX-PN examination. Several of the resources available to you are identified in the various steps of your remediation plan, and a description of how the resource(s) will be beneficial is provided. Any of these resources can be obtained at the Elsevier Health website at www.elsevierhealth.com.

As you prepare for this examination it is important to review nursing content areas, particularly the subject matter identified as an area requiring improvement on your performance report. Therefore, you need to use NCLEX-PN review resources. The resources that are available in the Pyramid to Success that contain nursing content are the *Saunders Comprehensive Review for the NCLEX-PN® Examination* and the *Saunders Instructor's Resource Package for the NCLEX-PN® Examination.* Following is a description of each resource.

Saunders Comprehensive Review for the NCLEX-PN® Examination:

- The book contains both nursing content of all areas of nursing including pharmacology, and practice questions.
- Nursing content areas include all of the areas identified in the NCLEX-PN test plan.
- The interactive CD-ROM contains more than 3500 practice questions and therefore provides you with practice questions on a computer.
- All practice questions are presented in either a multiple-choice format or an alternate test question format that is used in the NCLEX-PN examination.
- All practice questions provide a rationale for the correct and incorrect answer(s), a test-taking strategy, question codes based on the NCLEX-PN test plan categories and nursing content areas, content area to review if you answered the question incorrectly, and a reference source and page number.

Saunders Instructor's Resource Package for the NCLEX-PN® Examination:

- Ask your nursing faculty about his valuable resource!
- This resource may have been purchased by your nursing program for your use in preparing for the NCLEX-PN examination
- The CD-ROM contains 90 modules of specific nursing content reviews with colorful graphics, and a total of 3000 practice test questions.
- Each nursing review module is followed by a 20-question practice test that reflects the content of the module.
- All practice questions provide a rationale for the correct and incorrect answer(s), a test-taking strategy, question codes based on the NCLEX-PN test plan categories and nursing content areas, content area to review if you answered the question incorrectly, and a reference source and page number.

Step 6: Practice Test Questions Using the Study Mode on the CD-ROM

> Practicing test questions is a must!

Practicing test questions is a must! Practicing test questions yields a twofold reward. The first reward is that you will strengthen your knowledge base of nursing content. The second reward is that you will become skillful in using test-taking strategies. The more that you practice the more prepared you will be for this examination.

In addition to the *Saunders Comprehensive Review for the NCLEX-PN® Examination* one other extremely helpful resource for repeat test-takers is the *Saunders Q&A Review for the NCLEX-PN® Examination.* The reason that this resource is so helpful is that the book is uniquely designed to contain chapters with practice questions specific to each Client Needs area identified in the NCLEX-PN test plan. Therefore, if you are having difficulty with a specific Client Needs category of the test plan, you can refer to that specific Client Needs area in the book or on the CD-ROM and obtain practice questions that relate specifically to your area in need of improvement.

Because strengthening your nursing knowledge base and improving your test-taking skills are your goals, it is important that you use the NCLEX-PN review resources in the most effective manner. If you are using the CD-ROM in either the *Saunders Comprehensive Review for the NCLEX-PN® Examination* or the *Saunders Q&A Review for the NCLEX-PN® Examination,* it is best to access the Study Mode because you are given important information immediately after answering each question. This information includes a rationale for the correct and incorrect answer(s), a test-taking strategy, question codes based on the NCLEX-PN test plan categories and nursing content areas, content area to review if you answered the question incorrectly, and a reference source and page number. Therefore, your study efforts will be most productive in achieving your goals of strengthening your nursing knowledge base and improving your test-taking skills because you will gain knowledge and become skilled as you move along through your review.

Step 7: Take a Test Using the Quiz Mode on the CD-ROM

Take several 10-question quizzes.

Once you have reviewed nursing content and practiced test questions in the Study Mode, it is time to determine how you have improved your nursing knowledge and test-taking abilities. It is important to feel comfortable and reassured that you are ready for this examination because this will maintain that self-confidence in your ability to be successful and sustain your positive attitude.

Select the Quiz Mode on the CD-ROM in either the *Saunders Comprehensive Review for the NCLEX-PN® Examination* or the *Saunders Q&A Review for the NCLEX-PN® Examination.* The Quiz Mode will provide you with 10 randomly chosen test questions in a specific selected content area. You will need to answer all 10 questions before obtaining feedback on your performance—your score and specific feedback regarding your strengths and areas in need of review will be provided after completion of the quiz. Specific feedback includes a rationale for the correct and incorrect answer(s), a test-taking strategy, question codes based on the NCLEX-PN test plan categories and nursing content areas, content area to review if you answered the question incorrectly, and a reference source and page number.

Once you receive this feedback you will be able to identify any remaining content areas that need fine-tuning. If you note any remaining content areas that need fine-tuning, return to your *Saunders Comprehensive Review for the NCLEX-PN® Examination* and review these areas.

Step 8: Take a Test Using the Exam Mode on the CD-ROM

> Take several 100-question exams.

Taking several 100-question exams is the last step in your remediation process before you retake the examination. It is important to feel comfortable and reassured that you are ready to retake this examination because this will maintain that self-confidence in your ability to be successful and sustain your positive attitude.

Select the Exam Mode on the CD-ROM in either the *Saunders Comprehensive Review for the NCLEX-PN® Examination* or the *Saunders Q&A Review for the NCLEX-PN® Examination.* The Exam Mode will provide you with 100 randomly chosen test questions from the entire pool of test questions in the resource. This will simulate the integration of nursing content areas that occurs with the questions that appear on the NCLEX-PN. You will need to answer all 100 questions before obtaining feedback on your performance—your score and specific feedback regarding your strengths and areas in need of review will be provided after completion of the exam. Similar to the Quiz Mode, feedback includes a rationale for the correct and incorrect answer(s), a test-taking strategy, question codes based on the NCLEX-PN test plan categories and nursing content areas, content area to review if you answered the question incorrectly, and a reference source and page number.

Step 9: Review Any Content Areas That Still Need Some Fine-Tuning

If you have consistently demonstrated improvement in the scores that you received in the 100 question practice tests, then you know that it is time to retake the examination. If you are still having difficulty with improving your scores, then you know that you need to do additional content review and practice questions before you retake the examination. Review your performance report again and the practice test results that you printed out from all of the tests that you took from the CD-ROMs in the review resources. Again, identify the content areas in need of improvement and focus on these areas before retaking the NCLEX-PN examination. An additional resource for preparing for the examination is the *Saunders Review Cards for the NCLEX-PN® Examination.* This resource provides you with more than 900 practice test questions, including multiple-choice questions and the new alternate test items, such as fill-in-the-blank, multiple-response, prioritizing (ordered response), and image questions. This resource and any of the other NCLEX-PN resources can be used to help you fine-tune those areas in need of improvement.

Step 10: Retake the NCLEX-PN

It's time! Are you ready? Of course you are! As long as you followed your remediation plan and strengthened those content areas that needed improvement, you are ready! Now, what do you do?

Think positive!
Groom yourself for success on the day of the examination!
Maintain confidence and belief in yourself!
Meet the challenges of the day!
Retake the examination!
Become a licensed practical/vocational nurse!
And of course, don't forget to smile!

REFERENCES

National Council of State Boards of Nursing, Inc. *Test Plan for the National Council Licensure Examination for Licensed Practical/Vocational Nurses* (effective date: April 2005), National Council of State Boards of Nursing, Chicago, 2004.

National Council of State Boards of Nursing, Inc. Online: available at www.ncsbn.org.

Chapter 15

Tips for International Nurses

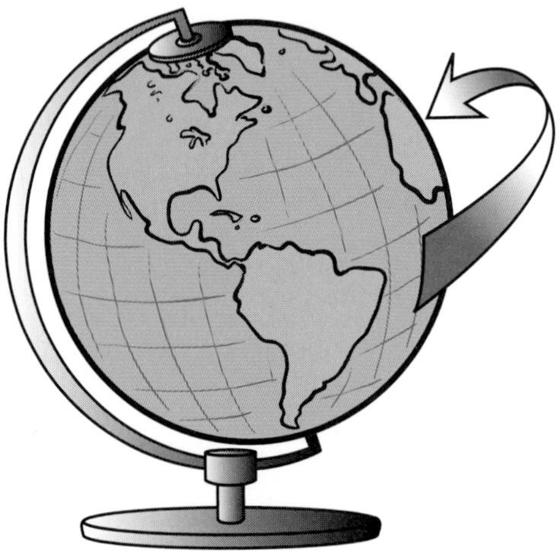

For an international or foreign-educated nurse, preparation to take the NCLEX-PN® examination involves basically four processes. These include meeting the requirements defined by the United States Immigration law, meeting the eligibility requirements defined by the National Council of State Boards of Nursing and the specific state board of nursing in the state that you intend to obtain licensure, registering to take the NCLEX-PN examination, and academic preparation for the NCLEX-PN examination.

EXAMINATION PREPARATION

Meeting the requirements defined by U.S. Immigration law
Meeting the eligibility requirements defined by the National Council of State Boards of Nursing and the state board of nursing
Registering to take the NCLEX-PN examination
Academic preparation for the NCLEX-PN examination

This chapter provides information regarding the certification processes that you will have to pursue to become a licensed practical/vocational nurse in the United States. An important factor to consider as you pursue this process is that some of the certification requirements may vary from state to state. Therefore, an important first step for you is to contact the board of nursing in the state in which you are planning to obtain licensure. State board of nursing contact information can be obtained through the National Council of State Boards of Nursing (NCSBN) website at www.ncsbn.org. Once you have accessed the NCSBN website, select the link titled "Boards of Nursing." In addition, you can write, call, or fax the NCSBN regarding the NCLEX-PN examination at NCSBN, 111 E. Wacker Drive, Suite 2900, Chicago, IL 60601; (312) 525-3600 voice; (312) 279-1032 fax.

WHAT DO YOU NEED TO DO TO MEET THE REQUIREMENTS DEFINED BY THE U.S. IMMIGRATION LAW?

You are required to obtain a VisaScreen™ certificate. The VisaScreen components include an educational analysis, license verification, assessment of proficiency in the English language, and an examination that tests nursing knowledge. All documents that verify eligibility must be submitted by the school or nursing program, licensure agency, or testing agency.

VisaScreen COMPONENTS

Educational analysis
License verification
Assessment of proficiency in the English language
An exam that tests nursing knowledge

The VisaScreen

U.S. immigration law requires certain health care professionals to successfully complete a screening program before receiving an occupational visa (Section 343 of the Illegal Immigration Reform and Immigration Responsibility Act of 1996). Therefore, you are required to obtain a VisaScreen certificate.

The Commission on Graduates of Foreign Nursing Schools (CGFNS) is the organization that offers this federal screening program. The International Commission on Health Care Professions (ICHP), a division of the CGFNS, administers the VisaScreen. Once each of the VisaScreen components have been successfully achieved, you will be presented with a VisaScreen certificate. Information related to the VisaScreen can be obtained through the CGFNS website at www.cgfns.org.

Educational Analysis

The educational analysis ensures that the applicant's education meets all statutory and regulatory requirements for the profession and is comparable with the education of a U.S. graduate seeking licensure.

The educational analysis component of the VisaScreen may require the following:

- Proof of completion of a senior secondary school education or high school education
- Proof of completion from a government-approved professional health care nursing program
- Documentation of completion of a specified number of clock and/or credit hours in specific theoretical and clinical areas while in nursing school

Licensure Verification

You must present all current and past licensure for review.

Proficiency in the English Language

You must submit proof of a passing score on an approved U.S. Department of Education and Health and Human Services English language proficiency examination. Acceptable English language proficiency examinations and the testing organizations are listed below.

Tests Administered by the Educational Testing Service (ETS) Worldwide

- Test of English as a Foreign Language (TOEFL)
- The Test of English for International Communication (TOEIC)
  Contact Information:
  Educational Testing Service (ETS)
  P.O. Box 6151
  Princeton, NJ 08541-6151
  Telephone: (609) 771-7100
  Email: toefl@ets.org
- International English Language Testing System (IELTS), jointly managed by British Council and IELTS Australia
  Contact Information:
  International English Language Testing System (IELTS)
  IELTS Administrator
  Cambridge Examinations and IELTS International
  100 East Corson Street, Suite 200
  Pasadena, CA 91103
  Telephone: (626) 564-2954
  Email: ielts@ceii.org
  Web site: www.ielts.org

Examination to Test Nursing Knowledge

An exam to test nursing knowledge includes the following:

1. A qualifying exam that is administered as part of the process for obtaining a CGFNS certificate tests nursing knowledge; therefore, a CGFNS certificate provides proof of adequate nursing knowledge. This qualifying exam is described later under "Components of the CGFNS Certification Program."
2. A foreign-educated nurse who is licensed and practicing nursing in the United States is also required to obtain a VisaScreen; if the nurse does not have a CGFNS certificate, the nurse may be granted eligibility to take the NCLEX examination to provide proof of nursing knowledge

WHAT ARE THE NATIONAL COUNCIL OF STATE BOARDS OF NURSING AND THE SPECIFIC STATE BOARD OF NURSING REQUIREMENTS?

> Find out what the National Council of State Boards of Nursing and the specific state board of nursing requires.

State requirements are developed based on the guidelines and requirements set by the NCSBN. Most states in the United States require that you receive certification from the CGFNS before you can be eligible to take the NCLEX examination. If the state in which you intend to obtain licensure does not require CGFNS certification, it may require submission of some of the same documents that CGFNS required. Therefore, in addition to what CGFNS requires, a state may require the following:

1. Proof of citizenship or lawful alien status
2. Official transcripts of educational credentials sent directly to the board of nursing from the school of nursing
3. Validation of theoretical instruction and clinical practice in a variety of nursing areas including medical nursing, surgical nursing, pediatric nursing, maternity and newborn nursing, and mental health nursing
4. Copy of nursing license and/or diploma
5. Proof of proficiency in the English language
6. Photographs of the applicant
7. Application fees

WHAT DOES THE COMMISSION ON GRADUATES OF FOREIGN NURSING SCHOOLS PROVIDE?

> CGFNS provides a certification program for nurses educated and licensed outside the United States.

The CGFNS provides a certification program for nurses educated and licensed outside the United States.

The certificate program offered by the CGFNS is a requirement of most state boards of nursing, and the certificate may be required before you can take the NCLEX examination. The certificate program ensures that you are eligible and qualified to meet licensure and other practice requirements in the United States, and it predicts your success on the NCLEX examination.

This program also assists you in obtaining your VisaScreen certificate. Additional information relating to CGFNS and its certification program can be obtained through the CGFNS website at www.cgfns.org.

WHAT ARE THE ELIGIBILITY REQUIREMENTS FOR THE COMMISSION ON GRADUATES OF FOREIGN NURSING SCHOOLS CERTIFICATION PROGRAM?

The CGFNS certification program is designed for nurses educated in nursing outside the United States who hold both an initial and current registration/licensure as a nurse. According to the CGFNS, the foreign-educated nurse must have obtained theoretical instruction and clinical practice in a variety of nursing areas, including medical nursing, surgical nursing, pediatric nursing, maternity and newborn nursing, and mental health nursing. If the nurse educated outside the United States does not meet these requirements, he or she is not eligible for the certification program.

WHAT ARE THE COMPONENTS OF THE COMMISSION ON GRADUATES OF FOREIGN NURSING SCHOOLS CERTIFICATION PROGRAM?

COMPONENTS OF THE CGFNS CERTIFICATION PROGRAM

Credentials review
Qualifying examination that tests nursing knowledge
English language proficiency exam

The CGFNS certification program contains three parts, and all parts must be successfully completed in order to be awarded a CGFNS certificate. The three parts include a credentials review, a qualifying examination that tests nursing knowledge, and an English language proficiency examination. The qualifying examination and the English language proficiency examination can be taken at various locations throughout the world. This provides you the opportunity to obtain the CGFNS certificate before traveling to the Unites States or other countries to take the NCLEX examination. These three parts of the certificate program are described in detail below.

Credentials Review

The CGFNS requires validation of education and a licensing history of the applicant to ensure that the applicant has the appropriate credentials to seek certification. CGFNS must receive transcripts and validation documents directly from the nursing program and licensing agency. Transcripts and validation documents will not be accepted from the applicant. The specific credentialing requirements are similar to those needed for the VisaScreen certificate and include the following:

1. Completed a senior secondary school education or high school education
2. Graduated from a government-approved nursing program
3. Obtained theoretical instruction and clinical practice in the areas of medical nursing, surgical nursing, pediatric nursing, maternity/newborn nursing, and mental health nursing
4. Hold a full and unrestricted current license or registration to practice in the country where his or her general nursing education was completed

Qualifying Examination

The qualifying examination tests your knowledge in nursing in a variety of areas such as adult health, pediatrics, maternity and newborn, and mental health. The examination is designed to ensure that you have the knowledge to provide nursing care to various client groups at the same level as recent U.S. nursing graduates.

English Language Proficiency Exam

You must take and pass an English language proficiency examination, which can be taken before or after the qualifying examination. This examination needs to be taken from a testing organization that is approved by CGFNS, and you must apply directly with the testing organization to take the examination. The examination scores must be sent directly to CGFNS from the testing organization. CGFNS will not accept test scores from the applicant. The types of English proficiency exams, approved testing organizations, and their contact information are listed earlier in this chapter under the heading "Proficiency in the English Language."

CGFNS identifies certain applicants as exempt from the English language proficiency requirement. In order for an applicant to be exempt, he or she must meet all of the following criteria: native language is English; country of nursing education is Australia, Canada (except Quebec), New Zealand, the United Kingdom; Trinidad and Tobago; and language of instruction and language of textbooks is English.

Once you have successfully met each of the three required components of the CGFNS certification program, CGFNS will issue a certificate of completion. Unless the state in which you intend to obtain licensure indicates additional requirements, and if you have received your VisaScreen certificate, you will be eligible to take the NCLEX examination.

HOW DO YOU REGISTER TO TAKE THE NATIONAL COUNCIL LICENSURE EXAMINATION FOR PRACTICAL/ VOCATIONAL NURSES?

If you are planning to take the NCLEX-PN examination in the United States, the initial step in the registration process is to submit an application to the state board of nursing in the state in which you intend to obtain licensure. You need to obtain information from the board of nursing regarding the specific registration process, because the process may vary from state to state. In most states, you may register for the examination through the Internet, by mail, or by telephone. It is important that you follow the registration instructions and complete the registration forms precisely and accurately. Registration forms not properly completed or not accompanied by the proper fees in the required method of payment, will be returned to you and will delay testing. There is a fee for taking the examination, and you may have to pay additional fees to the board of nursing in the state in which you are applying. You will be sent a confirmation indicating that your registration was received. If you do not receive a confirmation within 4 weeks of submitting your registration, you should contact the candidate services. Information regarding this contact can be obtained at the NCLEX candidate website (www.vue.com/nclex).

REGISTERING FOR THE EXAMINATION

You may register for the examination through the Internet (www.vue.com/nclex), by mail, or by telephone.

Once your eligibility to take the NCLEX examination has been verified by the board of nursing in the state in which licensure is requested, your registration form is processed and an Authorization to Test form will be sent to you. You cannot make an appointment until the board of nursing declares eligibility and you receive an Authorization to Test form. The examination will take place at Pearson Professional Centers and an appointment can be made through the Internet or by telephone. You can schedule an appointment at any Pearson Professional Center. You do not have to take the examination in the same state in which you are seeking licensure. A confirmation of your appointment will be sent to you. (See Chapters 1 and 2 for additional information regarding the NCLEX examination and testing procedures.)

IS THE NATIONAL COUNCIL LICENSURE EXAMINATION ADMINISTERED IN ANY LOCATIONS OUTSIDE OF THE UNITED STATES?

According to the NCSBN, as of January 2005, NCLEX testing abroad is available. The locations that provide this testing service are Seoul, South Korea; London, United Kingdom; and Hong Kong. Testing services abroad provides the nurse who is interested in becoming a licensed nurse in the United States an opportunity to pass the NCLEX examination before traveling to the United States.

HOW DO YOU PREPARE ACADEMICALLY TO TAKE THE NATIONAL COUNCIL LICENSURE EXAMINATION?

The challenge that is presented to you is one that requires patience and endurance. The positive result of your endeavor will certainly reward you professionally and give you the personal satisfaction of knowing you have become part of a family of skilled professionals, the licensed practical/vocational nurse. You have successfully completed the requirements to become eligible to take the NCLEX examination and now you have one more important goal to achieve, to pass the NCLEX examination.

Adequate preparation for the NCLEX examination is critical. The examination is difficult and it tests you on your competence to practice as a licensed practical/vocational nurse in the United States. So what does this mean in terms of what you need to do to prepare academically? Some of these critical points are as follows:

> Know what you need to know!

1. You need to be knowledgeable of nursing content in all areas of nursing as practiced in the United States. There may be some variations in the methods of delivering care from country to country, but you need to be familiar with the *American way of nursing care,* so to speak.
2. You need to know the roles and responsibilities of the licensed practical/vocational nurse practicing in the United States.
3. You need to understand the purpose and use of the nurse practice acts.
4. You need to understand words and acceptable abbreviations used in nursing in the United States.

5. You need to be knowledgeable about the communication process used in the United States and be able to use therapeutic communication techniques effectively.
6. You need to be knowledgeable about the medications that are used to treat health conditions in the United States and how to administer medications.
7. You need to understand each step of the clinical problem-solving process (nursing process).
8. You need to understand the NCLEX-PN test plan and the testing procedures.
9. You need to be familiar with the types of questions that are used in the NCLEX-PN examination.
10. You need to be skillful in the use of test-taking strategies to answer questions.
11. You need to know how to develop a study plan.
12. You need to know how to prepare yourself from a nonacademic perspective.
13. You need to know when you are adequately prepared to take the NCLEX-PN examination.

These are some of the critical points that you need to address as you prepare to take this examination. The task of preparing may seem overwhelming to you, but don't despair. An important step that you have already taken in preparing is that you are using this book and as a result are becoming familiar with the NCLEX-PN test plan, the examination process, the types of questions on the examination, nonacademic preparation strategies, and test-taking strategies. There are also additional resources available to you that will help you address all of the critical points related to this examination. It is vital that you use review resources to prepare because they will focus your review on essential content areas. Several of these review resources are described below along with suggestions regarding their use. As you decide on a review resource for preparation, think about your needs and determine which resource or resources will meet your needs. These review resources can be obtained at the Elsevier Health website at www.elsevierhealth.com.

> Review resources can be obtained at www.elsevierhealth.com.

Saunders Comprehensive Review for the NCLEX-PN® Examination

The *Saunders Comprehensive Review for the NCLEX-PN® Examination* is one valuable tool that contains both content and practice questions. Its accompanying interactive CD-ROM contains more than 3500 practice questions presented in multiple-choice format and in the alternate test question format that is used in the NCLEX-PN examination. When using this CD-ROM, it is best to access the Study Mode because you are given important information immediately after answering the question. This information includes the correct answer, rationale for the correct and incorrect options, the test-taking strategy for answering the question, content area to review if you answered the question incorrectly, and the reference source and page number. Therefore, you learn as you move along through your review. As you are studying, if you have difficulty with a specific topic, make a note of it and be sure to review the topic.

> *Saunders Comprehensive Review for the NCLEX-PN® Examination* contains nursing content and more than 3500 practice questions!

Saunders Q&A Review for the NCLEX-PN® Examination

One other extremely helpful resource is the *Saunders Q&A Review for the NCLEX-PN® Examination,* which includes a CD-ROM that contains more than 3000 practice questions. The reason that this resource is so helpful is that the book is uniquely designed to contain chapters with practice questions specific to each Client Needs area identified in the NCLEX-PN test plan. Therefore as you are reviewing, if you are having difficulty with a specific Client Needs category of the test plan, you can refer to that specific Client Needs area in the book or on the CD-ROM and obtain practice questions that relate specifically to your area in need of improvement.

As with the *Saunders Comprehensive Review for the NCLEX-PN® Examination,* when using this CD-ROM, it is best to access the Study Mode because you are given important information immediately after answering the question. This information includes the correct answer, rationale for the correct and incorrect options, the test-taking strategy for answering the question, content area to review if you answered the question incorrectly, and the reference source and page number. Therefore, you learn as you move along through your review.

> *Saunders Q&A Review for the NCLEX-PN® Examination* is uniquely designed to contain chapters with practice questions specific to each Client Needs area identified in the NCLEX-PN test plan.

Saunders Review Cards for the NCLEX-PN" Examination provides you with more than 900 practice test questions, including multiple-choice questions and the new alternate test items, such as fill-in-the-blank, multiple response, prioritizing (ordered response), and image questions. This resource and any of the other NCLEX-PN preparation resources will assist in strengthening your knowledge in nursing and your skills in test-taking.

Saunders Review Cards for the NCLEX-PN® Examination provides you with more than 900 practice NCLEX-PN test questions based on the test plan.

WISHING YOU SUCCESS!

Never lose sight of the goals that you want to achieve. Patience and dedication will contribute significantly to your achieving the status of licensed practical/vocational nurse. Remember, success is climbing a mountain, facing the challenge of obstacles, and reaching the top of the mountain. I wish you the best success in your career as a licensed practical/vocational nurse in the United States of America!

REFERENCES

Commission on Graduates of Foreign Nursing Schools, www.cgfns.org.
Commission on Graduates of Foreign Nursing Schools. Fact sheet (4/3/05), www.cgfns.org/fact-cert.shtml.
Commission on Graduates of Foreign Nursing Schools. VisaScreen™ (4/3/05), www.cgfns.org/prog-visa.shtml.
Commission on Graduates of Foreign Nursing Schools. Certification program (4/3/05), www.cgfns.org/prog-cert.shtml.
Educational Testing Service, Princeton, New Jersey, toefl@ets.org.
International English Language Testing System, ielts@ceii.org; www.ielts.org.
National Council of State Boards of Nursing, www.ncsbn.org.
National Council of State Boards of Nursing. (2005). *2005 NCLEX® for VisaScreen™ Candidate Bulletin.* Chicago: Author.
National Council of State Boards of Nursing. (2005). *2005 NCLEX® Examination Candidate Bulletin.* Chicago: Author.

"My first tip would be to do as many NCLEX review questions as possible. I did thousands and found that as I reviewed the material, not only did I become familiar with content that was not covered in school, but I began to see patterns to the material. This made it easier to reason through those questions I just didn't know. I highly recommend hand written review cards, not only for studying for the NCLEX exam, but for studying throughout nursing school. The cards were also portable and I could carry them with me. As I "mastered" a particular card I would take it out of the stack and concentrate on the material I didn't know as well. Our school's goal for its nursing students was to develop critical thinking skills. We were told that we could no longer memorize material; we had to be able to apply it. This is true to an extent, however, there were countless times during tests that I was able to draw on material memorized from review cards. I graduated with a 4.0. They served me well."

—Lori, Valencia Community College, Orlando, FL

"I recommend that if you are easily distracted by noises, you should request earplugs. There will be various noises in the room. Who wants to worry about blocking out noises when you are trying to concentrate on the test."

—Anissa, Piedmont Technical College, Greenwood, SC

Part 4 Practice Test

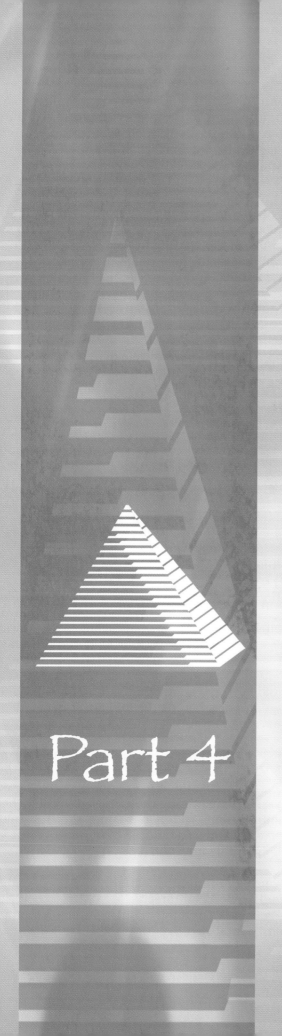

1. Flurbiprofen (Ocufen) is prescribed for a client with osteoarthritis. On a follow-up visit to the physician's office, the nurse asks the client if the medication has provided relief from which of the following?
   1 Indigestion
   2 Diarrhea
   3 Abdominal cramps
   4 Pain

Answer: 4

Rationale: Flurbiprofen is a nonsteroidal antiinflammatory medication that reduces inflammatory response and the intensity of pain stimulus that reaches sensory nerve endings. In the client with osteoarthritis, the intended effect is pain relief. Indigestion, diarrhea, and abdominal cramps are occasional side effects of the medication.

Test-Taking Strategy: Note the key words "provided relief from." Also, note that the question provides the client's diagnosis. Recalling the pathophysiology related to osteoarthritis will assist in directing you to option 4. Additionally options 1, 2, and 3 are similar in that they all address gastrointestinal symptoms. Review this medication and the test-taking strategies for answering pharmacology questions if you had difficulty with this question.

Level of Cognitive Ability: Analysis
Client Needs: Physiological Integrity
Integrated Process: Nursing Process/Evaluation
Content Area: Pharmacology

Reference

Hodgson, B. & Kizior, R. (2005). *Saunders nursing drug handbook 2005.* Philadelphia: Saunders, p. 458.

---

2. Select all nursing statements that indicate the use of a therapeutic communication technique.
   ___ "You will do just fine. You'll see."
   ___ "What would you like to discuss?"
   ___ "I wouldn't worry about that."
   ___ "Can you describe your feelings?"
   ___ "Can you tell me what the voices are saying?"

Answer:
"What would you like to discuss?"
"Can you describe your feelings?"
"Can you tell me what the voices are saying?"

Rationale: The nursing statement "What would you like to discuss?" is therapeutic and an open-ended question that invites the client to share personal feelings. The nursing statements "Can you describe your feelings?" and "Can you tell me what the voices are saying?" are therapeutic and are focused statements that are exploratory. The nursing statements "I wouldn't worry about that" and "You will do just fine. You'll see" are nontherapeutic and are statements that provide false reassurance.

Test-Taking Strategy: Read each nursing statement and focus on the issue, *use of therapeutic communication techniques*. Recalling the therapeutic and nontherapeutic techniques will assist in answering the question. Review therapeutic communication techniques and the test-taking strategies for answering communication questions if you had difficulty with this question.

Level of Cognitive Ability: Application
Client Needs: Psychosocial Integrity
Integrated Process: Communication and Documentation
Content Area: Mental Health

Reference

Morrison-Valfre, M. (2005). *Foundations of mental health care* (3rd ed). St. Louis: Mosby, p. 88.

3. Adalimumab (Humira) is added to the medication regimen for a client with severe rheumatoid arthritis. The nurse provides instructions to the client about the medication and tells the client that:
   1 the medication is used to slow the progression of joint damage but cannot be coadministered with an analgesic.
   2 the medication is used to slow the progression of joint damage and can be coadministered with an analgesic.
   3 the medication is available in an oral liquid form only.
   4 the medication never needs to be refrigerated.

Answer: 2

Rationale: Adalimumab is a disease-modifying antirheumatic drug (DMARD) and a monoclonal antibody that binds to and thereby neutralizes tumor necrosis factor (TNF). It reduces symptoms and slows the progression of joint damage. This medication can be used alone or in combination with methotrexate or other antirheumatic medicines. It is administered by subcutaneous injection. It should be stored in a cold environment at 2° to 8° C (36° to 46° F) and protected from light.

Test-Taking Strategy: Eliminate option 3 because of the absolute word "only" and option 4 because of the absolute word "never." Also note that options 1 and 2 indicate opposite statements; this may indicate that one of these options is correct. Note that the client has severe rheumatoid arthritis and that adalimumab is "added to the medication regimen." This will direct you to option 2. Review this medication and the test-taking strategies for answering pharmacology questions if you had difficulty with this question.

Level of Cognitive Ability: Application
Client Needs: Physiological Integrity
Integrated Process: Teaching/Learning
Content Area: Pharmacology

Reference

Lehne, R. (2004). *Pharmacology for nursing care* (5th ed). Philadelphia: Saunders, pp. 770t, 772.

---

4. A psychiatrist prescribes aripiprazole (Abilify) for a client with a diagnosis of schizophrenia. Which of the following nursing interventions is therapeutic?
   1 Administer the medication only after meals.
   2 Instruct the client that the medication may cause sedation and should be taken at bedtime.
   3 Advise the client to increase his usual exercise pattern threefold to help with medication absorption.
   4 Advise the client to limit his alcohol intake to one drink each day.

Answer: 2

Rationale: Aripiprazole is an antipsychotic agent that may be referred to as a dopamine system stabilizer (DDS). Because antipsychotics cause sedation, bedtime dosing helps promote sleep while decreasing daytime drowsiness. It may be administered with or without food and is well absorbed in the presence as well as in the absence of food. It is not necessary for the client to increase the usual exercise pattern to assist in absorption of the medication. Alcohol is avoided not limited.

Test-Taking Strategy: Noting that the client has schizophrenia will assist in determining that the medication is an antipsychotic. Eliminate option 1 because of the absolute word "only." Eliminate option 4, recalling that alcohol intake is avoided, not limited. From the remaining options eliminate option 3 because of the words "increase his usual exercise pattern threefold." Review this medication and the test-taking strategies for answering pharmacology questions if you had difficulty with this question.

Level of Cognitive Ability: Application
Client Needs: Physiological Integrity

Integrated Process: Teaching/Learning
Content Area: Pharmacology

Reference

Lehne, R. (2004). *Pharmacology for nursing care* (5th ed). Philadelphia: Saunders, pp. 284t, 293-294.

---

5. A client receiving therapy at a mental health clinic says to the nurse, "When I have a stressful day at work and when my boss is on my case all day, I go home and take my frustrations out on my children." The appropriate response to the client is which of the following?
   1 "Why do you do this? Can you think of another way to take out your frustrations?"
   2 "The only way to take out your frustrations is to join a health care center that provides equipment for weightlifting and boxing."
   3 "Is there someplace that you can go after work to relieve your frustrations before going home?"
   4 "Let's talk about some other ways that you can handle your frustrations."

Answer: 4
Rationale: The nursing response in option 4 provides the client the opportunity to problem-solve. Option 1 uses the word "why," which can make the client feel defensive and often implies criticism. Option 2 is incorrect because physical activity is not the only way to relieve frustrations. Additionally, this may not be appropriate for this client. Option 3 avoids the fact that the client needs to deal with the issue, taking frustrations out on the children.

Test-Taking Strategy: Use therapeutic communication techniques. Eliminate option 1 because of the word "why." Next eliminate option 2 because of the absolute word "only." From the remaining options, note that option 3 is similar to option 2 (options that are similar are incorrect) and that option 4 provides the client the opportunity to problem-solve. Review therapeutic communication techniques and the test-taking strategies for answering communication questions if you had difficulty with this question.

Level of Cognitive Ability: Application
Client Needs: Psychosocial Integrity
Integrated Process: Communication and Documentation
Content Area: Mental Health

Reference

Morrison-Valfre, M. (2005). *Foundations of mental health care* (3rd ed). St. Louis: Mosby, p. 88.

---

6. A physician orders 3000 mL of 0.9% normal saline solution to be administered intravenously over a 24-hour period. The nurse sets the flow rate to infuse at how many milliliters per hour?
   Answer: _________

Answer: 125
Rationale: Use the IV formula to determine milliliters per hour.

Formula:

$$\frac{\text{Total volume in mL}}{\text{Number of hours}} = \text{Number of mL per hour}$$

$$\frac{3000\text{ mL}}{24\text{ hours}} = 125\text{ mL per hour}$$

Test-Taking Strategy: Use the formula for calculating milliliters per hour. Remember, use a calculator, follow the formula, recheck your answer, and make sure that the answer makes sense before documenting the answer. Review the test-taking strategies for answering intravenous calculation questions if you had difficulty with this question.

Level of Cognitive Ability: Application
Client Needs: Physiological Integrity
Integrated Process: Nursing Process/Implementation
Content Area: Fundamental Skills

Reference

Kee, J. & Marshall, S. (2004). *Clinical calculations: with applications to general and specialty areas* (5th ed). Philadelphia: Saunders, pp. 204-205.

---

7. A female client hospitalized in the mental health unit for treatment of depression says to a female nurse, "Women always get put down. It's as if we are useless members of society." The appropriate nursing response is which of the following?

1 "Tell me how you feel as a woman."
2 "Yes, that does happen to women but it doesn't mean that women have to stand for that kind of treatment."
3 "I never let anyone make me feel as though I am useless!"
4 "Think about it. That's no longer true in today's society."

Answer: 1
Rationale: In option 1 the nurse uses the therapeutic technique of focusing and encourages the client to verbalize and expand on her feelings. In option 2 the nurse agrees with the client and then takes a forceful stance with regard to how the client would deal with these feelings. In option 3 the nurse provides an opinion; additionally this option uses the absolute word "never." In option 4 the nurse disagrees with the client.

Test-Taking Strategy: Use therapeutic communication techniques. Eliminate option 3 first because of the absolute word "never." Additionally, in this option the nurse provides an opinion, which is nontherapeutic. Next eliminate options 2 and 4. In option 2 the nurse agrees with the client, and in option 4 the nurse disagrees with the client. Review therapeutic communication techniques and the test-taking strategies for answering communication questions if you had difficulty with this question.

Level of Cognitive Ability: Application
Client Needs: Psychosocial Integrity
Integrated Process: Communication and Documentation
Content Area: Mental Health

Reference

Morrison-Valfre, M. (2005). *Foundations of mental health care* (3rd ed). St. Louis: Mosby, p. 88.

---

8. Erythromycin (EES) has been prescribed for a client with otitis media. To ensure optimal absorption, the nurse tells the client to take the medication:

1 on an empty stomach.
2 immediately after a meal.
3 just before eating.
4 with a snack such as peanut butter and crackers.

Answer: 1
Rationale: Erythromycin is an antibiotic. It may be taken without regard to meals but optimal absorption occurs when taken on an empty stomach. Therefore, options 2, 3, and 4 are incorrect.

Test-Taking Strategy: If you are unfamiliar with the medication identified in the question (erythromycin), noting that it is prescribed to treat otitis media provides the clue that it is an antibiotic. Focus on the issue, to ensure optimal absorption. Note that options 2, 3, and 4 are similar in that they all indicate taking the medication with food.

Review this medication and the test-taking strategies for answering pharmacology questions if you had difficulty with this question.

Level of Cognitive Ability: Application
Client Needs: Physiological Integrity
Integrated Process: Nursing Process/Implementation
Content Area: Pharmacology

Reference

Hodgson, B. & Kizior, R. (2005). *Saunders nursing drug handbook 2005.* Philadelphia: Saunders, p. 396.

---

9. A nurse employed in a mental health unit is meeting with a client for the first time. Which nursing statement should the nurse make to initiate the conversation?

1 "Have psychiatric medications ever been prescribed for you?"
2 "What would you like to discuss?"
3 "Are you feeling sad?'
4 "Have you ever been admitted to a mental health facility?"

Answer: 2

Rationale: The nursing statement in option 2 is an open-ended question and encourages conversation because it requires more than a one-word answer. In options 1, 3, and 4 the nurse attempts to obtain information from the client; however, these statements are close-ended in that the client can respond by a yes or no response. These statements do not encourage discussion.

Test-Taking Strategy: Use therapeutic communication techniques. Eliminate options 1, 3 and 4 because they are similar and all are close-ended questions. Review therapeutic communication techniques and the test-taking strategies for answering communication questions if you had difficulty with this question.

Level of Cognitive Ability: Application
Client Needs: Psychosocial Integrity
Integrated Process: Communication and Documentation
Content Area: Mental Health

Reference

Morrison-Valfre, M. (2005). *Foundations of mental health care* (3rd ed). St. Louis: Mosby, p. 88.

---

10. Metoprolol tartrate (Toprol-XL) has been prescribed for a client to treat hypertension. To enhance absorption the nurse tells the client to take the medication:

1 crushed in apple sauce.
2 with a meal.
3 with 8 ounces of grapefruit juice.
4 with 1 ounce of aluminum hydroxide (Amphojel).

Answer: 2

Rationale: Metoprolol tartrate is a beta adrenergic blocker that is used to treat hypertension. To enhance absorption, it is administered with or immediately after meals. Extended-release tablets should not be crushed. Administration of medication with grapefruit juice should be avoided because it affects absorption. Likewise antacids affect the absorption of medication.

Test-Taking Strategy: If you are unfamiliar with the medication identified in the question (metoprolol tartrate), noting that its name ends with the letters "lol" provides the clue that it is a beta adrenergic blocker. Noting the letters "XL" after the medication name provides the clue that the medication is extended release. Focus on the issue, to enhance optimal absorption, and use pharmacology guidelines to answer the question. Remember sustained (extended)-release tablets should not be crushed and that grapefruit juice and antacids are not administered with medication because these items affect absorption. Review this medication and the test-taking strategies for answering pharmacology questions if you had difficulty with this question.

Level of Cognitive Ability: Application
Client Needs: Physiological Integrity
Integrated Process: Nursing Process/Implementation
Content Area: Pharmacology

Reference

Hodgson, B. & Kizior, R. (2005). *Saunders nursing drug handbook 2005.* Philadelphia: Saunders, p. 704.

---

11. A nurse is having a conversation with a client hospitalized in a mental health unit. The client says to the nurse, "I work in a factory doing piecework and I am very competitive with the people that I work with." The appropriate nursing response is which of the following?

1 "In other words, you seem to be saying that you try to do better than your fellow employees."
2 "When you are being paid by piecework, then you need to be competitive."
3 "Why are you competitive? After all, you get paid based on the amount of work that you do."
4 "Do you find that your fellow employees are competitive also?"

Answer: 1
Rationale: Option 1 uses the therapeutic technique of paraphrasing. In paraphrasing, the nurse restates in different words what the client has said to confirm an understanding of what the client has said. In option 2 the nurse agrees with the client. In option 3 the nurse uses the word "why," which can make the client feel defensive and often implies criticism. Option 4 focuses on fellow employees, not the client.

Test-Taking Strategy: Use therapeutic communication techniques. Eliminate option 4 first because it does not focus on the client. Next eliminate option 3 because the nurse uses the word "why." From the remaining options eliminate option 2 because the nurse agrees with the client. Additionally, option 1 uses the therapeutic technique of paraphrasing. Review therapeutic communication techniques and the test-taking strategies for answering communication questions if you had difficulty with this question.

Level of Cognitive Ability: Application
Client Needs: Psychosocial Integrity
Integrated Process: Communication and Documentation
Content Area: Mental Health

Reference

Morrison-Valfre, M. (2005). *Foundations of mental health care* (3rd ed). St. Louis: Mosby, p. 88.

---

12. A physician's order reads morphine sulfate, gr 1/8 intramuscularly stat. The medication ampule reads morphine sulfate, 10 mg per mL. A nurse prepares how many milliliters to administer the correct dose?
Answer: __________

Answer: 0.75
Rationale: It is necessary to convert gr 1/8 to mg. After converting gr to mg, use the formula to calculate the correct dose.

Conversion:

$$60 \text{ mg: gr } 1 :: \times \text{ mg : gr } 1/8$$
$$1x = 1/8 \times 60/1$$
$$x = 60/8 = 7.5 \text{ mg}$$

Formula:

$$\frac{\text{Desired}}{\text{Available}} \times \text{mL} = \text{mL per dose}$$

$$\frac{7.5 \text{ mg}}{10 \text{ mg}} \times 1 \text{ mL} = 0.75 \text{ mL}$$

Test-Taking Strategy: In this medication calculation problem, it is necessary to first convert grains to milligrams. Next, use a calculator and follow the formula for the calculation of the correct dose. Recheck your work, and make sure that the answer makes sense. Review the test-taking strategies for answering medication calculation questions if you had difficulty with this question.

Level of Cognitive Ability: Application
Client Needs: Physiological Integrity
Integrated Process: Nursing Process/Implementation
Content Area: Fundamental Skills

Reference

Kee, J. & Marshall, S. (2004). *Clinical calculations: with applications to general and specialty areas* (5th ed.). Philadelphia: Saunders, p. 80.

---

13. A client says to the nurse, "Ever since my wife passed on, my life is empty and has no meaning." The appropriate nursing response is which of the following?

1 "What would your children think if they knew how you felt?"
2 "Most people who lose a loved one feel empty."
3 "Your life has no meaning?"
4 "Let's talk about the positive things that you have in your life."

Answer: 3

Rationale: In option 3 the nurse uses the therapeutic technique of restating. In this technique, the nurse explores more thoroughly topics that are significant to the client. Option 1 does not focus on the client's feelings. Rather, it focuses on the client's children. Option 2 generalizes and does not focus on the client. Option 4 avoids the client's feelings.

Test-Taking Strategy: Use therapeutic communication techniques. Eliminate options 1 and 4 first because they are similar and do not focus on the client's feelings. Next eliminate option 2 because it is a generalized statement and stereotypes the client. Option 3 uses the therapeutic technique of restating. Review therapeutic communication techniques and the test-taking strategies for answering communication questions if you had difficulty with this question.

Level of Cognitive Ability: Application
Client Needs: Psychosocial Integrity
Integrated Process: Communication and Documentation
Content Area: Mental Health

Reference

Morrison-Valfre, M. (2005). *Foundations of mental health care* (3rd ed). St. Louis: Mosby, p. 88.

14. A nurse is having a conversation with a client and responds to the client's statement by saying, "You say that your mother left you when you were 6 years old." The nurse is using which therapeutic communication technique?

1 Restating
2 Giving approval
3 Agreeing
4 Advising

Answer: 1

Rationale: In restating, the nurse repeats the main thought that the client expressed. This therapeutic communication technique indicates that the nurse is listening to the client. In this technique, the nurse validates, reinforces, or calls attention to something important that the client said. Giving approval, agreeing, and giving advice are nontherapeutic communication techniques.

Test-Taking Strategy: Focus on the issue, a therapeutic communication technique, and on the nursing statement. Note that the key words "You say that..." in the nursing statement will assist in identifying the technique that the nurse is using. Review therapeutic communication techniques and the test-taking strategies for answering communication questions if you had difficulty with this question.

Level of Cognitive Ability: Application
Client Needs: Psychosocial Integrity
Integrated Process: Communication and Documentation
Content Area: Mental Health

Reference

Morrison-Valfre, M. (2005). *Foundations of mental health care* (3rd ed). St. Louis: Mosby, p. 88.

---

15. A client says to the nurse, "My doctor ordered adefovir (Hepsera) for me so I guess I'll soon be cured." Which nursing response is therapeutic?

1 "Yes. Although it's relatively new and its results remain tentative, it does seem so."
2 "Yes, it will cure the disease but you will want to monitor for side effects and stop the medication immediately if any occur."
3 "Although this medication cannot cure your disease, it will control it."
4 "Yes, but just be certain to divide the dosage as the doctor has indicated in his instructions."

Answer: 3

Rationale: Adefovir is an antiviral that is used to treat clients with chronic hepatitis B exhibiting active viral replication and persistent increases of liver function blood levels. It controls the disease but does not cure it. Its mechanism is similar to acyclovir (Zovirax) and it is used cautiously in older adults and those who may have untreated human immunodeficiency virus infection. Nephrotoxicity is the primary concern with the use of this medication. It should not be stopped suddenly and may be administered once daily without regard to food.

Test-Taking Strategy: If you are unfamiliar with this medication note the letters "vir" in its name. This indicates that the medication is an antiviral. Note that options 1, 2, and 4 are similar in that they all indicate that the client will be cured of the disease. Option 3 is the option that is different. Review this medication and the test-taking strategies for answering pharmacology questions if you had difficulty with this question.

Level of Cognitive Ability: Application
Client Needs: Physiological Integrity
Integrated Process: Teaching/Learning
Content Area: Pharmacology

Reference

Lehne, R. (2004). *Pharmacology for nursing care* (5th ed). Philadelphia: Saunders, pp. 975-976.

16. A clinic nurse is collecting a medication history on a client being seen in the clinic for the first time. The nurse notes that the client takes terbutaline (Brethine) and asks the client about a history of which disorder that is treated with this medication?

1 Ulcerative colitis
2 Congestive heart failure
3 Asthma
4 Hypothyroidism

Answer: 3

Rationale: Terbutaline is an oral beta adrenergic agonist bronchodilator that is used to treat asthma. It is not used to treat ulcerative colitis, congestive heart failure, or hypothyroidism.

Test-Taking Strategy: Focus on the name of the medication. Recalling that most xanthine bronchodilators' medication names end with the letters "line" will direct you to option 3. Review this medication and the test-taking strategies for answering pharmacology questions if you had difficulty with this question.

Level of Cognitive Ability: Analysis
Client Needs: Physiological Integrity
Integrated Process: Nursing Process/Data Collection
Content Area: Pharmacology

Reference

Lehne, R. (2004). *Pharmacology for nursing care* (5th ed). Philadelphia: Saunders, p. 798.

---

17. A nurse is preparing to administer medications to a hospitalized client and notes that the client takes levothyroxine (Synthroid) daily. The nurse suspects that the client has a history of:

1 hypothyroidism.
2 hyperthyroidism.
3 hypotension.
4 hypertension.

Answer: 1

Rationale: Levothyroxine is a synthetic thyroid hormone used to treat hypothyroidism. It is not used to treat hyperthyroidism, hypotension, or hypertension.

Test-Taking Strategy: Focus on the name of the medication. Recalling that most thyroid medications contain the letters "thy" in their name will assist in eliminating options 3 and 4. From the remaining options, eliminate option 2 because it would be harmful to administer thyroid to a client who is in a hyperthyroid state. Review this medication and the test-taking strategies for answering pharmacology questions if you had difficulty with this question.

Level of Cognitive Ability: Analysis
Client Needs: Physiological Integrity
Integrated Process: Nursing Process/Data Collection
Content Area: Pharmacology

Reference

Hodgson, B. & Kizior, R. (2005). *Saunders nursing drug handbook 2005*. Philadelphia: Saunders, p. 632.

---

18. Sucralfate (Carafate) is prescribed for a client with a gastric ulcer. The nurse tells the client to take the medication:

1 1 hour before meals and at bedtime.
2 just after meals.
3 with meals and at bedtime.
4 with a snack at bedtime.

Answer: 1

Rationale: Sucralfate is an antiulcer medication and should be scheduled for administration 1 hour before meals and at bedtime. Administration at these times allows it to form a protective coating over the ulcer before food intake stimulates gastric acid production and mechanical irritation. The bedtime dose protects the stomach lining during sleep.

Test-Taking Strategy: Note the similarities in options 2, 3, and 4, and eliminate these options. Each of these options indicates taking the medication with a food item. Review this medication and the test-taking strategies for answering pharmacology questions if you had difficulty with this question.

Level of Cognitive Ability: Application
Client Needs: Health Promotion and Maintenance
Integrated Process: Teaching/Learning
Content Area: Pharmacology

Reference
Hodgson, B. & Kizior, R. (2005). *Saunders nursing drug handbook 2005.* Philadelphia: Saunders, p. 994.

---

19. Sulfasalazine (Azulfidine) is prescribed for a client with ulcerative colitis. The nurse determines that the medication is achieving the intended effect if the client reports which of the following?

1 Increased urinary output
2 Formed stools
3 Absence of nausea
4 Relief of headaches

Answer: 2
Rationale: Sulfasalazine is a sulfonamide and is used to treat acute ulcerative colitis and prevent recurrences. It acts by inhibiting prostaglandin synthesis, thus reducing inflammation. The intended effect that occurs as a result of reducing bowel inflammation is the relief of diarrhea and production of formed stools. Options 1, 3, and 4 are not intended effects of this medication.

Test-Taking Strategy: Focus on the issue, an intended effect of the medication. Noting that the client has ulcerative colitis will assist in directing you to option 2. Also remember that medications that include "sulf" in their names are sulfonamides; this will also assist in answering the question correctly. Review this medication and the test-taking strategies for answering pharmacology questions if you had difficulty with this question.

Level of Cognitive Ability: Analysis
Client Needs: Physiological Integrity
Integrated Process: Nursing Process/Evaluation
Content Area: Pharmacology

Reference
Skidmore-Roth, L. (2005). *Mosby's drug guide for nurses* (6th ed). St. Louis: Mosby, p. 805.

---

20. A nurse is reviewing the plan of care for a child with juvenile rheumatoid arthritis (JRA). The nurse determines that which of the following is a priority nursing diagnosis?

1 Disturbed Body Image
2 Risk for Bathing/Hygiene Self-Care Deficit
3 Risk for Injury
4 Acute Pain

Answer: 4
Rationale: All of the nursing diagnoses are appropriate for the child with JRA. The priority nursing diagnosis relates to pain. Acute pain needs to be managed before other problems can be addressed.

Test-Taking Strategy: Note the key word "priority." Use Maslow's hierarchy of needs theory, remembering that physiological needs (option 4) receive highest priority. Option 3 addresses safety and security needs. Options 1 addresses self-esteem needs. Option 2 identifies an at-risk (potential, not an actual), problem. Review care to the child with JRA and the test-taking strategies for answering prioritizing questions if you had difficulty with this question.

Level of Cognitive Ability: Analysis
Client Needs: Physiological Integrity
Integrated Process: Nursing Process/Planning
Content Area: Delegating/Prioritizing

Reference

Leifer, G. (2003). *Introduction to maternity & pediatric nursing* (4th ed). Philadelphia: Saunders, p. 580.

---

21. The nurse is checking for the presence of cyanosis in a dark-skinned client. The nurse checks which best site for the presence of cyanosis?

1 Soles of the feet
2 Backs of the hands
3 Conjunctivae of the eyes
4 Earlobes

Answer: 3

Rationale: In a dark-skinned client, the presence of cyanosis can be best seen in the areas where the epidermis is thin and pigmentation is lighter. These areas include the conjunctivae of the eyes, mucous membranes, and nailbeds. In a light-skinned client, cyanosis can be most easily detected in nail beds, earlobes, lips, mucous membranes, and palms and soles of the feet.

Test-Taking Strategy: Focus on the issue, cyanosis, and note the key word "best" and that the client is dark skinned. Eliminate options 1, 2, and 4 because these options are similar and identify body areas where the epidermis is thick. Review skin assessment techniques and the various test-taking strategies if you had difficulty with this question.

Level of Cognitive Ability: Application
Client Needs: Health Promotion and Maintenance
Integrated Process: Nursing Process/Data Collection
Content Area: Adult Health/Cardiovascular

Reference

Ignatavicius, D. & Workman, M. (2006). *Medical-surgical nursing: critical thinking for collaborative care* (5th ed). Philadelphia: Saunders, p. 1571.

---

22. A nurse is identifying the risk factors for a group of clients for acquiring pneumonia during hospitalization. The nurse determines that which client is at lowest risk?

1 An older client with diabetes mellitus
2 A client with human immunodeficiency virus (HIV)
3 A client with a spinal cord injury who is immobile
4 A postoperative client who is ambulating

Answer: 4

Rationale: The postoperative client who is ambulating is at lowest risk. This client has had no direct insult to the respiratory tract. Clients with HIV, an upper respiratory infection, or a chronic disease (e.g., heart, lung, or kidney disease, diabetes mellitus, or cancer) are more at risk for developing pneumonia. Clients on bed rest and immobilized are also at risk for developing pneumonia.

Test-Taking Strategy: This is a false response question. Note the key words, "lowest risk," which tells you that the correct option will be the client who does not have a significant risk for developing pneumonia. Focusing on these key words will direct you to option 4. Review the risk factors related to developing pneumonia and the test-taking strategies for answering false response questions if you had difficulty with this question.

Level of Cognitive Ability: Analysis
Client Needs: Health Promotion and Maintenance
Integrated Process: Nursing Process/Data Collection
Content Area: Adult Health/Respiratory

Reference

deWit, S. (2005). *Fundamental concepts and skills for nursing.* Philadelphia: Saunders, p. 750.

---

23. A physician orders 500 mL of normal saline to infuse intravenously over 5 hours. The drop factor is 10 drops (gtt) per 1 mL. A nurse sets the flow rate at how many drops per minute? (Round answer to the nearest whole number.)
Answer: ___________

Answer: 17
Rationale: Use the IV flow rate formula.

Formula:

$$\frac{\text{Total volume} \times \text{gtt factor}}{\text{Time in minutes}} = \text{gtt per min}$$

$$\frac{500 \text{ mL} \times 10 \text{ gtt}}{300 \text{ minutes}} = \frac{5000}{300} = 16.6, \text{ or } 17 \text{ gtt per minute}$$

Test-Taking Strategy: Use the formula for calculating IV flow rates. Remember, use a calculator, follow the formula, recheck your answer, and make sure that the answer makes sense before documenting it. Review the test-taking strategies for answering intravenous calculation questions if you had difficulty with this question.

Level of Cognitive Ability: Application
Client Needs: Physiological Integrity
Integrated Process: Nursing Process/Implementation
Content Area: Fundamental Skills

Reference

Kee, J. & Marshall, S. (2004). *Clinical calculations: with applications to general and specialty areas* (5th ed). Philadelphia: Saunders, pp. 204-205.

---

24. A client with an iron deficiency anemia is taking an iron supplement and tells the nurse that she is going to stop the medication because it causes constipation. The nurse appropriately responds by stating which of the following?

1 "Constipation is bothersome but it is much more important to take the medication."
2 "Constipation is most intense during initial therapy and be-

Answer: 2
Rationale: Constipation is a side effect of iron supplements but this side effect becomes less bothersome with continued use. Additionally there are measures to take to alleviate this side effect. Option 2 addresses the client's concern. In options 1 and 3 the nurse disapproves of the client's feelings. Additionally, the nurse lectures the client in these options. Option 4 places the client's issue on hold.

Test-Taking Strategy: Use therapeutic communication techniques. Eliminate option 3 because of the absolute word "never." Next eliminate option 4 because it places the

comes less bothersome with continued use."
3 "Never stop taking any medication without talking to the physician first."
4 "In time you will get used to this side effect."

client's issue on hold. From the remaining options, remembering to focus on the client's feeling and concerns will direct you to option 2. Review client teaching points for administering iron tablets and the test-taking strategies for answering communication questions if you had difficulty with this question.

Level of Cognitive Ability: Application
Client Needs: Psychosocial Integrity
Integrated Process: Communication and Documentation
Content Area: Pharmacology

References

Harkreader, H. & Hogan, M.A. (2004). *Fundamentals of nursing: caring and clinical judgment* (2nd ed). Philadelphia: Saunders, pp. 251, 255-257.

Lehne, R. (2004). *Pharmacology for nursing care* (5th ed). Philadelphia: Saunders, p. 584.

---

25. A client has been newly diagnosed with diabetes mellitus. The nurse plans to do which of the following as the first step in teaching the client about the disorder?
1 Gather all available resource materials
2 Plan for the evaluation of the session
3 Identify the client's knowledge and needs
4 Decide on the teaching approach

Answer: 3
Rationale: Determining what to teach a client begins with an assessment of the client's own knowledge and learning needs. Once these have been determined, the nurse can effectively plan a teaching approach, the actual content, and resource materials that may be needed. The evaluation is done after teaching is completed.

Test-Taking Strategy: Note the key word "first." Use the steps of the clinical problem-solving process (nursing process). Remember that data collection is the first step. Review teaching-learning principles and the test-taking strategies for answering prioritizing questions if you had difficulty with this question.

Level of Cognitive Ability: Application
Client Needs: Health Promotion and Maintenance
Integrated Process: Teaching/Learning
Content Area: Delegating/Prioritizing

Reference

Harkreader, H. & Hogan, M.A. (2004). *Fundamentals of nursing: caring and clinical judgment* (2nd ed). Philadelphia: Saunders, p. 262.

---

26. A client with heart disease says to the nurse, "I guess I'll never be able to eat ice cream again." The nurse responds by stating:
1 "There are lots of other foods you can eat."
2 "Ice cream has too much fat content so why would you even want to eat it?"
3 "You don't think you will be able to eat ice cream at all?"
4 "Why do you say that?"

Answer: 3
Rationale: The nurse appropriately responds by rephrasing the client's statement. Option 3 is a therapeutic response and rephrases the client's statement. Options 1, 2, and 4 are examples of nontherapeutic communication techniques. Options 1 and 2 give advice. Additionally, option 2 lectures the client. Option 4 requests an explanation from the client.

Test-Taking Strategy: Use therapeutic communication techniques. Option 3 is the only therapeutic response and rephrases the client's statement. Review therapeutic communication techniques and the test-taking strategies for answering communication questions if you had difficulty with this question.

Level of Cognitive Ability: Application
Client Needs: Psychosocial Integrity
Integrated Process: Communication and Documentation
Content Area: Fundamental Skills

Reference

Harkreader, H. & Hogan, M.A. (2004). *Fundamentals of nursing: caring and clinical judgment* (2nd ed). Philadelphia: Saunders, pp. 251, 255-257.

---

27. A client scheduled for a coronary artery bypass graft states to the nurse, "I'm not sure if I should have this surgery." The nurse makes which response to the client?

1 "Don't worry. Everything will be fine."
2 "It's your decision."
3 "Why don't you want to have this surgery?"
4 "Tell me what concerns you have about the surgery."

Answer: 4

Rationale: The nurse needs to gather more data and assist the client in exploring his or her feelings about the surgery. Options 1, 2, and 3 are nontherapeutic. Option 1 provides false reassurance. Option 2 is a blunt response and does not address the client's concern. Option 3 can make the client feel defensive.

Test-Taking Strategy: Use therapeutic communication techniques. Option 4 is the only option that addresses the client's concern. Review therapeutic communication techniques and the test-taking strategies for answering communication questions if you had difficulty with this question.

Level of Cognitive Ability: Application
Client Needs: Psychosocial Integrity
Integrated Process: Communication and Documentation
Content Area: Fundamental Skills

References

Harkreader, H. & Hogan, M.A. (2004). *Fundamentals of nursing: caring and clinical judgment* (2nd ed). Philadelphia: Saunders, pp. 251, 255-257.
Potter, P. & Perry, A. (2005). *Fundamentals of nursing* (6th ed). St. Louis: Mosby, p. 437.

---

28. A client states, "It will be so hard to wait for the results of this biopsy. I don't know what I will do if the results are positive." The nurse makes which response to the client?

1 "It's not good for you to worry."
2 "Most biopsies end up being negative so don't worry about it."
3 "You sound concerned about the results of this test."
4 "You are in good hands; even if it is positive, your doctor is the best."

Answer: 3

Rationale: The nurse needs to gather more data and assist the client in exploring his or her feelings about the results of the biopsy. The nurse should not disregard the client's feelings. Options 1, 2, and 4 are incorrect. These statements provide false reassurances and do not focus on the client's feelings.

Test-Taking Strategy: Use therapeutic communication techniques. Options 1, 2, and 4 are nontherapeutic, provide false reassurances, and do not focus on the client's feelings. Option 3 addresses the client's concern. Review therapeutic communication techniques and the test-taking strategies for answering communication questions if you had difficulty with this question.

Level of Cognitive Ability: Application
Client Needs: Psychosocial Integrity
Integrated Process: Communication and Documentation
Content Area: Fundamental Skills

References

Harkreader, H. & Hogan, M.A. (2004). *Fundamentals of nursing: caring and clinical judgment* (2nd ed). Philadelphia: Saunders, pp. 251, 255-257.

Potter, P. & Perry, A. (2005). *Fundamentals of nursing* (6th ed). St. Louis: Mosby, p. 437.

---

29. A client will be receiving long-term continuous total parenteral nutrition (TPN) at home. The nurse reviews the plan of care and determines that which nursing diagnosis is the priority?

1 Ineffective coping
2 Hopelessness
3 Social isolation
4 Risk for situational low self-esteem

Answer: 3

Rationale: The client will be receiving TPN long term and continuous at home. Therefore, the client will be socially isolated from stimuli outside the home. There are no data in the question to support options 1, 2, and 4.

Test-Taking Strategy: Focus on the data provided in the question and note the key words "long-term, continuous," and "at home." Eliminate options 1, 2, and 4 because there are no data in the question to support these options. Review care to the client receiving TPN and the various test-taking strategies if you had difficulty with this question.

Level of Cognitive Ability: Analysis
Client Needs: Psychosocial Integrity
Integrated Process: Nursing Process/Planning
Content Area: Fundamental Skills

Reference

deWit, S. (2005). *Fundamental concepts and skills for nursing.* Philadelphia: Saunders, p. 488.

---

30. A physician orders 1000 mL normal saline to infuse intravenously at a rate of 125 mL per hour. A nurse plans care knowing that it will take how many hours for 1 L to infuse?

Answer: ___________

Answer: 8

Rationale: It is necessary to determine that 1 L = 1000 mL. Next, use the formula for determining infusion time in hours.

Formula:

$$\frac{\text{Total volume to infuse}}{\text{mL per hour being infused}} = \text{Infusion time}$$

$$\frac{1000 \text{ mL}}{125 \text{ mL}} = 8 \text{ hours}$$

Test-Taking Strategy: Read the question carefully, noting that the question is asking about infusion time in hours. First, convert 1 L to milliliters. Next, use a calculator and use the formula for determining infusion time in hours.

Review the test-taking strategies for answering intravenous calculation questions if you had difficulty with this question.

Level of Cognitive Ability: Comprehension
Client Needs: Physiological Integrity
Integrated Process: Nursing Process/Planning
Content Area: Fundamental Skills

Reference
Kee, J. & Marshall, S. (2004). *Clinical calculations: with applications to general and specialty areas* (5th ed). Philadelphia: Saunders, p. 202.

---

31. A client has been taking fosinopril (Monopril). The nurse determines that the medication is having the intended effect if which of the following is noted?

1 Relief of diarrhea
2 Lowered pulse rate
3 Relief of headaches
4 Lowered blood pressure

Answer: 4
Rationale: Fosinopril is an angiotensin-converting enzyme (ACE) inhibitor that lowers blood pressure. It can cause excessive hypotension as an adverse effect of therapy. Other adverse effects of the medication are neutropenia and agranulocytopenia. Options 1, 2, and 3 are not intended effects of the medication.

Test-Taking Strategy: Note the key words "intended effect." Recalling that most ACE inhibitor medication names end with the letters "pril" and that these medications are used to treat hypertension will direct you to option 4. Review this medication and the test-taking strategies for answering pharmacology questions if you had difficulty with this question.

Level of Cognitive Ability: Analysis
Client Needs: Physiological Integrity
Integrated Process: Nursing Process/Evaluation
Content Area: Pharmacology

Reference
Hodgson, B. & Kizior, R. (2005). *Saunders nursing drug handbook 2005.* Philadelphia: Saunders, p. 473.

---

32. A nurse is caring for a client who is receiving a potassium-sparing diuretic. The nurse monitors for which side effect of the medication?

1 Hypernatremia
2 Hyperkalemia
3 Constipation
4 Dry skin

Answer: 2
Rationale: A potassium-sparing diuretic spares potassium, which means that potassium is retained in the body. Side effects of potassium-sparing diuretics usually include hyperkalemia, dehydration, hyponatremia, and lethargy. Although hypokalemia is a concern with the administration of most diuretics, hyperkalemia is a concern with the administration of a potassium-sparing medication. Additional side effects of these types of medications include nausea, vomiting, cramping, diarrhea, headache, ataxia, drowsiness, confusion, and fever.

Test-Taking Strategy: Note the key words "potassium-sparing," and focus on the issue, a side effect. Recalling that a potassium-sparing diuretic spares potassium will direct you to option 2. Review this medication and the test-taking strategies for answering pharmacology questions if you had difficulty with this question.

Level of Cognitive Ability: Analysis
Client Needs: Physiological Integrity
Integrated Process: Nursing Process/Data Collection
Content Area: Pharmacology

Reference
Lehne, R. (2004). *Pharmacology for nursing care* (5th ed). Philadelphia: Saunders, pp. 406-407.

---

33. A client is scheduled for a diagnostic procedure requiring the injection of a radiopaque dye. The nurse checks which most critical information before the procedure?

1 Intake and output
2 Baseline vital signs
3 Height and weight
4 History of allergy to iodine or shellfish

Answer: 4
Rationale: Procedures that involve the injection of a radiopaque dye require an informed consent. The risk for allergic reaction exists if the client has an allergy to iodine or shellfish. The risk of allergic reaction and possible anaphylaxis must be determined before the procedure. Although options 1, 2, and 3 identify information obtained before the procedure, these items are not the most critical one.

Test-Taking Strategy: Note the key words "most critical." Use the ABCs—airway, breathing, and circulation. The risk for an allergic reaction and anaphylaxis makes option 4 correct. Review the complications associated with injection of a radiopaque dye and the test-taking strategies for answering prioritizing questions if you had difficulty with this question.

Level of Cognitive Ability: Application
Client Needs: Physiological Integrity
Integrated Process: Nursing Process/Data Collection
Content Area: Delegating/Prioritizing

Reference
Black, J. & Hawks, J. (2005). *Medical-surgical nursing: clinical management for positive outcomes* (7th ed). Philadelphia: Saunders, p. 103

---

34. A physician orders potassium chloride (KCl) 12 mEq PO for an adult client to treat a low potassium level. The label on the medication bottle reads 20 mEq KCl per 15 mL. A nurse prepares how many mL of potassium chloride (KCl) to administer the correct dose of medication?
Answer: _________

Answer: 9
Rationale: Use the medication formula.

Formula:

$$\frac{\text{D (Desired)}}{\text{A (Available)}} \times \text{Q (Quantity)} = \text{X}$$

$$\frac{12 \text{ mEq}}{20 \text{ mEq}} \times 15 \text{ mL} = 9 \text{ mL}$$

Test-Taking Strategy: Use a calculator and follow the formula for the calculation of the correct dose. Label each figure, including the answer. Recheck your work and make sure that the answer makes sense. Review the test-taking strategies for answering medication calculation questions if you had difficulty with this question.

Level of Cognitive Ability: Application
Client Needs: Physiological Integrity
Integrated Process: Nursing Process/Implementation
Content Area: Fundamental Skills

Reference
Kee, J. & Marshall, S. (2004). *Clinical calculations: with applications to general and specialty areas* (5th ed). Philadelphia: Saunders, p. 80.

---

35. A client with acquired immunodeficiency syndrome (AIDS) is suspected of having cutaneous Kaposi's sarcoma. The nurse prepares the client for which test that will confirm the presence of this type of sarcoma?

1 Sputum culture
2 Liver biopsy
3 Punch biopsy of the cutaneous lesions
4 White blood cell count

Answer: 3
Rationale: Kaposi's sarcoma lesions begin as red, dark blue, or purple macules on the lower legs that change into plaques. These large plaques ulcerate or open and drain. The lesions spread by metastasis to the upper body then to the face and oral mucosa. It can move to the lymphatic system, lungs, and gastrointestinal (GI) tract. Late disease results in swelling and pain in the lower extremities, penis, scrotum, or face. Diagnosis is made by punch biopsy of cutaneous lesions and biopsy of pulmonary and GI lesions. Options 1, 2, and 4 are incorrect.

Test-Taking Strategy: Note the key word "confirm." Also, noting the relationship between the words "cutaneous" in the question and in the correct option will direct you to option 3. Review the procedure for diagnosing Kaposi's sarcoma and the various test-taking strategies if you had difficulty with this question.

Level of Cognitive Ability: Application
Client Needs: Physiological Integrity
Integrated Process: Nursing Process/Planning
Content Area: Adult Health/Immune

Reference
Linton, A. & Maebius, N. (2003). *Introduction to medical-surgical nursing* (3rd ed). Philadelphia: Saunders, p. 1032.

---

36. A nurse is caring for a client following an allogeneic liver transplant and who is receiving tacrolimus (Prograf). The nurse monitors the client for which adverse effect of the medication?

1 Decrease in urine output
2 Hypotension
3 Profuse sweating
4 Photophobia

Answer: 1
Rationale: Tacrolimus is an immunosuppressant medication used in the prophylaxis of organ rejection in clients receiving allogeneic liver transplants. Frequent side effects include headache, tremor, insomnia, paresthesia, diarrhea, nausea, constipation, vomiting, abdominal pain, and hypertension. Adverse and toxic effects include nephrotoxicity, neurotoxicity, and pleural effusion. Nephrotoxicity is characterized by increasing serum creatinine and blood urea nitrogen levels and a decrease in urine output. Neurotoxicity, including tremor, headache, and mental status changes, can occur commonly.

Test-Taking Strategy: Use medical terminology to identify the medication. Look at the medication name, Prograf. *Pro* means for and *graf* means graft. This assists you in identifying the action of the medication (to prevent transplant rejection) and classifying it as an immunosuppressant (which may in turn assist you in remembering the side effects and adverse and toxic effects of the medication). Review this medication and the test-taking strategies for answering pharmacology questions if you had difficulty with this question.

Level of Cognitive Ability: Analysis
Client Needs: Physiological Integrity
Integrated Process: Nursing Process/Data Collection
Content Area: Pharmacology

Reference
Hodgson, B. & Kizior, R. (2005). *Saunders nursing drug handbook 2005.* Philadelphia: Saunders, p. 1004.

---

37. An antepartum client is diagnosed with bacterial vaginosis. The nurse expects to note which of the following on data collection of the client?
1 Hematuria and hypertension
2 Itching and vaginal discharge
3 Proteinuria and hematuria
4 Costovertebral angle pain and hematuria

Answer: 2
Rationale: Clinical manifestations of bacterial vaginosis include pain, itching, and a thick white vaginal discharge. Proteinuria, hematuria, hypertension, and costovertebral angle pain are clinical manifestations associated with urinary tract infections.

Test-Taking Strategy: Focus on the information in the question. Note the relationship between the words "vaginosis" in the question and "vaginal" in option 2. Also remember when options contain two parts and each part is separated by the word "and" that all parts of the option must be correct. Review the clinical manifestations of bacterial vaginosis and the various test-taking strategies if you had difficulty with this question.

Level of Cognitive Ability: Analysis
Client Needs: Physiological Integrity
Integrated Process: Nursing Process/Data Collection
Content Area: Maternity/Antepartum

Reference
Leifer, G. (2005). *Maternity nursing* (9th ed). Philadelphia: Saunders, p. 231.

---

38. A nurse is caring for a client who has pheochromocytoma. The nurse monitors for the major symptom of pheochromocytoma when the nurse:
1 tests the client's urine for occult blood.
2 takes the client's weight.

Answer: 4
Rationale: Hypertension is the major symptom associated with pheochromocytoma. The blood pressure status is monitored by taking the client's blood pressure. Glycosuria, weight loss, and diaphoresis are clinical manifestations as well; however, hypertension is the major symptom. Hematuria (option 1) is not associated with this disorder.

3 palpates the client's skin for its temperature.
4 takes the client's blood pressure.

Test-Taking Strategy: Note the key word "major." Use the ABCs—airway, breathing, and circulation. A method of monitoring circulation is to take the blood pressure. Review the clinical manifestations associated with this disorder and the various test-taking strategies if you had difficulty with this question.

Level of Cognitive Ability: Application
Client Needs: Physiological Integrity
Integrated Process: Nursing Process/Data Collection
Content Area: Adult Health/Endocrine

Reference

Christensen, B. & Kockrow, E. (2003). *Adult health nursing* (4th ed). St. Louis: Mosby, p. 474.

---

39. A nurse is monitoring a client who was treated for an asthmatic attack. The nurse determines that the client's respiratory status has worsened if which of the following is noted?
1 Loud wheezing heard throughout the lung fields
2 Clear breath sounds
3 Wheezing heard only during exhalation
4 Diminished breath sounds

Answer: 4
Rationale: Diminished breath sounds are an indication of obstruction and possible impending respiratory failure. Wheezing is not a reliable manifestation to determine the severity of an asthma attack. Clear breath sounds indicates improvement and is a positive sign.

Test-Taking Strategy: Eliminate option 3 because of the absolute word "only." From the remaining options, focus on the key words "respiratory status has worsened." Use the ABCs—airway, breathing, and circulation. Remember that diminished breath sounds indicate obstruction and possibly respiratory failure. Review data collection of the client experiencing an asthma attack and the various test-taking strategies if you had difficulty with this question.

Level of Cognitive Ability: Analysis
Client Needs: Physiological Integrity
Integrated Process: Nursing Process/Data Collection
Content Area: Adult Health/Respiratory

Reference

Christensen, B. & Kockrow, E. (2003). *Adult health nursing* (4th ed). St. Louis: Mosby, p. 403.

---

40. A physician's office nurse is collecting data from a client who recently had a renal transplant. The nurse checks the client for which signs of acute graft rejection?
1 Hypotension, graft tenderness, and anemia
2 Hypertension, oliguria, thirst, and hypothermia
3 Fever, vomiting, hypotension, and copious amounts of dilute urine

Answer: 4
Rationale: Acute rejection usually occurs within the first 3 months after transplant, although it can occur for up to 2 years post-transplant. The client exhibits fever, hypertension, malaise, and graft tenderness. Options 1, 2, and 3 do not completely identify signs of acute rejection.

Test-Taking Strategy: Focus on the issue, acute graft rejection. Remember that when an option contains more than one part, all parts of the option need to be correct. Begin to answer this question by eliminating options 1 and 3 because hypotension is not part of the clinical picture with

4 Fever, hypertension, graft tenderness, and malaise

graft rejection. Select option 4 instead of option 2 because fever, not hypothermia, accompanies this complication. Review the signs of acute graft rejection and the various test-taking strategies if you had difficulty with this question.

Level of Cognitive Ability: Analysis
Client Needs: Physiological Integrity
Integrated Process: Nursing Process/Data Collection
Content Area: Adult Health/Renal

Reference

Linton, A. & Maebius, N. (2003). *Introduction to medical-surgical nursing* (3rd ed). Philadelphia: Saunders, pp. 791-792.

---

41. A nurse is assisting in caring for a client who has a fungal infection and is receiving amphotericin B (Fungizone) intravenously. Which of the following indicates that the client is experiencing an adverse or toxic effect from the medication?

1 Lethargy
2 Decreased urinary output
3 Muscle weakness
4 Confusion

Answer: 2

Rationale: Amphotericin B is an antifungal agent. Adverse reactions include nephrotoxicity evidenced by decreased urinary output. Cardiovascular toxicity as evidenced by hypotension and ventricular fibrillation, and anaphylactic reaction occur rarely. Vision and hearing alterations, seizures, hepatic failure, and coagulation defects also may occur. Options 1, 3, and 4 are not associated with an adverse effect.

Test-Taking Strategy: Focus on the information in the question. Noting that the client has a fungal infection will assist in determining that the medication is an antifungal one. Remembering that this medication causes nephrotoxicity, cardiovascular toxicity, and vision and hearing alterations leads you to option 2. Review this medication and the test-taking strategies for answering pharmacology questions if you had difficulty with this question.

Level of Cognitive Ability: Analysis
Client Needs: Physiological Integrity
Integrated Process: Nursing Process/Data Collection
Content Area: Pharmacology

Reference

Hodgson, B. & Kizior, R. (2005). *Saunders nursing drug handbook 2005.* Philadelphia: Saunders, p. 65.

---

42. Penicillin V potassium (Pen-Vee K) has been prescribed to treat a hospitalized client with a respiratory tract infection. Which priority action will the nurse take before administering the medication?

1 Call the pharmacy to order the medication
2 Ask the client about a history of allergies
3 Inform the client about the im-

Answer: 2

Rationale: Penicillin V potassium is an antibiotic. Before administering the medication the nurse performs a baseline assessment and questions the client about a history of allergies to penicillin or to a cephalosporin. Although the nurse would need to order the medication and teach the client about the adverse effects of the medication, determining allergies is the priority (the medication would not be given to the client if an allergy exists). Although deep-breathing exercises are important for a client with a respiratory infection, this action is not directly related to administering penicillin V potassium.

portance of deep-breathing exercises

4 Tell the client to report symptoms of a rash or itching immediately

Test-Taking Strategy: If you are unfamiliar with the medication identified in the question (penicillin V potassium), noting that it is prescribed for a respiratory infection provides the clue that it is an antibiotic. Note the key word "priority" and the issue of the question, the action that the nurse will take. Using pharmacology guidelines will direct you to option 2. Also, using the steps of the clinical problem-solving process (nursing process) will direct you to option 2 because it is the only option that addresses data collection. Options 1, 3, and 4 address implementation. Review this medication and the test-taking strategies for answering pharmacology questions if you had difficulty with this question.

Level of Cognitive Ability: Application
Client Needs: Physiological Integrity
Integrated Process: Nursing Process/Implementation
Content Area: Pharmacology

Reference

Hodgson, B. & Kizior, R. (2005). *Saunders nursing drug handbook 2005.* Philadelphia: Saunders, p. 841.

---

43. Normal saline solution 1000 mL is to be administered over 10 hours. The drop factor is 10 drops (gtt) per mL. A nurse sets the flow rate at how many drops per minute? (Round to the nearest whole number.)
Answer: _________

Answer: 17

Rationale: Use the IV flow rate formula.
Formula:

$$\frac{\text{Total volume} \times \text{gtt factor}}{\text{Time in minutes}} = \text{gtt per min}$$

$$\frac{1000 \text{ mL} \times 10 \text{ gtt}}{600 \text{ minutes}} = \frac{10000}{600} = 16.6, \text{ or } 17 \text{ gtt per minute}$$

Test-Taking Strategy: Use the formula for calculating IV flow rates. Remember, use a calculator, follow the formula, recheck your answer, and make sure that the answer makes sense before documenting it. Review the test-taking strategies for answering intravenous calculation questions if you had difficulty with this question.

Level of Cognitive Ability: Application
Client Needs: Physiological Integrity
Integrated Process: Nursing Process/Implementation
Content Area: Fundamental Skills

Reference

Kee, J. & Marshall, S. (2004). *Clinical calculations: with applications to general and specialty areas* (5th ed). Philadelphia: Saunders, pp. 204-205.

44. A physician's order reads levothyroxine (Synthroid), 150 mcg orally daily. The medication label reads Synthroid, 0.1 mg per tablet. A nurse administers how many tablet(s) to the client?
Answer: ________________

Answer: 1.5
Rationale: It is necessary to convert 150 mcg to mg. In the metric system, to convert smaller to larger, divide by 1000 or move the decimal 3 places to the left. Therefore, 150 mcg = 0.15 mg. Next, use the formula to calculate the correct dose.

Formula:

$$\frac{\text{Desired}}{\text{Available}} \times 1 \text{ tablet} = \text{Tablets per dose}$$

$$\frac{0.15 \text{ mg}}{0.1 \text{ mg}} \times 1 \text{ tablet} = 1.5 \text{ tablets}$$

Test-Taking Strategy: In this medication calculation problem, it is necessary to first convert micrograms to milligrams. Remember, use a calculator, follow the formula, recheck your answer, and make sure that the answer makes sense before documenting it. Review the test-taking strategies for answering medication calculation questions if you had difficulty with this question.

Level of Cognitive Ability: Application
Client Needs: Physiological Integrity
Integrated Process: Nursing Process/Implementation
Content Area: Fundamental Skills

Reference
Kee, J. & Marshall, S. (2004). *Clinical calculations: with applications to general and specialty areas* (5th ed). Philadelphia: Saunders, p. 80.

---

45. The nurse notes that a hospitalized client is receiving sotalol (Betapace). The nurse monitors the client for which side effect related to the medication?
1 Difficulty swallowing
2 Diaphoresis
3 Dry mouth
4 Bradycardia

Answer: 4
Rationale: Sotalol is a beta adrenergic blocking agent. Side effects include bradycardia, palpitations, difficulty breathing, irregular heartbeat, signs of congestive heart failure, and cold hands and feet. Gastrointestinal disturbances, anxiety and nervousness, and unusual tiredness and weakness also can occur. Options 1, 2, and 3 are not side effects.

Test-Taking Strategy: Focus on the issue, a side effect. Remember that medication names ending with the letters "lol" (sotalol) are beta-blockers, which are commonly used for cardiac disorders. The only option that is directly cardiac related is option 4. Review this medication and the test-taking strategies for answering pharmacology questions if you had difficulty with this question.

Level of Cognitive Ability: Analysis
Client Needs: Physiological Integrity
Integrated Process: Nursing Process/Data Collection
Content Area: Pharmacology

Reference
Hodgson, B. & Kizior, R. (2005). *Saunders nursing drug handbook 2005.* Philadelphia: Saunders, p. 983.

46. A nurse reviews the plan of care for a client in Buck's skin traction. The nurse identifies which nursing diagnosis as the priority?

1 Deficient Diversional Activity
2 Risk for Social Isolation
3 Risk for Impaired Skin Integrity
4 Risk for Loneliness

Answer: 3

Rationale: Buck's skin traction is a type of traction in which weights are attached to the skin with the use of a boot. The priority nursing diagnosis for the client is risk for Impaired Skin Integrity. Risk for altered neurovascular status is also a concern. Options 1, 2, and 4 may also be appropriate for the client in Buck's skin traction, but risk for Impaired Skin Integrity presents the greatest risk.

Test-Taking Strategy: Note the key word "priority." Use Maslow's Hierarchy of Needs theory. The only option that indicates a physiological need is option 3. Options 1, 2, and 4 indicate psychosocial needs. Review care to the client in Buck's skin traction and the test-taking strategies for answering prioritizing questions if you had difficulty with this question.

Level of Cognitive Ability: Analysis
Client Needs: Physiological Integrity
Integrated Process: Nursing Process/Planning
Content Area: Adult Health/Musculoskeletal

Reference
Christensen, B. & Kockrow, E. (2003). *Adult health nursing* (4th ed). St. Louis: Mosby, p. 153.

---

47. A client is being taught how to self-administer insulin. The client says to the nurse, "I'm not sure I will be able to do this." Which statement by the nurse is appropriate?

1 "What are your concerns about giving yourself insulin?"
2 "Don't worry. Everyone is unsure at first."
3 "You'll be fine once you get used to giving your own shots."
4 "Maybe your wife or daughter can give you your shot."

Answer: 1

Rationale: Option 1 restates the client's concern and provides the client the opportunity to verbalize. Options 2 and 3 indicate false reassurance, which invalidates the client's concern. Option 4 offers advice without knowing what the client's concerns really are.

Test-Taking Strategy: Use therapeutic communication techniques. Remembering to focus on the client's feelings will direct you to option 1. Review therapeutic communication techniques and the test-taking strategies for answering communication questions if you had difficulty with this question.

Level of Cognitive Ability: Application
Client Needs: Psychosocial Integrity
Integrated Process: Communication and Documentation
Content Area: Adult Health/Endocrine

Reference
Harkreader, H. & Hogan, M.A. (2004). *Fundamentals of nursing: caring and clinical judgment* (2nd ed). Philadelphia: Saunders, pp. 251, 255-257.

48. A physician orders 3000 mL of normal saline to infuse intravenously over 24 hours. The drop factor is 15 drops (gtt) per mL. The nurse prepares to set the flow rate at how many drops per minute? (Round to the nearest whole number.)
Answer: ____________

Answer: 31
Rationale: Use the IV flow rate formula.

Formula:

$$\frac{\text{Total volume} \times \text{gtt factor}}{\text{Time in minutes}} = \text{gtt per min}$$

$$\frac{3000 \text{ mL} \times 15 \text{ gtt}}{1440 \text{ minutes}} = \frac{45{,}000}{1440} = 31.2\text{, or } 31 \text{ gtt per minute}$$

Test-Taking Strategy: Use the formula for calculating IV flow rates. Remember, use a calculator, follow the formula, recheck your answer, and round to the nearest whole number before documenting it. Review the test-taking strategies for answering intravenous calculation questions if you had difficulty with this question.

Level of Cognitive Ability: Application
Client Needs: Physiological Integrity
Integrated Process: Nursing Process/Implementation
Content Area: Fundamental Skills

Reference
Kee, J. & Marshall, S. (2004). *Clinical calculations: with applications to general and specialty areas* (5th ed). Philadelphia: Saunders, pp. 204, 205.

---

49. Nitroglycerin (Nitro-Bid) is being administered to a client. The nurse monitors for which intended effect of the medication?
1 Headache
2 Flushing of the skin
3 Postural hypotension
4 Relief of chest pain

Answer: 4
Rationale: Nitroglycerin is an antianginal, antihypertensive, and coronary vasodilator. Its therapeutic or intended effect is to dilate coronary arteries, improve collateral blood flow to ischemic areas in the myocardium, and relieve chest pain. Flushing of the skin, postural hypotension, and headache are side effects of the medication.

Test-Taking Strategy: If you are unfamiliar with the medication identified in the question (nitroglycerin), noting that its name contains "nitr" provides the clue that it is a nitrate. Focus on the issue, an intended effect. Recalling that an intended effect is a desirable effect and the one that you would expect to occur, and that nitrates vasodilate will direct you to option 4. Review this medication and the test-taking strategies for answering pharmacology questions if you had difficulty with this question.

Level of Cognitive Ability: Analysis
Client Needs: Physiological Integrity
Integrated Process: Nursing Process/Evaluation
Content Area: Pharmacology

Reference
Hodgson, B. & Kizior, R. (2005). *Saunders nursing drug handbook 2005.* Philadelphia: Saunders, p. 780.

50. A nurse reviews the assessment data on a client with a head injury and notes that the client's intracranial pressure reading is 10 mm Hg. Based on this finding the nurse determines that the client's intracranial pressure reading:

1 is elevated.
2 is normal.
3 needs to be reduced with aggressive treatment measures.
4 requires notification of a registered nurse immediately.

Answer: 2

Rationale: The normal intracranial pressure readings are between 0 and 15 mm Hg, and pressures greater than 20 mm Hg are considered increased intracranial pressure. Therefore, options 1, 3, and 4 are incorrect.

Test-Taking Strategy: If you did not know the normal intracranial pressure reading, note that options 1, 3, and 4 are similar in that they indicate that the pressure is elevated and requires action and treatment. Review the normal intracranial pressure reading and the various test-taking strategies if you had difficulty with this question.

Level of Cognitive Ability: Analysis
Client Needs: Physiological Integrity
Integrated Process: Nursing Process/Data Collection
Content Area: Adult Health/Neurological

Reference

Linton, A. & Maebius, N. (2003). *Introduction to medical-surgical nursing* (3rd ed). Philadelphia: Saunders, p. 382.

---

51. The nurse is collecting cardiovascular data on a client. The nurse palpates which anatomical area to assess the popliteal pulse?
Answer: ________

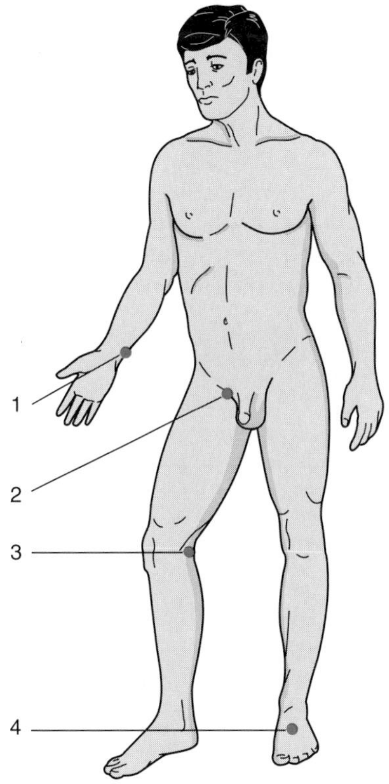

Answer: 3

Rationale: The popliteal pulse is located behind the knee. The ulnar pulse is located at the wrist. The femoral pulse is located in the groin area. The dorsalis pedis pulse is located on the top of the foot.

Test-Taking Strategy: Focus on the issue, the popliteal pulse. Use knowledge regarding anatomy of the body and pulse points to answer correctly. Review cardiovascular data collection techniques and the various test-taking strategies if you had difficulty with this question.

Level of Cognitive Ability: Application
Client Needs: Health Promotion and Maintenance
Integrated Process: Nursing Process/Data Collection
Content Area: Adult Health/Cardiovascular

Reference

deWit, S. (2005). *Fundamental concepts and skills for nursing.* Philadelphia: Saunders, p. 336.

52. The nurse notes documentation that a client's peripheral pulses are +3. The nurse determines that the pulses are:

1 full and brisk.
2 absent.
3 normal or average.
4 palpable but diminished.

Answer: 1

Rationale: Pulses are rated on a scale of 0 to +4 as follows: 0 = absent; +1 = palpable but diminished; +2 = normal or average; +3 = full and brisk; and +4 = full and bounding, often visible.

Test-Taking Strategy: Note the key words "peripheral pulses are +3." Recalling that pulses are rated on a scale of 0 to +4 will assist in directing you to option 1. Review the rating scale for checking pulses and the various test-taking strategies if you had difficulty with this question.

Level of Cognitive Ability: Analysis
Client Needs: Health Promotion and Maintenance
Integrated Process: Nursing Process/Data Collection
Content Area: Adult Health/Cardiovascular

Reference

deWit, S. (2005). *Fundamental concepts and skills for nursing.* Philadelphia: Saunders, p. 341.

---

53. A nurse is checking the extent of pitting edema in a client with congestive heart failure. The nurse gently presses a finger on the client's ankle and notes a barely perceptible pit. The nurse interprets this finding as which measurement of pitting edema?

1 1+
2 2+
3 3+
4 4+

Answer: 1

Rationale: The level of pitting edema is rated on a scale of 1+ to 4+. A barely perceptible pit is rated as 1+. A deeper pit that rebounds in a few seconds is rated as 2+. A deep pit that rebounds in 10 to 20 seconds is rated as 3+. A deeper pit that rebounds in greater than 30 seconds is rated as 4+.

Test-Taking Strategy: Note the key words "barely perceptible pit." Recalling that the level of pitting edema is rated on a scale of 1+ to 4+, with 1+ indicating the least amount of edema will direct you to option 1. Review the procedure for checking edema and the various test-taking strategies if you had difficulty with this question.

Level of Cognitive Ability: Analysis
Client Needs: Health Promotion and Maintenance
Integrated Process: Nursing Process/Data Collection
Content Area: Adult Health/Cardiovascular

Reference

Christensen, B. & Kockrow, E. (2003). *Adult health nursing* (4th ed). St. Louis: Mosby, p. 317.

---

54. A nurse is assisting in preparing a list of discharge instructions for a client who had a permanent pacemaker inserted. Select all instructions that the nurse should place on the list.

___ Avoid lifting more than 25 pounds until cleared by the physician.

Answer:

Monitor the insertion site for infection and bleeding.
Avoid contact sports.
Notify the physician if the radial pulse is outside of the range programmed in the pacemaker.

Rationale: The client is instructed to avoid lifting more than 10 pounds (not 25 pounds) until cleared by the physician. The client is instructed to monitor the insertion site

___ Monitor the insertion site for infection and bleeding.
___ The use of a cellular phone will never affect a pacemaker.
___ Avoid contact sports.
___ Notify the physician if the radial pulse is outside of the range programmed in the pacemaker.

for infection and bleeding and to take the radial pulse and to notify the physician if the radial pulse is outside of the range programmed in the pacemaker, because this may indicate pacemaker malfunction or battery depletion. Cellular phones should be used on the ear opposite the site of the pacemaker and should be carried away from the pacemaker site. Some cellular phones may not affect the pacemaker and the client is instructed to check with the manufacturer of the cellular phone. Contact sports are avoided to prevent injury to the pacemaker site.

Test-Taking Strategy: Read each instruction carefully. The instruction that indicates to avoid lifting more than 25 pounds until cleared by the physician can be eliminated because of the excessive amount of weight. The instruction that indicates that the use of a cellular phone will never affect a pacemaker can be eliminated because of the absolute word "never." Review instructions for a client with a permanent pacemaker and the various test-taking strategies if you had difficulty with this question.

Level of Cognitive Ability: Application
Client Needs: Health Promotion and Maintenance
Integrated Process: Teaching/Learning
Content Area: Adult Health/Cardiovascular

Reference

Phipps, W., Monahan, F., Sands, J., Marek, J., & Neighbors, M. (2003). *Medical-surgical nursing: health and illness perspectives* (7th ed). St. Louis: Mosby, p. 627.

---

55. A nurse is collecting data on a client who sustained a blunt chest injury and suspects the presence of flail chest. Which specific characteristic finding should the nurse note in this condition?

1 Slow deep respirations
2 Asymmetric chest movement
3 Loss of consciousness
4 Anxiety

Answer: 2

Rationale: Flail chest is a thoracic injury resulting in paradoxical (asymmetric) motion of the chest wall segments. The client also exhibits severe chest pain, oscillation of the mediastinum, increasing dyspnea, rapid shallow respirations, accessory muscle breathing, decreased breath sounds on auscultation, and cyanosis. Although the client may exhibit anxiety related to difficulty breathing, anxiety can occur in any respiratory disorder in which dyspnea is a problem. Loss of consciousness can occur in a head injury or if the respiratory condition deteriorated significantly.

Test-Taking Strategy: Note the key words "specific characteristic finding." Also note the relationship of the words "flail chest" in the question and words "asymmetric chest movement" in the correct option. Review the characteristics of flail chest and the various test-taking strategies if you had difficulty with this question.

Level of Cognitive Ability: Analysis
Client Needs: Physiological Integrity

Integrated Process: Nursing Process/Data Collection
Content Area: Adult Health/Respiratory

Reference
Linton, A. & Maebius, N. (2003). *Introduction to medical-surgical nursing* (3rd ed). Philadelphia: Saunders, pp. 197, 487-488.

---

56. A client seeks treatment for a fractured radius. There is an open wound on the arm through which jagged bone edges protrude. The nurse determines that the client has a:
1 greenstick fracture.
2 comminuted fracture.
3 open fracture.
4 simple fracture.

Answer: 3
Rationale: An open fracture (compound fracture) is one in which the skin or mucous membrane has been broken and the wound extends to the depth of the fractured bone. A greenstick fracture is an incomplete fracture, which occurs through part of the cross section of a bone; one side of the bone is fractured, and the other side is bent. A comminuted fracture is a complete fracture across the shaft of a bone, with splintering of the bone into fragments. A simple fracture is a fracture of the bone across its entire shaft, with some possible displacement but without breaking the skin.

Test-Taking Strategy: Note the key words "open" and "bone edges protrude." Note the relationship between these words and option 3. Review types of fractures and the various test-taking strategies if you had difficulty with this question.

Level of Cognitive Ability: Comprehension
Client Needs: Physiological Integrity
Integrated Process: Nursing Process/Data Collection
Content Area: Adult Health/Musculoskeletal

Reference
Christensen, B. & Kockrow, E. (2003). *Adult health nursing* (4th ed). St. Louis: Mosby, pp. 136-138.

---

57. A 4-year-old child is admitted to the hospital for surgery. The nurse asks the parents which priority question to identify the adequacy of support for the child's psychosocial needs?
1 "What signs and symptoms has your child been having?"
2 "Will a family member be able to stay with the child most of the time?"
3 "How much do you know about the surgery and its expected outcome?"
4 "What are your child's favorite toys?"

Answer: 2
Rationale: Separation from family is the most stressful aspect of hospitalization in young children. A primary goal is to prevent separation from family in children younger than the age of 5. Identifying support and the ability of family members to stay with the child takes priority over favorite toys or diversional activities. Options 1 and 3 relate to physiological needs.

Test-Taking Strategy: Focus on the issue, adequacy of support and the child's psychosocial needs. Options 1 and 3 relate to physiological needs, so eliminate these first. From the remaining options, use Maslow's Hierarchy of Needs theory to select the security issue instead of the diversional activity. Review psychosocial needs of a 4-year-old child and the test-taking strategies for answering prioritization questions if you had difficulty with this question.

Level of Cognitive Ability: Application
Client Needs: Psychosocial Integrity

Integrated Process: Nursing Process/Data Collection
Content Area: Child Health

Reference
Leifer, G. (2003). *Introduction to maternity & pediatric nursing* (4th ed). Philadelphia: Saunders, p. 483.

---

58. A nurse is collecting data on a child who has just returned from surgery in a hip spica cast. Which of the following is the priority?

1 The head of the bed is elevated
2 The hips are abducted
3 Circulation is adequate
4 The child is on the right side

Answer: 3

Rationale: The priority concern during the first few hours after a cast is applied is swelling, which may cause the cast to act as a tourniquet and constrict circulation. Therefore, ensuring that circulation is adequate is a high priority. Elevating the head of a bed of a child in a hip spica causes discomfort. Abducting the hips is not necessary because a hip spica cast immobilizes the hip and knee. Turning the child side to side at least every 2 hours is important because it allows the body cast to dry evenly and prevents complications related to immobility; however, it is not a higher priority than checking circulation.

Test-Taking Strategy: Note the key word "priority." Use the ABCs—airway, breathing, and circulation. Option 3 reflects circulation. Review care to the child in a hip spica cast and the test-taking strategies for answering prioritizing questions if you had difficulty with this question.

Level of Cognitive Ability: Application
Client Needs: Physiological Integrity
Integrated Process: Nursing Process/Implementation
Content Area: Child Health

Reference
Leifer, G. (2003). *Introduction to maternity & pediatric nursing* (4th ed). Philadelphia: Saunders, p. 332.

---

59. A nurse is caring for a client with a brainstem injury. The nurse monitors which of the following as the priority?

1 Respiratory rate and rhythm
2 Electrolyte results
3 Peripheral vascular status
4 Radial pulse rate

Answer: 1

Rationale: The respiratory center is located in the brainstem. Monitoring the respiratory status is critical in a client with a brainstem injury, although the nurse would also monitor laboratory results, pulse rate, and peripheral vascular status.

Test-Taking Strategy: Use the ABCs—airway, breathing, and circulation. Option 1 relates to airway. Also, recalling the anatomical location of the respiratory center will direct you to the correct option. Review care to the client with a brainstem injury and the test-taking strategies for prioritizing questions if you had difficulty with this question.

Level of Cognitive Ability: Application
Client Needs: Physiological Integrity
Integrated Process: Nursing Process/Data Collection
Content Area: Delegating/Prioritizing

Reference
Ignatavicius, D. & Workman, M. (2006). *Medical-surgical nursing: critical thinking for collaborative care* (5th ed). Philadelphia: Saunders, pp. 926, 1049.

---

60. A nurse is caring for a client with a diagnosis of rheumatoid arthritis who is receiving aspirin (acetylsalicylic acid, ASA) 5 g orally daily. The nurse recognizes which of the following as an adverse effect related to the medication?

1 Tinnitus
2 Urinary retention
3 Joint pain
4 Difficulty voiding

Answer: 1

Rationale: Aspirin is a nonsteroidal antiinflammatory drug. Adverse effects include gastrointestinal bleeding or gastric mucosal lesions, ringing in the ears (tinnitus), or generalized pruritus. Headache, dizziness, flushing, tachycardia, hyperventilation, sweating, and thirst are also adverse effects. Options 2, 3, and 4 are incorrect. Additionally, aspirin is administered to the client with rheumatoid arthritis to relieve joint pain.

Test-Taking Strategy: Focus on the issue, an adverse effect. Eliminate options 2 and 4 first because they are similar. Next eliminate option 3 because aspirin is administered to relieve joint pain. Lastly, remembering that aspirin can cause gastrointestinal disturbances and ototoxicity will direct you to the correct option. Review this medication and the test-taking strategies for pharmacology questions if you had difficulty with this question.

Level of Cognitive Ability: Analysis
Client Needs: Physiological Integrity
Integrated Process: Nursing Process/Data Collection
Content Area: Pharmacology

Reference
Hodgson, B. & Kizior, R. (2005). *Saunders nursing drug handbook 2005.* Philadelphia: Saunders, p. 88.

---

61. A child with hemophilia is brought into the emergency department after being hit on the neck with a baseball. The nurse should immediately check the child for:

1 spontaneous hematuria.
2 airway obstruction.
3 headache.
4 slurred speech.

Answer: 2

Rationale: Trauma to the neck may cause bleeding into the tissues of the neck, which may compromise the airway. Hematuria is a symptom of hemophilia, although it is not associated with neck injury. Headache and slurred speech are associated with head trauma and are not the priority in this situation.

Test-Taking Strategy: Note the key word "immediately." Use the ABCs—airway, breathing, and circulation. Airway is always a first priority. This directs you to option 2. Review care to the child with hemophilia and the test-taking strategies for answering prioritizing questions if you had difficulty with this question.

Level of Cognitive Ability: Application
Client Needs: Physiological Integrity
Integrated Process: Nursing Process/Data Collection
Content Area: Child Health

Reference

Wong, D. & Hockenberry, M. (2003). *Wong's nursing care of infants and children* (7th ed). St. Louis: Mosby, p. 1565.

---

62. A client received a thermal burn caused by the inhalation of steam. The client's mouth is edematous and the nurse notes blisters in the client's mouth. Based on these data, the nurse monitors the client most closely for:

1 difficulty swallowing.
2 pain.
3 fluid and electrolyte imbalances.
4 wheezing.

Answer: 4

Rationale: Thermal burns to the airway can occur with the inhalation of steam or explosive gases or with the aspiration of scalding liquids. Thermal burns to the upper airway result in edema in the mouth with mucosal blisters or ulcerations. The mucosal edema can lead to upper airway obstruction, manifested by wheezing, particularly during the first 24 to 48 hours after burn injury. The client should be maintained on NPO status after a burn injury. Although options 2 and 3 are components of care, they are not the priority.

Test-Taking Strategy: Note the key words "most closely." Use the ABCs—airway, breathing, and circulation. Wheezing relates to airway. Review care to the client with a thermal burn to the airway and the test-taking strategies for answering prioritizing questions if you had difficulty with this question.

Level of Cognitive Ability: Application
Client Needs: Physiological Integrity
Integrated Process: Nursing Process/Implementation
Content Area: Adult Health/Integumentary

Reference

Ignatavicius, D. & Workman, M. (2006). *Medical-surgical nursing: critical thinking for collaborative care* (5th ed). Philadelphia: Saunders, pp. 1628-1629.

---

63. A nurse is caring for a client who is receiving theophylline (Theo-Dur). The nurse reviews the client's laboratory results and determines that the drug plasma level is therapeutic if which value is noted?

1 5 mcg/mL
2 8 mcg/mL
3 15 mcg/mL
4 25 mcg/mL

Answer: 3

Rationale: Theophylline is a bronchodilator. The therapeutic serum level range is 10 to 20 mcg/mL. Options 1 and 2 identify low levels. Option 4 identifies an elevated level, requiring physician notification.

Test-Taking Strategy: Focus on the name of the medication and recall that most xanthine bronchodilator medication names end with the letters "line." Remember that the therapeutic serum level range is 10 to 20 mcg/mL. This will direct you to option 3. Review this drug plasma level and the test-taking strategies for answering pharmacology questions if you had difficulty with this question.

Level of Cognitive Ability: Analysis
Client Needs: Physiological Integrity
Integrated Process: Nursing Process/Data Collection
Content Area: Pharmacology

Reference

Lehne, R. (2004). *Pharmacology for nursing care* (5th ed). Philadelphia: Saunders, p. 803.

64. A client taking divalproex sodium (Depakote) for the management of seizure disorder reports to the laboratory for follow-up blood tests. The clinic nurse checks the results of which laboratory test to monitor for medication toxicity?

1 Liver function studies
2 Sedimentation rate
3 Glucose
4 Electrolytes

Answer: 1

Rationale: Divalproex sodium is an anticonvulsant that can cause fatal hepatotoxicity. The nurse checks the results of liver function studies to monitor for toxicity. Options 2, 3, and 4 are not associated with monitoring for medication toxicity.

Test-Taking Strategy: Focus on the key word "toxicity." Recall that toxicity occurs when the medication level in the body exceeds the therapeutic level either from overdosing or medication accumulation. Think about the organs involved in the absorption and elimination of medications. The body systems most often affected are the liver and the kidneys, although some medications are ototoxic or neurotoxic. Keeping these guidelines in mind, look for the option that relates to one of these body systems. This will direct you to option 1. Review this medication and the test-taking strategies for answering pharmacology questions if you had difficulty with this question.

Level of Cognitive Ability: Analysis
Client Needs: Physiological Integrity
Integrated Process: Nursing Process/Data Collection
Content Area: Pharmacology

Reference

Hodgson, B. & Kizior, R. (2005). *Saunders nursing drug handbook 2005.* Philadelphia: Saunders, p. 1094.

---

65. A nurse is caring for a client who has a history of cardiac disease involved in a motor vehicle crash. The nurse monitors the client focusing on which priority item?

1 Peripheral pulse rate
2 Apical heart rate
3 Body temperature
4 Bowel sounds

Answer: 2

Rationale: Monitoring the apical heart rate is a priority component of data collection in a client with cardiac disease. Monitoring the peripheral pulse rate is also important but is not as important as the apical heart rate. Bowel sounds and body temperature may be a component of data collection but are unrelated to the information in the question.

Test-Taking Strategy: Use the ABCs—airway, breathing, and circulation. This will direct you to the correct option. Also note the relationship of the words "cardiac disease" in the question and "heart" in the correct option. Review care to the client with a history of cardiac disease and the test-taking strategies for answering prioritizing questions if you had difficulty with this question.

Level of Cognitive Ability: Application
Client Needs: Physiological Integrity
Integrated Process: Nursing Process/Data Collection
Content Area: Adult Health/Cardiovascular

Reference

Christensen, B. & Kockrow, E. (2003). *Adult health nursing* (4th ed). St. Louis: Mosby, p. 321.

66. A nurse is monitoring a client with a tracheostomy tube for complications related to the tube. The nurse suspects tracheoesophageal fistula if which if the following is noted?

1. Abdominal distention
2. Excess mucus production
3. Abnormal skin and mucous membrane color
4. Use of accessory muscles to assist with breathing

Answer: 1

Rationale: Necrosis of the tracheal wall can lead to an artificial opening between the posterior trachea and esophagus. This problem is called tracheoesophageal fistula. The fistula allows air to escape into the stomach, causing abdominal distention. It also causes aspiration of gastric contents. Options 2, 3, and 4 are not findings associated with this complication.

Test-Taking Strategy: Use medical terminology to assist you in answering this question. A fistula is an artificial opening. *Tracheoesophageal* indicates trachea to esophagus. Based on this medical terminology, review the options. Think of air from the trachea moving to the esophagus. If this occurs, you would note abdominal distention. Review care to the client with a tracheostomy tube and the various test-taking strategies if you had difficulty with this question.

Level of Cognitive Ability: Analysis
Client Needs: Physiological Integrity
Integrated Process: Nursing Process/Data Collection
Content Area: Adult Health/Respiratory

Reference

Black, J. & Hawks, J. (2005). *Medical-surgical nursing: clinical management for positive outcomes* (7th ed). Philadelphia: Saunders, p. 1779.

---

67. A nurse suctioning a client through an endotracheal tube monitors the client for complications associated with the procedure. Which of the following indicates a complication?

1. A blood pressure of 128/88 mm Hg
2. An irregular heart rate
3. A reddish coloration in the client's face
4. A pulse oximetry level of 95%

Answer: 2

Rationale: The client should be monitored closely for complications related to suctioning. These include hypoxemia, cardiac irregularities resulting from vagal stimulation, mucosal trauma, and paroxysmal coughing. If complications occur during the procedure, especially cardiac irregularities, the procedure is stopped, and the client is reoxygenated.

Test-Taking Strategy: Eliminate options 1 and 4 first because they identify normal findings. From the remaining options, use the ABCs—airway, breathing, and circulation—to direct you to option 2. Review the complications of suctioning and the various test-taking strategies if you had difficulty with this question.

Level of Cognitive Ability: Analysis
Client Needs: Physiological Integrity
Integrated Process: Nursing Process/Data Collection
Content Area: Adult Health/Respiratory

Reference

Harkreader, H. & Hogan, M.A. (2004). *Fundamentals of nursing: caring and clinical judgment* (2nd ed). Philadelphia: Saunders, pp. 866-868.

68. A clinic nurse is checking the neurological status of a client. The nurse should check for new memory by asking the client:

1 to state the city of birth.
2 what type of transportation was used to get to the clinic.
3 what the client ate for lunch yesterday.
4 to repeat three unrelated words spoken to the client immediately and 5 minutes later.

Answer: 4

Rationale: Remote memory, or long-term memory, is tested by asking the client about something from the past (option 1). The nurse must be able to verify this information. Recent (recall) memory tests information within days, weeks, or months (options 2 and 3). New (immediate) memory is tested by asking the client to repeat three unrelated words that the examiner speaks. The client repeats them immediately so the nurse knows they have been heard correctly, and the nurse asks the client to repeat them again 5 minutes later.

Test-Taking Strategy: Note the key words "new memory." Each of the incorrect options can be eliminated by comparing which of the pieces of information would be *newest* to the client. This will direct you to option 4. Review neurological data collection techniques and the various test-taking strategies if you had difficulty with this question.

Level of Cognitive Ability: Application
Client Needs: Health Promotion and Maintenance
Integrated Process: Nursing Process/Data Collection
Content Area: Adult Health/Neurological

References

Christensen, B. & Kockrow, E. (2003). *Adult health nursing* (4th ed). St. Louis: Mosby, pp. 607-608.
Linton, A. & Maebius, N. (2003). *Introduction to medical-surgical nursing* (3rd ed). Philadelphia: Saunders, pp. 371-372.

---

69. A nurse is collecting data on a client with a disorder of the inner ear. Which question will the nurse ask the client to determine if the client is experiencing the most common symptom of this type of ear disorder?

1 "Do you have any hearing loss?"
2 "Do you have any itching around your ear?"
3 "Do you have any ringing in the ears?"
4 "Do you have any pain in the ear?"

Answer: 3

Rationale: Tinnitus is the most common complaint of clients with otological disorders, especially disorders involving the inner ear. Symptoms of tinnitus range from mild ringing in the ear that can go unnoticed during the day, to a loud roaring in the ear that can interfere with the client's thinking process and attention span. The client may experience some pain or hearing loss depending on the disorder, but these are not the most common symptoms. Itching around the ear may be associated with a disorder other than an inner-ear disorder.

Test-Taking Strategy: Focus on the issue, a disorder of the inner ear and note the key words "most common." Recalling the anatomy and physiology of the inner ear will assist in directing you to option 3. Review the characteristics of inner ear disorders and the various test-taking strategies if you had difficulty with this question.

Level of Cognitive Ability: Application
Client Needs: Physiological Integrity
Integrated Process: Nursing Process/Data Collection
Content Area: Adult Health/Ear

Reference

Christensen, B. & Kockrow, E. (2003). *Adult health nursing* (4th ed). St. Louis: Mosby, p. 591.

70. A client arrives at the health care clinic after sustaining an eye injury in which paint thinner splashed into the eye. The nurse should initially ask the client which of the following questions?

1 "Did you bring the container of paint thinner with you?"
2 "What time did the injury occur?"
3 "Did you flush the eye after the injury?"
4 "What brand of paint thinner caused the injury?"

Answer: 3

Rationale: Emergency care after a chemical burn to the eye includes irrigating the eye immediately with tap water or sterile normal saline or ocular irrigating solution if available. The irrigation should be maintained for at least 10 minutes. After this emergency treatment, visual acuity is assessed. The initial data collection should focus on the type of treatment that took place immediately after the injury.

Test-Taking Strategy: Note the key word "initially" and note the type of injury to the eye. Eliminate options 1 and 4 first because they are similar. From the remaining options, use Maslow's Hierarchy of Needs theory. The treatment of the injury is the priority. Review care to the client with an eye injury and the test-taking strategies for answering prioritizing questions if you had difficulty with this question.

Level of Cognitive Ability: Application
Client Needs: Physiological Integrity
Integrated Process: Nursing Process/Data Collection
Content Area: Adult Health/Eye

Reference
Linton, A. & Maebius, N. (2003). *Introduction to medical-surgical nursing* (3rd ed). Philadelphia: Saunders, p. 196.

---

71. A nurse is observing a client who is ambulating after a prolonged period of bed rest. The nurse determines that the client should immediately stop the activity if the client exhibits:

1 an increase in pulse rate from 78 to 80 beats per minute.
2 an increase in respiratory rate from 16 to 18 breaths per minute.
3 some arm and leg weakness.
4 shortness of breath and diaphoresis.

Answer: 4

Rationale: Bed rest decreases the client's strength and endurance. Shortness of breath and diaphoresis are systemic signs of fatigue indicating that the client should rest. Options 1, 2, and 3 are normal findings.

Test-Taking Strategy: Note the key words "immediately stop." Use the ABCs—airway, breathing, and circulation. Option 4 indicates that the client is not tolerating the activity from a cardiopulmonary standpoint. Options 1, 2, and 3 are expected effects. Review the effects of mobility and the various test-taking strategies if you had difficulty with this question.

Level of Cognitive Ability: Analysis
Client Needs: Physiological Integrity
Integrated Process: Nursing Process/Evaluation
Content Area: Adult Health/Musculoskeletal

Reference
Christensen, B. & Kockrow, E. (2003). *Foundations of nursing* (4th ed). St. Louis: Mosby, pp. 293-294.

72. A client who has been raped arrives at the emergency department. Which of these observations is most important for the nurse to consider when planning the immediate care for the client?

1 The victim states she "feels like it didn't happen."
2 The victim states that she "feels numb."
3 The victim states the rapist knows where she lives and has stated: "He will kill me if I tell anyone about the rape."
4 The victim states she knows the rapist well; in fact they had been dating for several weeks.

Answer: 3

Rationale: To provide for safety is the primary concern for the nurse. The priority statement by the victim is that the rapist will kill her. The victim who states she "feels like it didn't happen" or that she "feels numb" is most likely in the denial stage, which can be a helpful defense mechanism for the client. The fact that the rapist and the victim knew each other is a common phenomenon; in many situations of abuse, the victim does know the rapist.

Test-Taking Strategy: Note the key words "most important" and "immediate." Eliminate options 1 and 2 first because they are similar. From the remaining options use Maslow's Hierarchy of Needs theory. Option 3 is concerned with safety. Review care to the rape victim and the test-taking strategies for answering prioritizing questions if you had difficulty with this question.

Level of Cognitive Ability: Application
Client Needs: Physiological Integrity
Integrated Process: Nursing Process/Planning
Content Area: Mental Health

Reference

Morrison-Valfre, M. (2005). *Foundations of mental health care* (3rd ed). St. Louis: Mosby, pp. 273-274.

---

73. A nurse is assisting in monitoring a client with acute pulmonary emboli who is receiving a thrombolytic medication. Which finding indicates an adverse effect related to the medication and the need to notify a registered nurse immediately?

1 Positive peripheral pulses
2 A radial pulse rate of 58 beats per minute
3 A blood pressure of 140/90 mm Hg
4 Client complaints of back pain

Answer: 4

Rationale: A thrombolytic medication acts directly on the fibrinolytic system to convert plasminogen to plasmin, an enzyme that degrades fibrin clots, fibrinogen, and other plasma proteins. The nurse should monitor the client for bleeding during administration of this medication because severe internal hemorrhage can occur as an adverse effect. Signs of bleeding or internal hemorrhage include a drop in blood pressure, a rise in pulse, or complaints of abdominal or back pain. Positive peripheral pulses are a normal finding. If signs of bleeding occur, the nurse would notify a registered nurse immediately, who would then contact the physician.

Test-Taking Strategy: Eliminate option 1 first because it is a normal finding. Next note the key word "immediately." Recalling that bleeding is a concern with the use of a thrombolytic medication will assist in answering the question. Options 2 and 3 are not signs of bleeding or shock. If a client is bleeding internally, the client will complain of back or abdominal pain. Also, remember that a registered nurse is notified immediately if a client is experiencing a life-threatening situation. Review the adverse effects of thrombolytic medications and the various test-taking strategies if you had difficulty with this question.

Level of Cognitive Ability: Analysis
Client Needs: Physiological Integrity
Integrated Process: Nursing Process/Data Collection
Content Area: Pharmacology

Reference

Hodgson, B. & Kizior, R. (2005). *Saunders nursing drug handbook 2005.* Philadelphia: Saunders, p. 991.

---

74. A nurse is monitoring a newborn diagnosed with congenital hypothyroidism. The nurse expects to note which finding on data collection?

1 Excessive sleepiness
2 Hypertonic reflexes
3 Hyperactivity
4 Frequent, loose stools

Answer: 1

Rationale: Signs and symptoms of hypothyroidism may be nonspecific and may include feeding difficulty, prolonged jaundice, respiratory problems, hypotonia, constipation, large posterior fontanel, excessive sleepiness, large tongue, rare crying, dry and mottled skin, and slow deep tendon reflexes.

Test-Taking Strategy: Focus on the diagnosis, hypothyroidism. Recall that the physiological action of thyroid hormone is to regulate metabolism. Use medical terminology recalling that a condition that is *hypo* will reveal signs of depressed function. Also note that options 2, 3, and 4 indicate *hyper*activity of body systems. Review care to the newborn with congenital hypothyroidism and the various test-taking strategies if you had difficulty with this question.

Level of Cognitive Ability: Analysis
Client Needs: Physiological Integrity
Integrated Process: Nursing Process/Data Collection
Content Area: Maternity/Postpartum

Reference

Leifer, G. (2005). *Maternity nursing* (9th ed). Philadelphia: Saunders, p. 271.

---

75. A nurse is assisting in caring for a client with a diagnosis of acute lymphocytic leukemia who is receiving chemotherapy. The nurse reviews the client's laboratory results and determines that the client is experiencing an adverse effect of the chemotherapy if which of the following is noted?

1 White blood cell (WBC) count 5000 cells/L
2 Blood urea nitrogen (BUN) 15 mg/dL
3 Platelet count 200,000 mm^3
4 Alkaline phosphatase 25 units/dL

Answer: 4

Rationale: Adverse effects can occur from chemotherapy and can include effects such as hematological reactions, hepatotoxicity, neurotoxicity, and nephrotoxicity. The normal WBC count is 5000 to 10,000 cells/L. The normal platelet count is 150,000 to 450,000 mm^3. Normal BUN is 5 to 20 mg/dL. The normal alkaline phosphatase is 4.5 to 13 units/dL.

Test-Taking Strategy: Focus on the issue, an adverse effect. Review the laboratory values presented in the options and note that the only abnormal laboratory value is the alkaline phosphatase. Review these normal laboratory values and the various test-taking strategies if you had difficulty with this question.

Level of Cognitive Ability: Analysis
Client Needs: Physiological Integrity

Integrated Process: Nursing Process/Data Collection
Content Area: Pharmacology

Reference

Pagana, K. & Pagana, T. (2003). *Mosby's diagnostic and laboratory test reference* (6th ed). St. Louis: Mosby, pp. 36-37.

---

76. A nurse is caring for a client with a tracheostomy tube and is monitoring the client for subcutaneous emphysema. The nurse identifies this complication by noting which of the following?

1 Crackling sounds heard in the upper lobes bilaterally
2 A puffy and crackling sensation on palpation of the tissues surrounding the tracheostomy site
3 Signs of respiratory distress
4 Dyspnea

Answer: 2
Rationale: Subcutaneous emphysema occurs when air escapes from the tracheostomy incision into the tissues, dissects fascial planes under the skin, and accumulates around the face, neck, and upper chest. These areas appear puffy and slight finger pressure produces a crackling sound and sensation. Generally this is not a serious condition, as the air will eventually be absorbed. Options 1, 3, and 4 are not signs of subcutaneous emphysema but could be signs of other complications.

Test-Taking Strategy: Eliminate options 3 and 4 first because they are similar. Next note the word "subcutaneous" in the question and the relationship of this word to the description in option 2. Review the characteristics of subcutaneous emphysema and the various test-taking strategies if you had difficulty with this question.

Level of Cognitive Ability: Analysis
Client Needs: Physiological Integrity
Integrated Process: Nursing Process/Data Collection
Content Area: Adult Health/Respiratory

Reference

Linton, A. & Maebius, N. (2003). *Introduction to medical-surgical nursing* (3rd ed). Philadelphia: Saunders, p. 497.

---

77. A nurse is caring for a client with chronic stable angina who is receiving amlodipine (Norvasc). Which of the following indicates to the nurse that the client is experiencing an adverse effect of the medication?

1 Bradycardia
2 Hypotension
3 Constipation
4 Abdominal cramping

Answer: 2
Rationale: Amlodipine is a calcium channel blocker. Adverse or toxic effects may produce excessive peripheral vasodilation and marked hypotension with reflex tachycardia. Frequent side effects include peripheral edema, headache, and flushing. Constipation and abdominal cramping are not associated with this medication.

Test-Taking Strategy: Focus on the issue, an adverse effect. Note the name of the medication and recall that most calcium channel blocker medication names end with the letters "pine" and that these medications are used to treat hypertension. This will direct you to option 2. Review this medication and the various test-taking strategies if you had difficulty with this question.

Level of Cognitive Ability: Analysis
Client Needs: Physiological Integrity

Integrated Process: Nursing Process/Evaluation
Content Area: Pharmacology

Reference

Hodgson, B. & Kizior, R. (2005). *Saunders nursing drug handbook 2005.* Philadelphia: Saunders, p. 59.

---

78. A mother tells the clinic nurse that she doesn't want her child to receive any immunizations because she has heard that they cause serious illnesses. The nurse makes which appropriate statement to the mother?

1 "Why are you afraid? Children are immunized every day without a problem."
2 "There will be a slight discomfort at the time of the injection, but that is all that will happen."
3 "I can see you are very concerned about your child. What do you think might happen after an immunization is given?"
4 "Are you afraid the child is going to die from the injection?"

Answer: 3

Rationale: Option 3 acknowledges the mother's concern, which provides an opportunity for the mother to respond to the nurse's open-ended question. Options 1, 2, and 4 are nontherapeutic. Option 1 can make the mother feel defensive, devalues the mother's feelings, and requires an explanation from the mother. Option 2 provides false reassurance. Option 4 is an attempt to verify an assumption not supported in the question.

Test-Taking Strategy: Use therapeutic communication techniques. The correct option demonstrates empathy and helps the mother focus on specific fears so that the nurse can clarify information. Remember to focus on the client's feelings. Review therapeutic communication techniques and the test-taking strategies for answering communication questions if you had difficulty with this question.

Level of Cognitive Ability: Application
Client Needs: Psychosocial Integrity
Integrated Process: Communication and Documentation
Content Area: Child Health

Reference

Harkreader, H. & Hogan, M.A. (2004). *Fundamentals of nursing: caring and clinical judgment* (2nd ed). Philadelphia: Saunders, pp. 251, 255-257.

---

79. A nurse is reviewing the laboratory results of a client with cancer and notes that the calcium level is 14 mg/dL. The nurse determines that this calcium level is consistent with which oncological emergency?

1 Syndrome of inappropriate antidiuretic hormone (SIADH)
2 Spinal cord compression
3 Superior vena cava syndrome
4 Hypercalcemia

Answer: 4

Rationale: One potentially life-threatening complication of cancer is hypercalcemia, which is characterized by calcium levels greater than 11 mg/dL. Although spinal cord compression and superior vena cava syndrome are also oncological emergencies, they are not characterized by high calcium levels. SIADH is also an oncological emergency but is characterized by hyponatremia.

Test-Taking Strategy: Note the similarity of the calcium level in the question and the word "hypercalcemia" in the correct option. Review the significance of an elevated calcium level and the various test-taking strategies if you had difficulty with this question.

Level of Cognitive Ability: Analysis
Client Needs: Physiological Integrity
Integrated Process: Nursing Process/Data Collection
Content Area: Adult Health/Oncology

Reference

Pagana, K. & Pagana, T. (2003). *Mosby's diagnostic and laboratory test reference* (6th ed). St. Louis: Mosby, pp. 207-208.

---

80. A nurse is caring for a client admitted to the hospital with a musculoskeletal injury. The nurse monitors for the major symptom associated with neurovascular compromise by:

1 counting the client's apical pulse for 1 full minute.
2 observing for drainage on the dressing of the affected extremity.
3 taking the client's blood pressure on the unaffected side.
4 determining if pain is experienced with passive motion of the affected extremity.

Answer: 4

Rationale: Neurovascular compromise in a client with a musculoskeletal injury is created by increased pressure within a compartment. The pressure occurs because fascia is unable to expand when muscle swelling occurs. The only option that addresses neurovascular compromise is option 4.

Test-Taking Strategy: Focus on the key words "major symptom" and "neurovascular compromise." The only option that addresses neurovascular compromise is option 4. Review the signs of neurovascular compromise and the various test-taking strategies if you had difficulty with this question.

Level of Cognitive Ability: Application
Client Needs: Physiological Integrity
Integrated Process: Nursing Process/Data Collection
Content Area: Adult Health/Musculoskeletal

Reference

Lewis, S., Heitkemper, M., & Dirksen, S. (2004). *Medical-surgical nursing: assessment and management of clinical problems* (6th ed). St. Louis: Mosby, p. 1672.

---

81. A postpartum mother complains of severe pain and an intense feeling of swelling and pressure in the vaginal area. The nurse immediately checks the client's:

1 episiotomy site for drainage.
2 rectum for hemorrhoids.
3 vulva for a hematoma.
4 vagina for lacerations.

Answer: 3

Rationale: Hematoma is suspected when pain or pressure in the vaginal area is reported by the client. Massive hemorrhage can occur into the tissues, resulting in hypovolemia and shock. Options 1, 2, and 4 are not associated with the client's complaint.

Test-Taking Strategy: Note the key word "immediately" and focus on the client's complaints. Note that option 3 indicates a bleeding disorder, which is a priority. Review postpartum data collection techniques and the various test-taking strategies if you had difficulty with this question.

Level of Cognitive Ability: Application
Client Needs: Physiological Integrity
Integrated Process: Nursing Process/Data Collection
Content Area: Maternity/Postpartum

Reference

Lowdermilk, D. & Perry, A. (2004). *Maternity & women's health care* (8th ed). St. Louis: Mosby, p. 1037.

82. A nurse is caring for a client receiving hemodialysis who has an internal arteriovenous fistula. The nurse expects to note which finding if the fistula is patent?

1 White fibrin specks noted in the fistula
2 Palpation of a thrill over the site of the fistula
3 Lack of a bruit at the site of the fistula
4 Warmth and redness at the site of the fistula

Answer: 2

Rationale: An internal arteriovenous fistula is created through a surgical procedure in which an artery in the arm is anastomosed to a vein. The fistula is internal. To determine patency, the nurse palpates over the fistula for a thrill and auscultates for a bruit. The nurse would not note white fibrin specks in the fistula, because the fistula is internal. Warmth and redness may indicate a potential inflammatory process.

Test-Taking Strategy: Focus on the issue, a patent fistula. Option 1 can be eliminated first because the nurse would not note white fibrin specks in the fistula, because the fistula is internal. Next eliminate option 4 because warmth and redness may indicate a potential inflammatory process. From the remaining options, recall that the presence of a bruit or a thrill indicates a patent fistula. Review care to the client with an internal arteriovenous fistula and the various test-taking strategies if you had difficulty with this question.

Level of Cognitive Ability: Analysis
Client Needs: Physiological Integrity
Integrated Process: Nursing Process/Data Collection
Content Area: Adult Health/Renal

Reference

Christensen, B. & Kockrow, E. (2003). *Adult health nursing* (4th ed). St. Louis: Mosby, p. 443.

---

83. A nurse is collecting data on a client with a diagnosis of Meniere's disease who is being admitted to the hospital. The nurse asks the client which of the following questions that will elicit information specific to the attacks that occur with this disease?

1 "Do you have a feeling of fullness in your ear?"
2 "Are you having any headaches?"
3 "Do you have any visual problems?"
4 "Do you have difficulty sleeping at night?"

Answer: 1

Rationale: Meniere's disease results from a disturbance in the fluid of the endolymphatic system. The cause of the disturbance is unknown. Attacks may be preceded by a feeling of fullness in the ear, or by tinnitus. Headaches are not associated with this disorder. Options 3 and 4 are also unrelated to Meniere's disease.

Test -Taking Strategy: Focus on the disease and recall that this disorder is associated with the ear. This will direct you to option 1 because this is the only option that relates to the ear. Review Meniere's disease and the various test-taking strategies if you had difficulty with this question.

Level of Cognitive Ability: Application
Client Needs: Physiological Integrity
Integrated Process: Nursing Process/Data Collection
Content Area: Adult Health/Ear

Reference

Linton, A. & Maebius, N. (2003) *Introduction to medical-surgical nursing* (3rd ed.). Philadelphia: Saunders, p. 1089.

84. A nurse administers a fatal dose of morphine sulfate to a client. During the subsequent investigation of error, it is determined that the nurse did not check the client's respiratory rate before administering the medication. Failure to adequately check the client is addressed under which function of the nurse practice act?

1 Defining the specific educational requirements for licensure in the state
2 Describing the scope of practice of licensed and unlicensed care providers
3 Recommending specific terms of incarceration for nurses who violate the law
4 Identifying the process for disciplinary action if standards of care are not met

Answer: 4
Rationale: In the situation, acceptable standards of care were not met (the nurse failed to adequately check the client before administering a medication). Option 4 refers specifically to the situation described in the question, whereas options 1, 2, and 3 do not.

Test-Taking Strategy: Note the relationship between the words "failure to adequately check the client" in the question and "standards of care are not met" in option 4. Review the legal implications related to medication errors and the various test-taking strategies if you had difficulty with this question.

Level of Cognitive Ability: Analysis
Client Needs: Safe, Effective Care Environment
Integrated Process: Nursing Process/Data Collection
Content Area: Leadership/Management

Reference
Harkreader, H. & Hogan, M.A. (2004). *Fundamentals of nursing: caring and clinical judgment* (2nd ed). Philadelphia: Saunders, pp. 22-23.

---

85. A nurse is providing instructions to a client with glaucoma about prescribed treatment measures for the disorder. The nurse tells the client that the goal of treatment is:

1 maintaining intraocular pressure at a reduced level.
2 producing mydriasis in the eyes.
3 increasing the formation of aqueous humor.
4 promoting dilation of the pupil of the eyes.

Answer: 1
Rationale: The goal of treatment of the client with glaucoma is to maintain intraocular pressure at a reduced level to prevent further damage to intraocular structures. Medications are used to create miosis (constriction of the pupil) and to reduce formation of the aqueous humor by the ciliary body.

Test-Taking Strategy: Eliminate options 2 and 4 first because they are similar. Next recalling that glaucoma is a condition that is characterized by increased intraocular pressure will assist in eliminating option 3. Also note that option 1 is the umbrella (global) option. Review instructions for the client with glaucoma and the various test-taking strategies if you had difficulty with this question.

Level of Cognitive Ability: Application
Client Needs: Physiological Integrity
Integrated Process: Teaching/Learning
Content Area: Adult Health/Eye

Reference
Linton, A. & Maebius, N. (2003). *Introduction to medical-surgical nursing* (3rd ed). Philadelphia: Saunders, p. 1067.

---

86. A nurse receives a telephone call from the laboratory and is told that a client with bladder cancer and bone metastasis has a calcium level of 15 mg/dL. Which nursing action is appropriate?

1 Notify a registered nurse.
2 Document the results on the nursing worksheet.

Answer: 1
Rationale: Hypercalcemia is a serum calcium level greater than 11 mg/dL. It most often occurs in clients who have bone metastasis, and is a late manifestation of extensive malignancy. The presence of cancer in the bone causes the bone to release calcium into the bloodstream. Hypercalcemia is an oncological emergency and a registered nurse should be notified, who will then contact the physician. Options 2, 3, and 4 are incorrect.

3 Ask the dietary department to send additional calcium-containing foods on the client's meal trays.
4 File the report in the client's record.

Test-Taking Strategy: Eliminate options 2 and 4 first because they are similar actions. From the remaining options, knowing that the calcium level identified in the question indicates an elevated one will assist in eliminating option 3. Remember, a registered nurse and physician are notified if an emergency or life-threatening situation occurs. Review the normal calcium level and the various test-taking strategies if you had difficulty with this question.

Level of Cognitive Ability: Application
Client Needs: Physiological Integrity
Integrated Process: Nursing Process/Implementation
Content Area: Adult Health/Oncology

Reference

Linton, A. & Maebius, N. (2003). *Introduction to medical-surgical nursing* (3rd ed). Philadelphia: Saunders, p. 783.

---

87. A nurse notes excessive bleeding on the dressing of a client who underwent enucleation. Based on this finding which nursing action is appropriate?

1 Document the finding.
2 Reinforce the dressing.
3 Mark the amount of staining with a black pen and continue to monitor the drainage.
4 Notify a registered nurse.

Answer: 4

Rationale: Postoperative nursing care includes observing the dressing and reporting any swelling or excessive bleeding. The nurse should notify a registered nurse, who then notifies the surgeon if the client is bleeding. Although the nurse would document the findings and may reinforce the dressing until the surgeon arrives, these actions are not the most appropriate. Option 3 delays necessary intervention to the client who is bleeding.

Test-Taking Strategy: Note the words "excessive bleeding on the dressing." Remember a registered nurse and physician are notified if the client experiences an emergency or life-threatening occurrence. Review care to the client following enucleation and the various test-taking strategies if you had difficulty with this question.

Level of Cognitive Ability: Application
Client Needs: Physiological Integrity
Integrated Process: Nursing Process/Implementation
Content Area: Adult Health/Eye

Reference

Christensen, B. & Kockrow, E. (2003). *Adult health nursing* (4th ed). St. Louis: Mosby, p. 582.

---

88. A nurse is observing a nursing assistant talking to a client who is hearing impaired. The nurse intervenes if the nursing assistant does which of the following during communication with the client?

1 The nursing assistant is facing the client when speaking.
2 The nursing assistant is speaking clearly to the client.

Answer: 3

Rationale: When communicating with a hearing-impaired client, the nurse should speak in a normal tone to the client and not shout. The nurse should talk directly to the client while facing the client, and speak clearly. If the client does not seem to understand what is said, the nurse should express the statement differently. Moving closer to the client and toward the better ear may facilitate communication, but the nurse should avoid talking directly into the impaired ear.

3 The nursing assistant is speaking directly into the impaired ear.
4 The nursing assistant is speaking in a normal tone.

Test-Taking Strategy: Note the key words "the nurse intervenes." These words indicate a false response question and indicate that you are looking for the option that indicates an incorrect action by the nursing assistant. Noting the words "directly into the impaired ear" will direct you to option 3. Review care to the hearing-impaired client and the various test-taking strategies if you had difficulty with this question.

Level of Cognitive Ability: Application
Client Needs: Safe, Effective Care Environment
Integrated Process: Nursing Process/Implementation
Content Area: Leadership/Management

Reference
Harkreader, H. & Hogan, M.A. (2004). *Fundamentals of nursing: caring and clinical judgment* (2nd ed). Philadelphia: Saunders, pp. 989-990.

---

89. A nurse is assisting in developing a plan of care for a manic client and suggests a nursing diagnosis of Disturbed Thought Processes. Which activity related to this nursing diagnosis should the nurse suggest for the client initially?
1 Writing
2 Playing cards with another client
3 Playing checkers with another client
4 Playing a board game with another client

Answer: 1
Rationale: When the client is manic, solitary activities requiring a short attention span, or mild physical exertion activities such as writing, painting, fingerpainting, woodworking, or walks with the staff are best initially. Solitary activities minimize stimuli and mild physical activities release tension constructively. When less manic, the client may join one or two other clients in quiet nonstimulating activities. Competitive games should be avoided because they can stimulate aggression and cause increased psychomotor activity.

Test-Taking Strategy: Note the similarity in options 2, 3, and 4 in that they all involve activities with another individual. Option 1 is the only solitary activity that will minimize stimuli. Review care to the manic client and the various test-taking strategies if you had difficulty with this question.

Level of Cognitive Ability: Application
Client Needs: Psychosocial Integrity
Integrated Process: Nursing Process/Planning
Content Area: Mental Health

Reference
Stuart, G. & Laraia, M. (2005). *Principles & practice of psychiatric nursing* (8th ed). St. Louis: Mosby, pp. 355-356.

---

90. Select all nursing interventions to be included in a plan of care for a client with schizophrenia who is experiencing disturbed thought processes.
___ Schedule frequent one-hour sessions with the client.
___ Demonstrate an attitude of caring and concern.
___ Set goals for the client.
___ Help the client identify the dif-

Answer:
Demonstrate an attitude of caring and concern.

Help the client identify the difference between reality and internal thought processes.

Establish a nurse-client relationship contract mutually agreed on by the nurse and client.

Rationale: The establishment of a trusting relationship is the basis to developing open communication with the ference between reality and internal thought processes.

___ Establish a nurse-client relationship contract mutually agreed on by the nurse and client.

client. The nurse should schedule brief (5- to 10-minute) frequent contacts with the client because the client with disturbed thought processes cannot tolerate extended intrusive interactions and functions best in a structured environment. Demonstrating an attitude of caring and concern is basic to any nurse-client relationship. The nurse should establish mutual goals with the client and help the client identify reality.

Test-Taking Strategy: Focus on the client situation and look for key words in the interventions. Eliminate the intervention that reads "Schedule frequent one-hour sessions with the client" because of the words "one-hour." Also eliminate the intervention that reads "Set goals for the client" because basic and fundamental principles of a nurse-client relationship indicate that goals should be mutually set between the nurse and client. Review care to the client experiencing disturbed thought processes and the various test-taking strategies if you had difficulty with this question.

Level of Cognitive Ability: Application
Client Needs: Psychosocial Integrity
Integrated Process: Nursing Process/Planning
Content Area: Mental Health

Reference

Stuart, G. & Laraia, M. (2005). *Principles & practice of psychiatric nursing* (8th ed). St. Louis: Mosby, p. 116.

---

91. A client has received electroconvulsive therapy (ECT). The nurse implements which activity first in the post-treatment area?

1 Monitors the client's vital signs
2 Discusses the treatment
3 Provides frequent reassurance to the client
4 Encourages the client to eat

Answer: 1
Rationale: The nurse first monitors vital signs and then orients the client. The nursing interventions outlined in options 2, 3, and 4 follow accordingly. Additionally the nurse would assess for the return of a gag reflex before encouraging the client to eat.

Test-Taking Strategy: Note the key word "first." Use the ABCs—airway, breathing, and circulation—to direct you to option 1. Review care to the client receiving electroconvulsive therapy and the test-taking strategies for answering prioritizing questions if you had difficulty with this question.

Level of Cognitive Ability: Application
Client Needs: Physiological Integrity
Integrated Process: Nursing Process/Implementation
Content Area: Delegating/Prioritizing

Reference

Stuart, G. & Laraia, M. (2005). *Principles & practice of psychiatric nursing* (8th ed). St. Louis: Mosby, p. 607.

92. A client is admitted to the emergency department with complaints of severe, radiating chest pain. Admission orders include oxygen by nasal cannula at 4 L/min; troponins, creatine phosphokinase (CPK), and isoenzymes; a chest radiograph; and a 12-lead electrocardiogram (ECG). Number in order of priority how the nurse will implement the physician's orders. (Number 1 is the first action and Number 4 is the last action.)

___ Obtain the 12-lead ECG.
___ Call the laboratory to order the stat bloodwork.
___ Call radiology to order the chest radiograph.
___ Apply the oxygen to the client.

Answer: 2341

Rationale: The initial action is to apply oxygen, because the client may be experiencing myocardial ischemia. The ECG can provide evidence of cardiac damage and the location of myocardial ischemia and would be obtained next. The nurse would then obtain bloodwork because it can assist in determining the choice of treatment. Although the chest radiograph may show cardiac enlargement, it does not influence the immediate treatment.

Test-Taking Strategy: Note the key word "priority." Remember that the immediate goal of therapy is to prevent myocardial ischemia. Use the ABCs—airway, breathing, and circulation—and the procedures for determining treatment to answer this question. Review care to the client with chest pain and the test-taking strategies for answering prioritizing questions if you had difficulty with this question.

Level of Cognitive Ability: Application
Client Needs: Physiological Integrity
Integrated Process: Nursing Process/Implementation
Content Area: Delegating/Prioritizing

Reference

Christensen, B. & Kockrow, E. (2003). *Adult health nursing* (4th ed). St. Louis: Mosby, p. 310.

---

93. A nurse is observing a nursing student auscultating the breath sounds of a client. The nurse intervenes if the nursing student did which of the following?

1 Asked the client to lie flat on the right side and then on the left side
2 Asked the client to breathe slowly and deeply through the mouth
3 Placed the stethoscope directly on the client's skin
4 Used the diaphragm of the stethoscope

Answer: 1

Rationale: The client ideally should sit up and breathe slowly and deeply through the mouth. The diaphragm of the stethoscope, which is warmed before use, is placed directly on the client's skin, not over a gown or clothing.

Test-Taking Strategy: Note the key words "nurse intervenes." These words indicate a false response question and that you are looking for the option that identifies an incorrect action by the nursing student. Noting the words "lie flat" will direct you to option 1. Review the procedure for auscultating breath sounds and the various test-taking strategies if you had difficulty with this question.

Level of Cognitive Ability: Application
Client Needs: Safe, Effective Care Environment
Integrated Process: Nursing Process/Implementation
Content Area: Leadership/Management

Reference

Potter, P. & Perry, A. (2005). *Fundamentals of nursing* (6th ed). St. Louis: Mosby, p. 720.

94. An experienced licensed practical nurse is observing a new nurse insert a nasal trumpet airway into a client. The experienced licensed practical nurse intervenes if the new nurse does which of the following?

1 Checks the nose for septal deviation
2 Uses a nasal trumpet that is slightly larger than the nares
3 Lubricates the nasal trumpet with a water-soluble lubricant jelly containing a local anesthetic
4 Inserts the nasal trumpet gently following the contour of the nasopharyngeal passageway

Answer: 2

Rationale: The nurse should select a nasal trumpet airway that is slightly smaller than the nares and slightly larger than the suction catheter to be used to suction the client. Options 1, 3, and 4 are correct actions for inserting a nasal trumpet airway.

Test-Taking Strategy: Note the key words "nurse intervenes." These words indicate a false response question and indicate that you are looking for the option that indicates an incorrect action by the new nurse. Noting the words "slightly larger than the nares" and visualizing this procedure will direct you to option 2. Review the procedure for inserting a nasal trumpet and the various test-taking strategies if you had difficulty with this question.

Level of Cognitive Ability: Application
Client Needs: Safe, Effective Care Environment
Integrated Process: Nursing Process/Implementation
Content Area: Leadership/Management

Reference

Harkreader, H. & Hogan, M.A. (2004). *Fundamentals of nursing: caring and clinical judgment* (2nd ed). Philadelphia: Saunders, p. 876.

---

95. A client asks a nurse about the use of a complementary or alternative measure that will assist in promoting sleep. The nurse suggests which of the following?

1 Acupuncture sessions
2 Herbal therapy
3 Muscle relaxation techniques
4 Traditional Chinese medicine sessions

Answer: 3

Rationale: A simple relaxation technique such as muscle relaxation can help reduce any existing anxiety and promote sleep. Acupuncture is an invasive procedure that stimulates certain points on the body by the insertion of special needles to modify the perception of pain, normalize physiological functions, or treat or prevent disease. Traditional Chinese medicine focuses on restoring and maintaining a balanced flow of vital energy with interventions that include acupressure, acupuncture, herbal therapies, diet, meditation, tai chi, and qigong (exercise that focuses on breathing, visualization, and movement). Herbal therapy involves the use of herbs (plant or a plant part). Some herbs have been determined to be safe, yet some, even in small amounts, can be toxic and the nurse would not recommend their use to a client. If the client is taking prescription medications, the client should consult with the health care provider regarding the use of herbs because serious herb-medication interactions can occur.

Test-Taking Strategy: Note the relationship between the words "promoting sleep" and option 3. Also note that options 1, 2, and 4 are similar in that they include invasive measures. Review complementary and alternative therapies that will assist in promoting sleep and the various test-taking strategies if you had difficulty with this question.

Level of Cognitive Ability: Application
Client Needs: Physiological Integrity

Integrated Process: Teaching/Learning
Content Area: Fundamental Skills

Reference
Potter, P. & Perry, A. (2005). *Fundamentals of nursing* (6th ed). St. Louis: Mosby, p. 1217.

---

96. A nurse is caring for a child who sustained a head injury from a fall. The nurse avoids which of the following in the care of the child?
1 Elevating the head of the bed
2 Restricting oral fluids
3 Coughing and deep breathing
4 Performing frequent neurological checks

Answer: 3
Rationale: A child with a head injury is at risk for increased intracranial pressure (ICP). Elevating the head of the bed decreases fluid retention in cerebral tissue and promotes drainage. Fluids may be restricted to reduce the chance of fluid overload and resultant increased ICP. Hypoxia and Valsalva's maneuver associated with coughing both acutely elevate intracranial pressure. Neurological checks should be performed frequently to monitor for increased ICP.

Test-Taking Strategy: Note the key word "avoids" and recall that a head injury places the child at risk for increased ICP. From this point identify the option that would cause an increase in the intracranial pressure. This will direct you to option 3. Review care to the child who sustained a head injury and the various test-taking strategies if you had difficulty with this question.

Level of Cognitive Ability: Application
Client Needs: Physiological Integrity
Integrated Process: Nursing Process/Implementation
Content Area: Child Health

Reference
Price, D. & Gwin, J. (2005). *Thompson's pediatric nursing* (9th ed). Philadelphia: Saunders, pp. 201-203.

---

97. A client with a diagnosis of sickle cell crisis is being admitted to the hospital. The nurse anticipates that which priority intervention will be prescribed?
1 Oxygen administration
2 Red blood cell transfusions
3 Laboratory studies
4 Genetic counseling

Answer: 1
Rationale: Oxygen, intravenous fluids, and pain medication are the primary interventions for treating sickle cell crisis. Red blood cell transfusions may also be prescribed. Laboratory studies may also be prescribed but are not the priority in the care of the client. Genetic counseling is recommended, but not during the acute phase of illness.

Test-Taking Strategy: Note the key word "priority." Option 4 can be eliminated first using Maslow's Hierarchy of Needs theory because this option addresses a psychosocial need, not a physiological one. From the remaining options use the ABCs—airway, breathing, and circulation—to direct you to option 1. Review care to the client in sickle cell crisis and the test-taking strategies for questions that require prioritizing if you had difficulty with this question.

Level of Cognitive Ability: Analysis
Client Needs: Physiological Integrity

Integrated Process: Nursing Process/Planning
Content Area: Delegating/Prioritizing

Reference
Christensen, B. & Kockrow, E. (2003). *Adult health nursing* (4th ed). St. Louis: Mosby, p. 265.

---

98. A nurse is planning the client assignments for the day and most appropriately assigns which client to the nursing assistant?

1 A client scheduled for transfer to the hospital for surgery
2 A client on strict bed rest
3 A client with dyspnea who is receiving oxygen therapy
4 A client with a gastrostomy tube who requires tube feedings every 4 hours

Answer: 2
Rationale: The nurse is legally responsible for client assignments and must assign tasks based on the guidelines of nursing practice acts and the job descriptions of the employing agency. A client scheduled for transfer to the hospital for surgery, a client with dyspnea who is receiving oxygen therapy, or a client with a gastrostomy tube who requires tube feedings every 4 hours has both physiological and psychosocial needs that require care by a licensed nurse. The nursing assistant has been trained to care for a client on bed rest. The nurse provides instructions to the nursing assistant, but the tasks required are within the role description of a nursing assistant.

Test-Taking Strategy: Note that the question asks for the assignment to be delegated to the nursing assistant. When asked questions related to delegation, think about the role description of the employee and the needs of the client. This will direct you to option 2. Review the principles for planning client assignments and the test-taking strategies for answering delegation questions if you had difficulty with this question.

Level of Cognitive Ability: Application
Client Needs: Safe, Effective Care Environment
Integrated Process: Nursing Process/Implementation
Content Area: Delegating/Prioritizing

Reference
Potter, P. & Perry, A. (2005). *Fundamentals of nursing* (6th ed). St. Louis: Mosby, p. 379.

---

99. A client receiving a blood transfusion suddenly develops signs of a blood transfusion reaction. Number in order of priority the actions that the nurse will take. Number 1 is the first nursing action and Number 5 is the last action.

___ Document the occurrence.
___ Stop the blood transfusion and notify a registered nurse.
___ Maintain a patent intravenous line with normal saline solution.
___ Send the blood bag and tubing to the blood bank for examination.

Answer: 51243
Rationale: If a transfusion reaction is suspected, the transfusion is stopped and a registered nurse is immediately notified, who will then contact the physician. Normal saline solution is infused intravenously pending further physician orders. This maintains a patent intravenous access line and aids in maintaining the client's intravascular volume. The physician and blood bank are notified immediately. The nurse would monitor the client's vital signs and urine output, recheck the blood bag's identifying numbers and tags, treat symptoms per physician's orders, send the blood bag and tubing to the blood bank for examination, collect required blood and urine samples, and document the occurrence on the transfusion report and in the client's chart.

___ Monitor the client's vital signs and urine output.

Test-Taking Strategy: The best strategy to use to answer this question is to visualize the occurrence. Stopping the blood is the first action and because the intravenous line needs to remain patent, normal saline solution needs to be infused. Next, use the ABCs—airway, breathing, and circulation—to determine that the client's vital signs need to be monitored. From the remaining interventions, select documentation last because all interventions, including that the nurse sent the blood bag and tubing to the blood bank for examination, need to be documented. Review interventions if a transfusion reaction occurs and the test-taking strategies for answering prioritizing questions if you had difficulty with this question.

Level of Cognitive Ability: Application
Client Needs: Physiological Integrity
Integrated Process: Nursing Process/Implementation
Content Area: Delegating/Prioritizing

Reference
Christensen, B. & Kockrow, E. (2003). *Adult health nursing* (4th ed). St. Louis: Mosby, p. 665.

---

100. A nurse reviews the serum laboratory study results for a client taking chlorothiazide (Diuril) and monitors for which most frequent medication side effect?
1 Hyperphosphatemia
2 Hypocalcemia
3 Hypernatremia
4 Hypokalemia

Answer: 4
Rationale: The client taking a potassium-wasting diuretic such as chlorothiazide should be monitored for decreased potassium levels. Other fluid and electrolyte imbalances that occur with use of this medication include hyponatremia, hypercalcemia, hypomagnesemia, and hypophosphatemia.

Test-Taking Strategy: Focus on the name of the medication and recall that most thiazide diuretic medication names end with the letters "zide." Remember that thiazide diuretics are potassium wasting and hypokalemia is a concern. Review this medication and the test-taking strategies for answering pharmacology questions if you had difficulty with this question.

Level of Cognitive Ability: Application
Client Needs: Physiological Integrity
Integrated Process: Nursing Process/Data Collection
Content Area: Pharmacology

Reference
Skidmore-Roth, L. (2005). *Mosby's drug guide for nurses* (6th ed). St. Louis: Mosby, p. 179.

---

101. A client is taking amiloride hydrochloride (Midamor) daily. The nurse gives the client which of the following instructions about its use?
1 Take the dose in the morning with breakfast.
2 Take the dose on an empty stomach.

Answer: 1
Rationale: Amiloride is a potassium-sparing diuretic used to treat edema or hypertension. A daily dose should be taken in the morning to avoid nocturia. The dose should be taken with food to increase bioavailability.

Test-Taking Strategy: Eliminate options 2, 3, and 4 because they are similar in that they all indicate taking the

3 Take the dose between lunch and dinner.
4 Take the dose at bedtime.

medication dose without food. Review this medication and the test-taking strategies for answering pharmacology questions if you had difficulty with this question.

Level of Cognitive Ability: Application
Client Needs: Physiological Integrity
Integrated Process: Teaching/Learning
Content Area: Pharmacology

Reference
Skidmore-Roth, L. (2005). *Mosby's drug guide for nurses* (6th ed). St. Louis: Mosby, p. 39.

---

102. A client is started on tolbutamide (Orinase) once daily. The nurse observes for which intended effect of this medication?
1 Decreased blood pressure
2 Decreased blood glucose
3 Weight loss
4 Resolution of infection

Answer: 2
Rationale: Tolbutamide is an oral hypoglycemic agent that is taken in the morning. It is not used to decrease blood pressure, enhance weight loss, or treat infection.

Test-Taking Strategy: Note the key words "intended effect." Focus on the name of the medication and recall that most second-generation sulfonylurea medication names end with the letters "mide." Remember that sulfonylureas are used to treat diabetes mellitus. Review this medication and the test-taking strategies for answering pharmacology questions if you had difficulty with this question.

Level of Cognitive Ability: Analysis
Client Needs: Physiological Integrity
Integrated Process: Nursing Process/Evaluation
Content Area: Pharmacology

Reference
Lehne, R. (2004). *Pharmacology for nursing care* (5th ed). Philadelphia: Saunders, p. 608.

---

103. A nurse is providing instructions to a client about quinapril hydrochloride (Accupril). The nurse tells the client:
1 to take the medication with food only.
2 to rise slowly from a lying to a sitting position.
3 to discontinue the medication if nausea occurs.
4 that a therapeutic effect will be seen immediately.

Answer: 2
Rationale: Quinapril hydrochloride is an angiotensin-converting enzyme (ACE) inhibitor used in treating hypertension. The client should be instructed to rise slowly from a lying to a sitting position and to permit the legs to dangle from the bed momentarily before standing, to reduce the hypotensive effect. The medication may be given without regard to food. The client should be instructed to take a noncola carbonated beverage and salted crackers or dry toast if nauseated. A full therapeutic effect may take place in 1 to 2 weeks.

Test-Taking Strategy: Eliminate option 1 because of the absolute word "only" and option 4 because of the word "immediately." Next, focus on the name of the medication and recall that most ACE inhibitor medication names end with the letters "pril" and that these medications are used to treat hypertension. This will direct you to option 2. Review this medication and the test-taking strategies for answering pharmacology questions if you had difficulty with this question.

Level of Cognitive Ability: Application
Client Needs: Physiological Integrity
Integrated Process: Teaching/Learning
Content Area: Pharmacology

Reference

Hodgson, B. & Kizior, R. (2005). *Saunders nursing drug handbook 2005.* Philadelphia: Saunders, p. 916.

---

104. The nurse notes that a client is receiving ganciclovir sodium (Cytovene). The nurse suspects that the client is receiving this medication for the treatment of:

1 cytomegalovirus retinitis.
2 pancreatitis.
3 urolithiasis.
4 nephrotic syndrome.

Answer: 1

Rationale: Ganciclovir sodium is an antiviral medication used to treat cytomegalovirus retinitis (CMV) in immunocompromised clients, CMV gastrointestinal infections, and pneumonitis, and to prevent CMV disease in transplant clients. It is not used to treat pancreatitis, urolithiasis, or nephrotic syndrome.

Test-Taking Strategy: Focus on the name of the medication. Recalling that most antiviral medication names contain the letters "vir" will direct you to option 1. Review this medication and the test-taking strategies for answering pharmacology questions if you had difficulty with this question.

Level of Cognitive Ability: Analysis
Client Needs: Physiological Integrity
Integrated Process: Nursing Process/Data Collection
Content Area: Pharmacology

Reference

Hodgson, B. & Kizior, R. (2005). *Saunders nursing drug handbook 2005.* Philadelphia: Saunders, pp. 483-484.

---

105. A nurse has just finished suctioning a client's tracheostomy. The nurse evaluates the effectiveness of the procedure by checking which item?

1 Respiratory rate
2 Oxygen saturation level
3 Breath sounds
4 Capillary refill

Answer: 3

Rationale: After suctioning a client with or without an artificial airway, the breath sounds are auscultated to determine the extent to which the airways have been cleared of respiratory secretions. The other methods are not as precise indicators as breath sounds for this purpose.

Test-Taking Strategy: Note that this question is an evaluation-type question. Focus on the issue and the effectiveness of suctioning. Recall that the purpose of suctioning is to clear the airways of secretions—this will direct you to option 3. Review the procedure for suctioning and the various test-taking strategies if you had difficulty with this question.

Level of Cognitive Ability: Analysis
Client Needs: Physiological Integrity

Integrated Process: Nursing Process/Evaluation
Content Area: Adult Health/Respiratory

Reference

Harkreader, H. & Hogan, M.A. (2004). *Fundamentals of nursing: caring and clinical judgment* (2nd ed). Philadelphia: Saunders, p. 867.

---

106. A licensed practical nurse is assisting a registered nurse in carrying out emergency care measures for a postoperative client who is suspected of having a pulmonary embolism. The licensed practical nurse prepares to implement which of the following physician orders first?

1 Obtaining an arterial blood gas specimen
2 Applying oxygen
3 Starting an intravenous line
4 Obtaining an electrocardiogram

Answer: 2

Rationale: The client needs immediate oxygen as a result of hypoxemia, which is most often accompanied by respiratory distress and cyanosis. The client should have an intravenous line for administration of emergency medications such as morphine sulfate. An electrocardiogram is useful in determining the presence of possible right ventricular hypertrophy and an arterial blood gas specimen is drawn to assess oxygenation, respiratory, and metabolic status. All of the interventions listed are appropriate, but the client needs the oxygen first.

Test-Taking Strategy: Note the key word "first." Use the ABCs—airway, breathing, and circulation. This will direct you to option 2. Review care to the client experiencing pulmonary embolism and the test-taking strategies for answering prioritizing questions if you had difficulty with this question.

Level of Cognitive Ability: Application
Client Needs: Physiological Integrity
Integrated Process: Nursing Process/Implementation
Content Area: Delegating/Prioritizing

Reference

Christensen, B. & Kockrow, E. (2003). *Adult health nursing* (4th ed). St. Louis: Mosby, p. 392.

---

107. A nurse is collecting data about a client's cigarette smoking habit. The client admits to smoking 3 packs per day for the past 10 years. The nurse documents that the client has a smoking history of how many pack-years?
Answer: ______________

Answer: 30

Rationale: The standard method for quantifying smoking history is to multiply the number of packs smoked per day by the number of years of smoking. The number is recorded as the number of pack-years. The calculation for the number of pack-years for the client who has smoked 3 packs per day for 10 years is: 3 packs $\times$ 10 years = 30 pack-years.

Test-Taking Strategy: Focus on the information in the question. This question requires simple multiplication of the number of packs of cigarettes smoked per day by the number of years of smoking. Use a calculator to multiply and then verify your answer before documenting it. Review respiratory data collection procedures and the various test-taking strategies if you had difficulty with this question.

Level of Cognitive Ability: Comprehension
Client Needs: Health Promotion and Maintenance

Integrated Process: Nursing Process/Data Collection
Content Area: Adult Health/Respiratory

Reference

Lewis, S., Heitkemper, M., & Dirksen, S. (2004). *Medical-surgical nursing: assessment and management of clinical problems* (6th ed). St. Louis: Mosby, p. 552.

---

108. A newborn is diagnosed with imperforate anus and the parents ask the nurse to describe this abnormality. The nurse bases the response on which characteristic of the disorder?

1 Absence of the anus in its normal position in the perineum
2 Invagination of a section of the intestine into the distal bowel
3 The infrequent and difficult passage of dry stools
4 The presence of fecal incontinence

Answer: 1

Rationale: Imperforate anus (anal atresia, anal agenesis) is the incomplete development or absence of the anus in its normal position in the perineum. Option 2 describes intussusception. Option 3 describes constipation. Option 4 describes encopresis. Constipation can affect any child at any time, although it peaks at age 2 to 3 years. Encopresis generally affects preschool and school-age children.

Test-Taking Strategy: Noting the relationship between the disorder imperforate anus and the words "absence of the anus" in option 1 will direct you to this option. Also, noting that the question addresses a newborn will direct you to the correct option. Review the characteristics of this disorder and the various test-taking strategies if you had difficulty with this question.

Level of Cognitive Ability: Application
Client Needs: Physiological Integrity
Integrated Process: Teaching/Learning
Content Area: Maternity/Postpartum

Reference

Wong, D. & Hockenberry, M. (2003). *Wong's nursing care of infants and children* (7th ed). St. Louis: Mosby, pp. 466, 469.

---

109. A nurse is called by a group of neighbors to the scene of a house fire where a person escaped but sustained burns to the face and neck and is having slight trouble breathing. The nurse takes which priority action while waiting for emergency medical services to arrive?

1 Places a wet towel over the victim's face and places the client in a supine position
2 Keeps the client standing and supports the client while he leans up against a tree for support
3 Assists the client to a comfortable position and monitors for airway patency

Answer: 3

Rationale: The client requires continued monitoring by the nurse to ensure that his condition does not deteriorate, or to provide assistance if it does. Although the client is having only slight trouble breathing and is managing his own airway at this time, inhalation injury could cause laryngeal edema and subsequent airway obstruction. A supine position can make breathing more difficult for the client and can enhance edema development. Option 2 does nothing to assist the client and could cause added fatigue if the client becomes weak or has difficulty standing. Option 4 is unnecessary if the client is already breathing.

Test-Taking Strategy: Focus on the data in the question and use the ABCs—airway, breathing, and circulation. This will direct you to option 3. Review care to the burn client and the test-taking strategies for answering prioritizing questions if you had difficulty with this question.

4 Places the client in a supine position and begins rescue breathing

Level of Cognitive Ability: Application
Client Needs: Physiological Integrity
Integrated Process: Nursing Process/Implementation
Content Area: Adult Health/Integumentary

Reference

Ignatavicius, D. & Workman, M. (2006). *Medical-surgical nursing: critical thinking for collaborative care* (5th ed). Philadelphia: Saunders, p. 1627.

---

110. A mental health nurse is performing an initial interview with a depressed client who has suicidal ideation and is being admitted to the mental health unit. Following the interview, which nursing intervention is carried out first?

1. Isolate the client from other clients in the nursing unit.
2. Provide the client with diversional activities.
3. Communicate the client's risk for suicide to all team members.
4. Develop a plan of activities for the client.

Answer: 3

Rationale: The first priority intervention for the suicidal individual is to communicate the risk for suicide to all team members. The plan of activities (options 2 and 4) would take second priority. Client isolation is inappropriate. The client should be placed on one-on-one supervision if the client is suicidal.

Test-Taking Strategy: Note the key word "first." Eliminate options 2 and 4 because they are similar. From the remaining options, the priority item is communication to other members of the health care team, with the ultimate aim to increase client safety. Review care to the client with suicidal ideation and the test-taking strategies for answering prioritizing questions if you had difficulty with this question.

Level of Cognitive Ability: Application
Client Needs: Safe, Effective Care Environment
Integrated Process: Nursing Process/Implementation
Content Area: Mental Health

Reference

Morrison-Valfre, M. (2005). *Foundations of mental health care* (3rd ed). St. Louis: Mosby, p. 281.

---

111. A nurse is caring for a client with pancreatic cancer who is scheduled for a radical pancreaticoduodenectomy. The nurse best meets the psychosocial needs of the client by:

1. giving the client time to be alone to think about the outcome of the surgery.
2. ensuring that the client has been visited by a member of the clergy.
3. giving the client information about the surgery.
4. exploring the meaning of the surgery with the client.

Answer: 4

Rationale: The nurse should explore the meaning of the surgery in terms of pain, body image changes, fear, and dying from the client's perspective. It is then possible for the nurse to work effectively with the client. Option 4 is a direct action by the nurse that can best meet the client's need because it addresses the client's feelings. Options 1, 2, and 3 do not address the client's feelings.

Test-Taking Strategy: Note the key word "best." Use therapeutic communication techniques and the clinical problem-solving process (nursing process) to answer the question. Only option 4 addresses both data collection and the client's feelings. Review therapeutic communication techniques and the test-taking strategies for answering prioritizing questions if you had difficulty with this question.

Level of Cognitive Ability: Application

Client Needs: Psychosocial Integrity
Integrated Process: Caring
Content Area: Adult Health/Oncology

References

Christensen, B. & Kockrow, E. (2003). *Adult health nursing* (4th ed). St. Louis: Mosby, p. 246.

Potter, P. & Perry, A. (2005). *Fundamentals of nursing* (6th ed). St. Louis: Mosby, p. 437.

---

112. An antepartum client at 32 weeks of gestation positioned herself supine on the examination table to await the obstetrician. The nurse enters the examination room and the client says, "I'm feeling a little lightheaded and sick to my stomach." The nurse recognizes that the client may be experiencing vena cava syndrome (hypotensive syndrome) and takes which immediate action?

1 Gives the client an emesis basin
2 Places a cool cloth on the client's forehead
3 Places a folded towel or sheet under the client's right hip
4 Calls the obstetrician to see the client

Answer: 3

Rationale: Lying supine (on the back) applies additional gravity pressure on the abdominal blood vessels (iliac vessels, inferior vena cava, and ascending aorta), increasing compression and impeding blood flow and cardiac output. This results in hypotension, dizziness, nausea, pallor, clammy (cool, damp) skin, and sweating. Raising one hip higher than the other reduces the pressure on the vena cava, restoring the circulation and relieving the symptoms. Although an emesis basin and a cool cloth placed on the forehead may be helpful, these are not the immediate actions. It is not necessary to call the obstetrician immediately unless the client's complaints are unrelieved following repositioning.

Test-Taking Strategy: Note the key word "immediate." Focus on the information in the question and the goals of care. In other words, think about what complications that you want to prevent. Remember that if a question requires you to prioritize and one of the options relates to positioning a client, that option may be the correct one. Review care to the client experiencing vena cava syndrome and the test-taking strategies for answering prioritizing questions if you had difficulty with this question.

Level of Cognitive Ability: Application
Client Needs: Physiological Integrity
Integrated Process: Nursing Process/Implementation
Content Area: Maternity/Antepartum

Reference

Leifer, G. (2003). *Introduction to maternity & pediatric nursing* (4th ed). Philadelphia: Saunders, p. 55.

---

113. A postoperative client is angry after an argument on the telephone with her son and tells the nurse about her conversation. Which statement by the nurse is therapeutic?

1 "All mothers have arguments with their children."
2 "That's not very kind of your son. Doesn't he realize that you are trying to recuperate from surgery?"

Answer: 3

Rationale: Option 3 provides an opportunity for the client to further share and discuss feelings. Option 1 is a stereotypical comment. Options 2 and 4 seem to console the client, but they indicate that the nurse has taken "a side" in the argument, which is nontherapeutic.

Test-Taking Strategy: Use therapeutic communication techniques. Remember to address the client's concerns or feelings and elicit further information from the client. This will direct you to option 3. Review therapeutic communica-

3 "You seem quite upset."
4 "You need to focus your energy on building your strength."

tion techniques and the test-taking strategies for answering communication questions if you had difficulty with this question.

Level of Cognitive Ability: Application
Client Needs: Psychosocial Integrity
Integrated Process: Communication and Documentation
Content Area: Mental Health

Reference
Morrison-Valfre, M. (2005). *Foundations of mental health care* (3rd ed). St. Louis: Mosby, p. 88.

---

114. A client who had a mitral valve replacement is having a slow recovery. The client states, "I need to get better so that I can go hunting this season. If I'm not going to get better, I would be better off dead." Which response by the nurse is therapeutic?
1 "Can you tell me more about the way you feel?"
2 "Try to be a bit more positive."
3 "There is plenty of hunting seasons ahead of you. Let's focus on what you need to do now to get better."
4 "I know what you are saying. My husband is an avid hunter."

Answer: 1
Rationale: Option 1 encourages the client to share his or her fears. All of the incorrect options represent a block to communication because they do not acknowledge the client's feelings or concerns and they put the client's feelings on hold.

Test-Taking Strategy: Use therapeutic communication techniques. Option 1 addresses the client's feelings, is nonjudgmental, and promotes further communication. Remember the client's feelings are the priority. Review therapeutic communication techniques and the test-taking strategies for answering communication questions if you had difficulty with this question.

Level of Cognitive Ability: Application
Client Needs: Psychosocial Integrity
Integrated Process: Communication and Documentation
Content Area: Adult Health/Cardiovascular

Reference
Harkreader, H. & Hogan, M.A. (2004). *Fundamentals of nursing: caring and clinical judgment* (2nd ed). Philadelphia: Saunders, pp. 251, 255-257.

---

115. Levothyroxine sodium (Synthroid) is prescribed for a client with hypothyroidism. The nurse tells the client that this medication will result in:
1 decreased body temperature.
2 reduced gastric acid production.
3 increased energy level.
4 faster weight gain.

Answer: 3
Rationale: Levothyroxine sodium is a synthetically prepared thyroid hormone that increases body metabolism and the client's energy level. It promotes weight loss and increases body temperature. It does not affect gastric acid production.

Test-Taking Strategy: Note that the question indicates the client's diagnosis. Also recall that many thyroid hormone medications contain "thy" in their name. Remember, if the medication is used to treat hypothyroidism, the medication effects must be the opposite of the disease symptoms. This will direct you to option 3. Review this medication and the test-taking strategies for answering pharmacology questions if you had difficulty with this question.

Level of Cognitive Ability: Application
Client Needs: Physiological Integrity
Integrated Process: Teaching/Learning
Content Area: Adult Health/Endocrine

Reference

Hodgson, B. & Kizior, R. (2005). *Saunders nursing drug handbook 2005.* Philadelphia: Saunders, p. 632.

---

116. A client is admitted to the hospital after a high-voltage electrical injury. The client has dark-colored urine and urinalysis results are positive for myoglobin. The nurse places highest priority on which nursing action?

1 Monitoring the urine output and examining the urine for color, odor, and the presence of particulate matter
2 Obtaining a nasogastric tube and lubricant from the supply area in preparation for insertion
3 Ambulating the client frequently
4 Reassuring the client that the injury will resolve without residual effects

Answer: 1

Rationale: To prevent myoglobin from precipitating in the renal tubules, fluid intake is increased orally or by the intravenous route to maintain an adequate urine output of 30 to 50 mL or 0.5 mL/kg/hour in an adult client. There are no data in the question that indicate that a nasogastric tube is needed. Even so, this action is not the priority. A client with an acute injury would not be ambulated frequently. Option 4 is incorrect because it provides false reassurance.

Test-Taking Strategy: Note the key word "priority." Also note the relationship between the abnormal urine sample finding in the question and option 1. Also, option 3 can be eliminated because of the word "frequently." Option 4 can be eliminated using Maslow's Hierarchy of Needs theory because it is unrelated to a physiological need. Review care to the client who sustained a high-voltage electrical injury and the test-taking strategies for answering prioritizing questions if you had difficulty with this question.

Level of Cognitive Ability: Application
Client Needs: Physiological Integrity
Integrated Process: Nursing Process/Implementation
Content Area: Adult Health/Integumentary

References

Ignatavicius, D. & Workman, M. (2006). *Medical-surgical nursing: critical thinking for collaborative care* (5th ed). Philadelphia: Saunders, pp. 1629-1630.
Lewis, S., Heitkemper, M., & Dirksen, S. (2004). *Medical-surgical nursing: assessment and management of clinical problems* (6th ed). St. Louis: Mosby, pp. 517-518.

---

117. A woman is treated in the emergency department for a broken clavicle and a black eye. The woman reports that she sustained the injury from falling off of a stepstool while trying to change window curtains. If the nurse suspects physical abuse by the client's husband, which statement best encourages the client to share this information with the nurse?

Answer: 1

Rationale: The best approach to asking a woman about violence is to approach the client in a caring and nonthreatening manner. Options 2 and 3 are confrontational, and option 4 assumes that the client desires a restraining order. Option 2 is also incorrect because it is a judgmental statement that is likely to put the client on the defensive. Only option 1 allows the client the right to reject or accept further intervention by the nurse and is a caring response.

1 "At times I see women who have been hurt by their husband. Have you been hurt by anyone?"
2 "You're black eye sure doesn't seem as though it could have happened by accident."
3 "That black eye looks awfully painful. Did your husband hit you?"
4 "If your husband is abusing you, you can take him to court or get a restraining order."

Test-Taking Strategy: Use therapeutic communication techniques. Option 1 is the only therapeutic statement, is supportive and displays caring, and provides the client the opportunity to talk about the situation if she so desires. Review care to the client suspected of abuse and the test-taking strategies for answering communication questions if you had difficulty with this question.

Level of Cognitive Ability: Application
Client Needs: Psychosocial Integrity
Integrated Process: Caring
Content Area: Mental Health

Reference
Morrison-Valfre, M. (2005). *Foundations of mental health care* (3rd ed). St. Louis: Mosby, pp. 88, 268.

---

118. A nurse is caring for a woman who has just undergone an emergency cesarean section. In preparing to discuss postoperative and home care measures the nurse should first:
1 determine the client's ability to take in and process information.
2 make referrals to community agencies and support groups as needed.
3 provide comprehensive information about recovery and child care.
4 provide routine information according to standard teaching protocols.

Answer: 1
Rationale: The residual physical and psychological effects of emergency cesarean section can interfere with the client's ability to concentrate and learn new information. Therefore the nurse should first determine the anxiety level, level of consciousness, and ability to take in and process information. Teaching is likely to be ineffective if the client is not able to process information.

Test-Taking Strategy: Note the key word "first." Use the clinical problem-solving process (nursing process) and teaching/learning principles to answer the question. Recalling that data collection is the first step in the nursing process will direct you to option 1. Review home care measures for the client following an emergency cesarean section and the test-taking strategies for answering prioritizing questions if you had difficulty with this question.

Level of Cognitive Ability: Application
Client Needs: Health Promotion and Maintenance
Integrated Process: Nursing Process/Implementation
Content Area: Maternity/Postpartum

Reference
Leifer, G. (2005). *Maternity nursing* (9th ed). Philadelphia: Saunders, p. 252.

---

119. A client is scheduled for electroconvulsive therapy. The client says to the nurse, "I'm so afraid that it will hurt, and will make me worse off than I am." The nurse makes which therapeutic statement to the client?
1 "Can you tell me what you understand about the procedure?"

Answer: 1
Rationale: Option 1 is a therapeutic response that explores the client's feelings, determines the level of client understanding about the procedure, and displays caring. Option 2 does not address the client's fears and puts the client's feelings on hold. Option 3 diminishes the client's feelings by directing attention away from the client and to the doctor's importance. Option 4 demeans the client and does not encourage further sharing by the client.

2 "Those are very normal fears, but please be assured that everything will be okay."
3 "Try not to worry. This is a well-known and easy procedure for the doctor."
4 "Your fears are a sign that you really should have this procedure."

Test-Taking Strategy: Use therapeutic communication techniques, and remember to focus on the client's feelings and concerns. Option 1 is the only option that addresses the client's feelings, encourages client verbalization, and displays caring. Review therapeutic communication techniques and the test-taking strategies for answering communication questions if you had difficulty with this question.

Level of Cognitive Ability: Application
Client Needs: Psychosocial Integrity
Integrated Process: Caring
Content Area: Mental Health

Reference

Morrison-Valfre, M. (2005). *Foundations of mental health care* (3rd ed). St. Louis: Mosby, pp. 88, 218.

---

120. A 16-year-old client who underwent emergency surgery for a ruptured appendix refuses to allow the nurse to change the abdominal dressing, saying, "Go away. There is nothing wrong with this dressing." Which nursing response is best?
1 "I promise to do this really quickly, and then I will leave you alone."
2 "I'll draw the curtain and expose only the area on your abdomen that is needed. Can I go ahead with that?"
3 "You can refuse the dressing change at this time, but your friends can't visit you until it is done."
4 "Please don't be upset with me. I am just doing my job."

Answer: 2
Rationale: The primary developmental need of the hospitalized adolescent is maintenance of privacy, modesty, and control. The correct option strives to meet these needs. Options 1 and 4 do not address the client's concerns, and option 3 contains a threat.

Test-Taking Strategy: Note the key words "16-year-old client." Remember the developmental issues of the adolescent when answering this question. Also, use therapeutic communication techniques. Option 2 is the only option that focuses on the client's feelings and needs. Review therapeutic communication techniques and the test-taking strategies for answering communication questions if you had difficulty with this question.

Level of Cognitive Ability: Application
Client Needs: Health Promotion and Maintenance
Integrated Process: Communication and Documentation
Content Area: Child Health

References

Harkreader, H. & Hogan, M.A. (2004). *Fundamentals of nursing: caring and clinical judgment* (2nd ed). Philadelphia: Saunders, pp. 251, 255-257.
Price, D. & Gwin, J. (2005). *Thompson's pediatric nursing* (9th ed). Philadelphia: Saunders, p. 300.

---

121. A nurse is teaching a client with left-sided weakness how to safely use a cane. The nurse tells the client to hold the cane with the:
1 left hand, 6 inches lateral to the left foot.
2 left hand, placing the cane in front of the left foot.
3 right hand, 6 inches lateral to the right foot.

Answer: 3
Rationale: The client is taught to hold the cane on the opposite side of the weakness because with normal walking the opposite arm and leg move together (called reciprocal motion). A client with left-sided weakness would hold the cane in the right hand. The cane is placed 6 inches lateral to the fifth toe. Options 1, 2, and 4 are incorrect.

Test-Taking Strategy: Visualize the procedure for walking with a cane. Recalling that the cane is held at the client's

4 right hand, placing the cane in front of the right foot.

side, not in front, helps you to eliminate options 2 and 4 first. Knowing that the correct method is to have the cane positioned on the stronger side helps you to eliminate option 1. Review the procedure for teaching a client how to use a cane and the various test-taking strategies if you had difficulty with this question.

Level of Cognitive Ability: Application
Client Needs: Safe, Effective Care Environment
Integrated Process: Teaching/Learning
Content Area: Adult Health/Musculoskeletal

Reference

Harkreader, H. & Hogan, M.A. (2004). *Fundamentals of nursing: caring and clinical judgment* (2nd ed). Philadelphia: Saunders, p. 793.

---

122. A nurse is assisting in caring for a client 1 day after gastrectomy. The client has a nasogastric (NG) tube and the nurse notes that the tube is draining brown-tinged secretions. Which of the following is the appropriate nursing intervention?

1 Notify a registered nurse immediately.
2 Document the findings.
3 Reposition the client.
4 Irrigate the NG tube.

Answer: 2

Rationale: After gastrectomy, drainage from the NG tube is normally bloody for 24 hours and then changes to brown tinged and then to yellow or clear. The nurse should document this finding. There is no need to notify a registered nurse immediately because this finding is expected. Although the client is repositioned in the postoperative period, this action is unrelated to the data in the question. After gastrectomy, an NG tube should not be irrigated without specific physician's orders to do so.

Test-Taking Strategy: Focus on the key words "1 day after gastrectomy." Recalling that the gastrointestinal drainage would be brown tinged at this time will direct you to option 2. Review the expected findings following gastrectomy and the various test-taking strategies if you had difficulty with this question.

Level of Cognitive Ability: Application
Client Needs: Physiological Integrity
Integrated Process: Nursing Process/Implementation
Content Area: Adult Health/Gastrointestinal

Reference

Phipps, W., Monahan, F., Sands, J., Marek, J., & Neighbors, M. (2003). *Medical-surgical nursing: health and illness perspectives* (7th ed). St. Louis: Mosby, p. 1048.

---

123. A nurse has provided instructions to the mother of a child with a urinary tract infection about measures to prevent reinfection. Which statement by the mother indicates a need for further instructions?

1 "I should wipe my child from front to back after urination or a bowel movement."

Answer: 3

Rationale: The parents should be taught to wipe the child from front to back after urination or a bowel movement to avoid moving bacteria from the anus to the urethra. Fluid intake, including water, should be encouraged. The child should avoid holding urine, should urinate as needed, and should empty the bladder with each voiding. Bubble baths are avoided secondary to possible urethral irritation.

2 "I should increase my child's fluid intake."
3 "I should encourage my child to hold the urine and to urinate at least four times a day."
4 "I should avoid the use of bubble baths with my child."

Test-Taking Strategy: Note the key words "need for further instructions." This question is a false response one. Therefore you are looking for the option that indicates that further teaching needs to be done. Careful reading of the options and applying principles related to prevention of urinary tract infections will direct you to option 3. Review client instructions related to a urinary tract infection and the various test-taking strategies if you had difficulty with this question.

Level of Cognitive Ability: Comprehension
Client Needs: Health Promotion and Maintenance
Integrated Process: Nursing Process/Evaluation
Content Area: Child Health

References

Price, D. & Gwin, J. (2005). *Thompson's pediatric nursing* (9th ed). Philadelphia: Saunders, p. 245.
Wong, D. & Hockenberry, M. (2003). *Nursing care of infants and children* (7th ed). St. Louis: Mosby, p. 1268.

---

124. The nurse notes that a new postoperative client is experiencing tachycardia and tachypnea. The nurse takes the client's blood pressure and notes that it is 88/60 mm Hg. The nurse takes which immediate action?
1 Checks the hourly urine output
2 Checks the intravenous site for infiltration
3 Elevates the client's feet, keeping the head slightly elevated
4 Turns the client on the right side

Answer: 3
Rationale: The client is exhibiting signs of shock and requires emergency intervention. Placing the client flat or with the head slightly elevated and elevating the feet increases venous return and subsequently blood pressure. The nurse also notifies a registered nurse, who will then contact the physician. The nurse also verifies the client's volume status by checking the urine output and whether the intravenous fluid is running. Turning the client onto the right side will not assist the client in this situation.

Test-Taking Strategy: Focus on the information in the question and note the key word "immediate." After determining that this is an emergency situation, look for the option that supports the ABCs—airway, breathing, circulation. Because only option 3 supports the client's immediate physiological needs, the nurse should take this action immediately. Review care to the postoperative client and the test-taking strategies for answering prioritizing questions if you had difficulty with this question.

Level of Cognitive Ability: Application
Client Needs: Physiological Integrity
Integrated Process: Nursing Process/Implementation
Content Area: Adult Health/Cardiovascular

Reference

Linton, A. & Maebius, N. (2003). *Introduction to medical-surgical nursing* (3rd ed). Philadelphia: Saunders, p. 253.

125. The nurse tells a client scheduled to have a lumbar puncture that he will be placed in a knee-chest position for the procedure. When the client asks the nurse why this position is necessary, the nurse responds that it:

1 provides for greater client comfort.
2 prevents leakage of fluid from the brain.
3 allows for a smaller needle to be used.
4 increases the spacing between the vertebrae.

Answer: 4

Rationale: The anatomy of the vertebral column is such that curving the structure provides for more open spacing in the L3-L5 area. The choice of the size of the needle for puncture does not depend on position. Also, client position is not related to cerebrospinal fluid leakage. Pillows and support of the nursing staff aid in client comfort.

Test-Taking Strategy: Note the issue, the purpose of a knee-chest position. Visualizing this position will direct you to the correct option. Review this procedure and the various test-taking strategies if you had difficulty with this question.

Level of Cognitive Ability: Application
Client Needs: Physiological Integrity
Integrated Process: Nursing Process/Implementation
Content Area: Adult Health/Neurological

References

Chernecky, C. & Berger, B. (2004). *Laboratory tests and diagnostic procedures* (4th ed). Philadelphia: Saunders, p. 739.
Christensen, B. & Kockrow, E. (2003). *Adult health nursing* (4th ed). St. Louis: Mosby, p. 610.

---

126. A client comes to the hospital emergency department and verbalizes complaints of severe right lower abdominal pain characteristic of appendicitis. The client does not have any health insurance. The nurse understands that legally the hospital must:

1 refer the client to the nearest public hospital.
2 have a physician see the client before admission.
3 provide uncompensated care in emergency situations.
4 respect the family's requests to admit their family member to the hospital.

Answer: 3

Rationale: Federal law and many state laws require that hospitals must provide emergency care. The client can be transferred only after the client has been medically screened and stabilized. The client must give consent for the transfer and there must be a facility that will accept the client. Options 1, 2, and 4 do not fully address the legal requirements for emergency care.

Test-Taking Strategy: Note the key words "does not have any health insurance" and the word "legally." Noting that the situation presented is an emergency will direct you to option 3. Option 3 is the option that addresses the legal scope of providing emergency care. Review the legal issues related to providing emergency care and the various test-taking strategies if you had difficulty with this question.

Level of Cognitive Ability: Comprehension
Client Needs: Safe, Effective Care Environment
Integrated Process: Nursing Process/Planning
Content Area: Leadership/Management

References

Brent, N. (2001). *Nurses and the law* (2nd ed). Philadelphia: Saunders, pp. 366-368.
Potter, P. & Perry, A. (2005). *Fundamentals of nursing* (6th ed). St. Louis: Mosby, p. 43.

127. While caring for a client in labor, the nurse suspects an umbilical cord prolapse. The nurse should immediately:

1 adjust the bed to the Trendelenburg position.
2 encourage the woman to push with each contraction.
3 set up for an emergency cesarean section.
4 calmly reassure the woman and her partner that all possible measures are being taken.

Answer: 1

Rationale: Adjusting the bed into Trendelenburg (mattress flat, foot of bed elevated) position uses gravity to reverse the direction of the pressure, keeping the presenting part off the umbilical cord. In addition, the knee-chest, or modified Sims' position can be used. Pushing with contractions is contraindicated because it will push the presenting part against the cord. Not all prolapsed cords require a cesarean section. The nurse should reassure the woman and her partner after placing the woman in the Trendelenburg position.

Test-Taking Strategy: Note the key word "immediately" and visualize the situation. Eliminate option 4 first using Maslow's Hierarchy of Needs theory because it does not address a physiological need. From the remaining options, select the option that addresses the physiological safety of the primary client (the fetus). Also, remember in a prioritizing question if repositioning is indicated in one of the options, that option may be correct. Review immediate interventions for umbilical cord prolapse and the test-taking strategies for answering prioritizing questions if you had difficulty with this question.

Level of Cognitive Ability: Application
Client Needs: Physiological Integrity
Integrated Process: Nursing Process/Implementation
Content Area: Maternity/Intrapartum

Reference

Leifer, G. (2005). *Maternity nursing* (9th ed). Philadelphia: Saunders, p. 248.

---

128. A nurse hears a cardiac monitor alarm, rushes into the client's room, and notes a straight line on the monitor screen. The nurse takes which action first?

1 Calls a code
2 Turns up the amplitude on the monitor
3 Checks the client
4 Confirms the rhythm using a different cardiac lead

Answer: 3

Rationale: If the monitor alarm sounds, the nurse should first check the clinical status of the client to see if the problem is an actual dysrhythmia or a malfunction of the monitoring system. Options 1, 2, and 4 are not the first actions.

Test-Taking Strategy: Note the key word "first." Use the steps of the clinical problem-solving process (nursing process). Remember, data collection is the first step, so check the client first. Review care to the client on a cardiac monitor and the test-taking strategies for answering prioritizing questions if you had difficulty with this question.

Level of Cognitive Ability: Application
Client Needs: Physiological Integrity
Integrated Process: Nursing Process/Implementation
Content Area: Adult Health/Cardiovascular

References

Christensen, B. & Kockrow, E. (2003). *Adult health nursing* (4th ed). St. Louis: Mosby, p. 293.
Lewis, S., Heitkemper, M., & Dirksen, S. (2004). *Medical-surgical nursing: assessment and management of clinical problems* (6th ed). St. Louis: Mosby, pp. 864-865.

129. A nurse is preparing to care for a woman victimized by physical abuse. The nurse should appropriately plan to first:

1 talk to the woman about the fact that she might have provoked the abuse.
2 support the woman and facilitate access to a safe environment.
3 establish firm time lines for the woman to make necessary changes in her life situation.
4 reinforce that dealing with the psychological aspects is of the highest priority.

Answer: 2
Rationale: The nurse must provide emotional support to the client and measures to ensure a safe environment. Option 1 fosters the notion that the client is at fault. In options 3 and 4 the nurse may be making unreasonable demands, which could cause further distress for the client.

Test-Taking Strategy: Note the key word "first." Use Maslow's Hierarchy of Needs theory to assist in directing you to option 2. Remember that if a physiological need does not exist in one of the options, then a safety need is the priority. Also, option 2 provides support to the client. Review care to the client victimized by physical abuse and the test-taking strategies for answering prioritizing questions if you had difficulty with this question.

Level of Cognitive Ability: Application
Client Needs: Safe, Effective Care Environment
Integrated Process: Caring
Content Area: Mental Health

Reference
Morrison-Valfre, M. (2005). *Foundations of mental health care* (3rd ed). St. Louis: Mosby, p. 275.

---

130. A nurse is assigned to care for an obstetric client with acquired immunodeficiency syndrome (AIDS). The nurse develops a plan of care for the client and includes which priority client goal in the plan?

1 The client will not have sexual relations during the remainder of the pregnancy.
2 The client will not develop an opportunistic infection during the remainder of the pregnancy.
3 The client knows about local AIDS support groups.
4 The client moves through the grief process.

Answer: 2
Rationale: AIDS is caused by the retrovirus human immunodeficiency virus (HIV) that invades T lymphocytes. This disables the body's ability to fight infection. Nursing goals are directed toward the prevention of infections. Sexual relations are not contraindicated if protective devices are properly used. Options 3 and 4 are the focus of interventions, not goals.

Test-Taking Strategy: Note the key word "priority." Focusing on the issue, client goals, will assist in eliminating options 3 and 4. Option 1 is unrealistic, is unnecessary if protective devices are properly used, and may be a goal that the client will not adhere to. Also use Maslow's Hierarchy of Needs theory and note that option 2 addresses a physiological need. Review care to the obstetric client with AIDS and the test-taking strategies for answering prioritizing questions if you had difficulty with this question.

Level of Cognitive Ability: Application
Client Needs: Safe, Effective Care Environment
Integrated Process: Nursing Process/Planning
Content Area: Maternity/Antepartum

Reference
Leifer, G. (2005). *Maternity nursing* (9th ed). Philadelphia: Saunders, p. 339.

131. An older woman is admitted to the acute psychiatric unit with a diagnosis of moderate depression. The client is unclean, her hair is uncombed, and she is inappropriately dressed. She is accompanied by her adult daughter, who is very upset about her mother's lack of interest in her appearance. The nurse appropriately alleviates the daughter's concern by telling her that:

1 hygiene is not important to those who are depressed.

2 the nurse will assist her mother in meeting hygiene needs until she is able to resume self-care.

3 client self-esteem needs take priority over appearances.

4 group peer pressure on the unit will soon have her mother attending to her hygiene needs.

Answer: 2

Rationale: Both the client and family should know that the nurse will assist the client until the client can resume self-care activities. The client is experiencing psychomotor retardation and decreased energy at this time and requires assistance. Options 1, 3, and 4 will not alleviate the daughter's concern.

Test-Taking Strategy: Focus on the issue, alleviating the daughter's concern. Use Maslow's Hierarchy of Needs theory. Only option 2 addresses the client's physiological needs. Review care to the client with depression and the various test-taking strategies if you had difficulty with this question.

Level of Cognitive Ability: Application
Client Needs: Psychosocial Integrity
Integrated Process: Caring
Content Area: Mental Health

Reference

Morrison-Valfre, M. (2005). *Foundations of mental health care* (3rd ed). St. Louis: Mosby, pp. 215, 221

---

132. An emergency department nurse prepares to care for a client with a suspected fracture of the right radial bone. The nurse should initially do which of the following?

1 Obtain an x-ray of the right arm

2 Place a plastic cast on the right arm

3 Place the right arm in a sling and arrange for an orthopedic consultation

4 Check for distal pulses and the neurovascular status of the right arm

Answer: 4

Rationale: The initial intervention is to check for distal pulses and the neurovascular status of the affected extremity. A physician is responsible for obtaining a radiograph and applying a cast. It may be appropriate to place the extremity in a sling, but this is not the initial action.

Test-Taking Strategy: Note the key word "initially." Use both the steps of the clinical problem-solving process (nursing process) and the ABCs—airway, breathing, and circulation—to answer the question. Option 4 addresses data collection and circulation. Review care to the client with a fracture and the test-taking strategies for answering prioritizing questions if you had difficulty with this question.

Level of Cognitive Ability: Application
Client Needs: Physiological Integrity
Integrated Process: Nursing Process/Implementation
Content Area: Adult Health/Musculoskeletal

References

Christensen, B. & Kockrow, E. (2003). *Adult health nursing* (4th ed). St. Louis: Mosby, p. 143.
Phipps, W., Monahan, F., Sands, J., Marek, J., & Neighbors, M. (2003). *Medical-surgical nursing: health and illness perspectives* (7th ed). St. Louis: Mosby, p. 1478.

133. A nurse finds a hospitalized client lying on the floor after sustaining a fall and hitting his head on the bedside table. The client's breathing is shallow and a pulse is present. The nurse takes which action first?

1 Gets the client back to bed
2 Checks vital signs and level of consciousness
3 Calls a code
4 Calls the client's family

Answer: 2

Rationale: Because the client is breathing and has a pulse, the nurse needs to check the client before taking any other action. Level of consciousness and vital signs should be determined particularly in a client who sustained a head injury. The client is not moved until the extent of the injuries is determined. The nurse notifies a registered nurse, who then contacts the physician. Calling a code is not indicated at this time.

Test-Taking Strategy: Note the key word "first." Focus on the data in the question and note that the client is breathing and has a pulse. Next, use the steps of the clinical problem-solving process (nursing process). Only option 2 addresses data collection. Review care to the client who sustains a fall and the test-taking strategies for answering prioritizing questions if you had difficulty with this question.

Level of Cognitive Ability: Application
Client Needs: Physiological Integrity
Integrated Process: Nursing Process/Implementation
Content Area: Adult Health/Neurological

Reference

Christensen, B. & Kockrow, E. (2003). *Adult health nursing* (4th ed). St. Louis: Mosby, p. 648.

---

134. A client with chronic renal failure returns to the nursing unit after receiving his second hemodialysis treatment, and the nurse monitors the client closely for signs of disequilibrium syndrome. Which of the following is a sign of this syndrome?

1 Irritability
2 Mental confusion
3 Tachycardia
4 Hypothermia

Answer: 2

Rationale: Disequilibrium syndrome most often occurs in clients who are new to hemodialysis. It is characterized by headache, mental confusion, decreasing level of consciousness, nausea, vomiting, twitching, and possible seizure activity. It results from rapid removal of solutes from the body during hemodialysis, and a higher residual concentration gradient in the brain due to the blood-brain barrier. Water goes into cerebral cells because of the osmotic gradient, causing brain swelling and onset of symptoms. It is prevented by dialyzing for shorter times or at reduced blood flow rates. The signs in options 1, 3, and 4 are not associated with disequilibrium syndrome.

Test-Taking Strategy: Focusing on the name of the syndrome will assist in directing you to option 2. This is the only option that addresses a neurological sign. Review the signs of disequilibrium syndrome and the various test-taking strategies if you had difficulty with this question.

Level of Cognitive Ability: Analysis
Client Needs: Physiological Integrity
Integrated Process: Nursing Process/Data Collection
Content Area: Adult Health/Renal

Reference

Linton, A. & Maebius, N. (2003). *Introduction to medical-surgical nursing* (3rd ed). Philadelphia: Saunders, p. 784.

135. A nurse is preparing a client who will have spinal anesthesia for surgery. The nurse places highest priority on documenting and reporting which of the following items to a registered nurse?

1 Blood pressure of 126/78 mm Hg
2 Pulse rate of 78 beats per minute
3 Voided 300 mL
4 Presence of weakness in the left lower extremity

Answer: 4

Rationale: It is important to document and report any preoperative weakness or impaired movement of a lower extremity in the client who is to have spinal anesthesia because it causes temporary paralysis of the lower extremities. When the client's function returns, the preoperative weakness or impairment will not be misinterpreted as a complication of anesthesia. Options 1, 2, and 3 may be documented and reported, but they are not the highest priority.

Test-Taking Strategy: Note the key words "spinal anesthesia" and "highest priority." Note the relationship between the words "spinal anesthesia" and option 4. Also note that the data in options 1, 2, and 3 are normal findings. Review care to the preoperative client and the test-taking strategies for answering prioritizing questions if you had difficulty with this question.

Level of Cognitive Ability: Analysis
Client Needs: Physiological Integrity
Integrated Process: Nursing Process/Implementation
Content Area: Fundamental Skills

Reference

Harkreader, H. & Hogan, M.A. (2004). *Fundamentals of nursing: caring and clinical judgment* (2nd ed). Philadelphia: Saunders, pp. 1211, 1217.

---

136. A client experiencing delusions of being poisoned is admitted to the hospital after not eating or drinking for several days. The client shows no evidence of dehydration and malnutrition at this time. The nurse prepares a plan of care for the client and includes which client need as the priority?

1 Physiological needs
2 Safety and security needs
3 Self-esteem needs
4 Love and belonging needs

Answer: 2

Rationale: Maintaining safety is an important consideration when working with clients who have delusions. There are no data in the question to indicate that options 1, 3, and 4 require immediate attention.

Test-Taking Strategy: Note the key words "priority" and "shows no evidence of dehydration and malnutrition." Use Maslow's Hierarchy of Needs theory. Safety takes precedence if a physiological need does not exist. This will direct you to option 2. Review care to the client experiencing delusions and the test-taking strategies for answering prioritizing questions if you had difficulty with this question.

Level of Cognitive Ability: Application
Client Needs: Safe, Effective Care Environment
Integrated Process: Nursing Process/Planning
Content Area: Mental Health

References

Harkreader, H. & Hogan, M.A. (2004). *Fundamentals of nursing: caring and clinical judgment* (2nd ed). Philadelphia: Saunders, pp. 195-196.
Morrison-Valfre, M. (2005). *Foundations of mental health care* (3rd ed). St. Louis: Mosby, p. 332.

137. A nurse enters the room of a client with diabetes mellitus and finds the client difficult to arouse. The client's skin is cool and clammy and the pulse rate is elevated from the client's baseline. The nurse immediately:

1 obtains equipment needed to prepare an intravenous insulin solution.
2 gives the client a glass of orange juice.
3 prepares for the administration of an intravenous bolus dose of 50% dextrose.
4 checks the client's capillary blood glucose.

Answer: 4
Rationale: The client's signs and symptoms are consistent with hypoglycemia. The nurse must first obtain a blood glucose reading, and then report it to a registered nurse, who will contact the physician for subsequent orders. The nurse should not give a client fluid or food if the client is not alert because of the risk of aspiration. The physician may prescribe an intravenous bolus dose of 50% dextrose if needed, but preparing for this intervention is not the immediate action. Option 1 is implemented as needed in the treatment of hyperglycemia.

Test-Taking Strategy: Note the key word "immediately" and focus on the data in the question. Use the steps of the clinical problem-solving process (nursing process) and note that only option 4 addresses data collection. Review care to the client experiencing hypoglycemia and the test-taking strategies for answering prioritizing questions if you had difficulty with this question.

Level of Cognitive Ability: Application
Client Needs: Physiological Integrity
Integrated Process: Nursing Process/Implementation
Content Area: Adult Health/Endocrine

Reference
Christensen, B. & Kockrow, E. (2003). *Adult health nursing* (4th ed). St. Louis: Mosby, p. 488.

---

138. A nurse is caring for an older client who has hyperparathyroidism with severe osteoporosis. The nurse identifies which nursing diagnosis in the plan of care as the priority for this client?

1 Risk for Injury
2 Risk for Situational Low Self-Esteem
3 Social Isolation
4 Risk for Loneliness

Answer: 1
Rationale: The individual with hyperparathyroidism with severe osteoporosis is at risk for pathological fractures because of bone demineralization (option 1). Thus safety is a priority. No data in the question indicate that options 2, 3, and 4 are of concern.

Test-Taking Strategy: Focus on the client's diagnosis and note the key word "priority." Use Maslow's Hierarchy of Needs theory. Recall that if a physiological need is not identified in one of the options, then safety is the priority. Note that options 2, 3, and 4 are similar in that they address a psychosocial need. Review care to the client with hyperparathyroidism with severe osteoporosis and the test-taking strategies for answering prioritizing questions if you had difficulty with this question.

Level of Cognitive Ability: Analysis
Client Needs: Safe, Effective Care Environment
Integrated Process: Nursing Process/Planning
Content Area: Adult Health/Endocrine

Reference
Christensen, B. & Kockrow, E. (2003). *Adult health nursing* (4th ed). St. Louis: Mosby, p. 469.

139. Oxygen via nasal cannula at 4 L/min is prescribed for a hospitalized client. The nurse avoids which action in the care of the client?

1 Applies water-soluble lubricant to the nares
2 Instructs the client and family about the purpose of the oxygen
3 Humidifies the oxygen
4 Instructs the client to breathe only through the nose

Answer: 4

Rationale: The nasal cannula provides for lower concentrations of oxygen and can even be used with mouth breathers because movement of air through the oropharynx pulls oxygen from the nasopharynx. It is not necessary to instruct a client to breathe only through the nose. Options 1, 2, and 3 are correct interventions.

Test-Taking Strategy: Note the key word "avoids." This is a false response question and indicates that you need to look for the incorrect nursing action. Noting that option 4 contains the absolute word "only" will direct you to this option. Review care to the client receiving oxygen and the various test-taking strategies if you had difficulty with this question.

Level of Cognitive Ability: Application
Client Needs: Physiological Integrity
Integrated Process: Nursing Process/Implementation
Content Area: Fundamental Skills

Reference

Christensen, B. & Kockrow, E. (2003). *Foundations of nursing* (4th ed). St. Louis: Mosby, p. 452.

---

140. A nurse notes that the client has a nursing diagnosis of Ineffective Airway Clearance documented in the plan of care. The nurse plans to use which of the following indicators as the best guide to determine when the client needs suctioning?

1 Apical heart rate
2 Respiratory rate
3 Inability to expectorate mucus
4 Arterial blood gas results

Answer: 3

Rationale: Suctioning is indicated when the client cannot expectorate mucus after using a variety of other assistive methods. The need for suctioning is best determined by listening for coarse gurgling or bubbling respirations, or by hearing abnormal breath sounds with auscultation. The other options could be affected by factors other than the accumulation of secretions.

Test-Taking Strategy: Note the key word "best." Also, focus on the issue, the need for suctioning, and note the nursing diagnosis. Note the relationship of these items and option 3. Review suctioning procedures and the various test-taking strategies if you had difficulty with this question.

Level of Cognitive Ability: Analysis
Client Needs: Physiological Integrity
Integrated Process: Nursing Process/Planning
Content Area: Adult Health/Respiratory

Reference

deWit, S. (2005). *Fundamental concepts and skills for nursing.* Philadelphia: Saunders, p. 509.

---

141. The nurse checks the stoma of a postoperative client who had a creation of a colostomy performed and notes that it is a dark, dusky color. The nurse takes which immediate action?

Answer: 4

Rationale: The color of a stoma should be a moist, beefy red. A dark, dusky stoma indicates ischemia, requiring notification of a registered nurse, who will then contact the surgeon. Options 1, 2, and 3 are incorrect actions.

1 Changes the ostomy bag
2 Irrigates the colostomy
3 Orders a larger size ostomy bag
4 Notifies a registered nurse

Test-Taking Strategy: Note the key words "immediate" and "dark, dusky color." Recalling that a dark, dusky color indicates ischemia and that if this occurs it presents an emergency situation will direct you to option 4. Remember that if an emergency situation exists, the correct option may be the option that indicates notification of a registered nurse. Review care to the client following colostomy and the various test-taking strategies and strategies for answering prioritizing questions if you had difficulty with this question.

Level of Cognitive Ability: Application
Client Needs: Physiological Integrity
Integrated Process: Nursing Process/Implementation
Content Area: Adult Health/Gastrointestinal

Reference

Linton, A. & Maebius, N. (2003). *Introduction to medical-surgical nursing* (3rd ed). Philadelphia: Saunders, p. 350.

---

142. A nurse witnesses a motor vehicle crash in which a pedestrian is hit by a car. The nurse suspects that the client has a fractured leg. Which of the following is the appropriate nursing action?

1 Stay with the victim and encourage the victim to remain still.
2 Assist the victim to get up and walk to the sidewalk so that he or she is safe.
3 Leave the victim to call an ambulance.
4 Try to manually reduce the fracture.

Answer: 1
Rationale: The client with a suspected fracture is not moved unless it is dangerous to remain in that spot. The nurse should remain with the client and have someone else call for emergency help. A fracture is not reduced at the scene and is not performed by the nurse. The site of the fracture is immobilized to prevent further injury before moving the client.

Test-Taking Strategy: Note the key word "appropriate." Focus on the issue, a fractured leg. Eliminate options 2 and 4 first because they could result in further injury to the client. From the remaining options, focus on the client's needs, and remember that it is best for the nurse to remain with the client and have someone else call for emergency assistance. Review emergency interventions for a fracture and the various test-taking strategies if you had difficulty with this question.

Level of Cognitive Ability: Application
Client Needs: Physiological Integrity
Integrated Process: Nursing Process/Implementation
Content Area: Adult Health/Musculoskeletal

Reference

Lewis, S., Heitkemper, M., & Dirksen, S. (2004). *Medical-surgical nursing: assessment and management of clinical problems* (6th ed). St. Louis: Mosby, p. 1665.

---

143. A client with hypercholesterolemia is instructed to limit intake of dietary cholesterol. The nurse tells the client to select which of the following meat choices because it is lowest in fat?

1 Baked chicken
2 Pork spareribs

Answer: 1
Rationale: The best meat choices to lower intake of cholesterol include lean cuts of beef with the fat trimmed, lamb, pork (except spareribs), veal (except ground), skinless poultry, and shellfish. Meats that have larger amounts of cholesterol include prime grades of beef, pork spareribs, goose, duck, organ meats (liver, brain, kidney), sausage, bacon, luncheon meats, frankfurters, caviar, and fried meats.

3 Broiled duck
4 Fried turkey

Test-Taking Strategy: Note the key words "lowest in fat." Noting the word "baked" in option 1 and the relationship of the key words to option 1 will direct you to this option. Review dietary measures for the client with hypercholesterolemia and the various test-taking strategies if you had difficulty with this question.

Level of Cognitive Ability: Application
Client Needs: Health Promotion and Maintenance
Integrated Process: Teaching/Learning
Content Area: Adult Health/Cardiovascular

Reference

Peckenpaugh, N. (2003). Nutrition essentials and diet therapy (9th ed). Philadelphia: Saunders, p. 232.

---

144. A nurse provides dietary instructions to a client with hypertension. The nurse determines that the client understands the instructions if the client states that it is acceptable to eat which food item?
1 Hot dogs
2 Turkey
3 Salad with bleu cheese dressing
4 Corned beef hash

Answer: 2
Rationale: A client with hypertension needs to avoid foods that are high in sodium. Foods that are high in sodium include bacon, hot dogs, luncheon meat, chipped or corned beef, kosher meat, smoked or salted meat or fish, peanut butter, and a variety of shellfish. Processed foods, canned foods, cheese, and many salad dressings are also high in sodium.

Test-Taking Strategy: Eliminate options 1 and 4 first because they are similar and because hot dogs and corned beef are highly processed meats and are high in sodium. Option 3 is also eliminated because bleu cheese dressing is high in sodium. Review dietary instructions for the client with hypertension and the various test-taking strategies if you had difficulty with this question.

Level of Cognitive Ability: Comprehension
Client Needs: Health Promotion and Maintenance
Integrated Process: Nursing Process/Evaluation
Content Area: Adult Health/Cardiovascular

Reference

Nix, S. (2005). *Williams' basic nutrition & diet therapy* (12th ed). St. Louis: Mosby, pp. 356-360.

---

145. A nurse is collecting data from a client with a diagnosis of bulimia nervosa who has problems with nutrition. The nurse should obtain information from the client about which of the following first?
1 Feelings about self and body weight
2 Previous and current coping skills
3 Lack of control
4 Eating patterns, food preferences, concerns about eating

Answer: 4
Rationale: The nurse would first identify eating patterns, food preferences, and concerns about eating when caring for the client with bulimia nervosa. Obtaining information about the client's feelings about self and body weight, previous and current coping skills, and lack of control would also be obtained but are secondary to eating patterns and food preferences.

Test-Taking Strategy: Note the key word "first." Use Maslow's Hierarchy of Needs theory to prioritize. Option 4 is the only option that relates to a physiological need. Review care for the client with bulimia nervosa and the test-taking strategies for answering prioritizing questions if you had difficulty with this question.

Level of Cognitive Ability: Application
Client Needs: Physiological Integrity
Integrated Process: Nursing Process/Data Collection
Content Area: Delegating/Prioritizing

Reference

Morrison-Valfre, M. (2005). *Foundations of mental health care* (3rd ed). St. Louis: Mosby, p. 240.

---

146. The wife of a victim who sustains an eye injury calls the emergency department and speaks to a nurse. The wife reports that her husband was hit in the eye area by a piece of board while building a shed in the backyard. The nurse advises the wife to immediately:

1 apply ice to the affected eye.
2 call an ambulance.
3 irrigate the eye with cool water.
4 bring the husband to the emergency department.

Answer: 1
Rationale: Treatment for a contusion ideally begins at the time of injury, and includes applying ice to the site. The husband should also receive a thorough eye examination to rule out the presence of other injuries, but this is not the immediate action. Irrigating the eye with cool water may be implemented for injuries that involve a splash of an irritant into the eye. It is not necessary to call an ambulance.

Test-Taking Strategy: Eliminate options 2 and 4 first because they are similar. From the remaining options, focusing on the type of injury sustained will direct you to option 1. Review initial treatment following an eye contusion and the various test-taking strategies if you had difficulty with this question.

Level of Cognitive Ability: Application
Client Needs: Physiological Integrity
Integrated Process: Nursing Process/Implementation
Content Area: Adult Health/Eye

References

Ignatavicius, D. & Workman, M. (2006). *Medical-surgical nursing: critical thinking for collaborative care* (5th ed). Philadelphia: Saunders, p. 1105.
Lewis, S., Heitkemper, M., & Dirksen, S. (2004). *Medical-surgical nursing: assessment and management of clinical problems* (6th ed). St. Louis: Mosby, p. 445.

---

147. A nurse is preparing the parents of a newborn with respiratory distress syndrome for an initial visit to the neonatal intensive care unit. The nurse plans which action that will best facilitate parent-newborn bonding?

1 Explain the equipment used and how it will assist their newborn
2 Encourage the parents to touch their newborn
3 Identify specific care-taking tasks that may be assumed by the parents

Answer: 2
Rationale: The best action that promotes bonding is to encourage the parents to touch their newborn. Options 1 and 3 may be frightening because of the newborn's condition and the unfamiliarity of high-risk newborn care practices. Option 4 is inappropriate. Asking parents to read literature does not enhance the parent-newborn bond.

Test-Taking Strategy: Focus on the issue, the action that will best facilitate parent-newborn bonding. Note the relationship of the issue to option 2. Option 2 is the only option that addresses touch, which is directly related to bonding. Review parent-newborn bonding concepts and the various test-taking strategies if you had difficulty with this question.

4 Give the parents literature to read about respiratory distress syndrome

Level of Cognitive Ability: Application
Client Needs: Psychosocial Integrity
Integrated Process: Caring
Content Area: Maternity/Postpartum

Reference
Leifer, G. (2005). *Maternity nursing* (9th ed). Philadelphia: Saunders, p. 207.

---

148. A nurse is preparing to care for a client admitted to the mental health unit with a diagnosis of dementia and notes a nursing diagnosis of Self-Care Deficit in the plan of care. The nurse plans for which outcome in caring for the client?

1 The client will be oriented to place by the time of discharge.
2 The client will correctly identify objects in his or her room by the time of discharge.
3 The client will be free of hallucinations by the time of discharge.
4 The client will feed self with cueing within 24 hours.

Answer: 4

Rationale: Option 4 identifies an outcome directly related to the client's ability to care for self. Options 1, 2, and 3 are not related to self-care deficit.

Test-Taking Strategy: Note the relationship between the nursing diagnosis Self-Care Deficit and option 4. Also use Maslow's Hierarchy of Needs theory. Option 4 is the only option that addresses a physiological need. Review care to the client with dementia and the various test-taking strategies if you had difficulty with this question.

Level of Cognitive Ability: Application
Client Needs: Physiological Integrity
Integrated Process: Nursing Process/Planning
Content Area: Mental Health

Reference
Morrison-Valfre, M. (2005). *Foundations of mental health care* (3rd ed). St. Louis: Mosby, p. 174.

---

149. The nurse is called by a physical therapist to the room of a client experiencing a seizure. The nurse does which of the following to ensure the client's safety?

1 Wiggle a bite stick (airway) between the client's clenched teeth
2 Restrain the client to prevent bruising
3 Draw the curtain around the bedside area
4 Turn the client to the side if possible

Answer: 4

Rationale: Nursing management during a seizure includes easing the client to the floor if out of bed and loosening clothing such as a belt, tie, or collar. The client is turned to the side whenever possible to allow drainage of secretions from the mouth. A bite stick (airway) is never forced between the teeth of a client during a seizure; this could damage the teeth and gums. The client is not restrained because the strong muscle contractions during seizure activity could cause injury. The curtain should be drawn, but it is done for privacy, not to prevent injury.

Test-Taking Strategy: Focus on the issue, client safety. Use the ABCs—airway, breathing, and circulation—to direct you to option 4. Also eliminate options 1 and 2 because they could harm the client and option 3 because it relates to privacy, not safety. Review care to the client experiencing a seizure and the various test-taking strategies if you had difficulty with this question.

Level of Cognitive Ability: Application
Client Needs: Safe, Effective Care Environment

Integrated Process: Nursing Process/Implementation
Content Area: Adult Health/Neurological

Reference
Christensen, B. & Kockrow, E. (2003). *Adult health nursing* (4th ed). St. Louis: Mosby, p. 624.

---

150. A nurse is providing information to the family of a client with left-sided unilateral neglect about caring for the client. The nurse tells the family that it would be least helpful to do which of the following?

1 Approach the client from the right side.
2 Encourage the client to scan the environment.
3 Move the commode and chair to the left side.
4 Place bedside articles on the left side.

Answer: 1
Rationale: Unilateral neglect is an unawareness of the paralyzed side of the body, which increases the client's risk for injury. The nurse's role is to refocus the client's attention to the affected side. Personal care items, belongings, bedside chair, and commode are all placed on the affected side. The client is taught to scan the environment to become aware of that half of the body, and is approached on the affected side by family and staff as well.

Test-Taking Strategy: Note the key words "least helpful" and note that the client has "left-sided unilateral neglect." Remember that options that are similar are not likely to be correct; therefore eliminate options 3 and 4. From the remaining options, recall that unilateral neglect is an unawareness of the paralyzed side of the body and that it is necessary to refocus the client's attention to the affected side. Review care to the client with unilateral neglect and the various test-taking strategies if you had difficulty with this question.

Level of Cognitive Ability: Application
Client Needs: Safe, Effective Care Environment
Integrated Process: Nursing Process/Implementation
Content Area: Adult Health/Neurological

Reference
Christensen, B. & Kockrow, E. (2003). *Adult health nursing* (4th ed). St. Louis: Mosby, p. 640.

---

151. A nurse is reviewing the diagnostic tests prescribed for a client and notes that a lupus erythematosus cell preparation (LE cell prep) has been ordered. The nurse determines that this test is used to screen primarily for which disorder?

1 Histoplasmosis
2 Systemic lupus erythematosus (SLE)
3 Human immunodeficiency virus (HIV)
4 Progressive systemic sclerosis

Answer: 2
Rationale: The LE cell prep may be performed on a client suspected of having SLE or to screen for progressive systemic sclerosis. However, it is primarily used to screen for SLE. The other options are not associated with this diagnostic test.

Test-Taking Strategy: Note the key word "primarily." Also note the relationship between the word "lupus" in the question and in the correct option. Review the purpose of an LE cell prep and the various test-taking strategies if you had difficulty with this question.

Level of Cognitive Ability: Analysis
Client Needs: Physiological Integrity
Integrated Process: Nursing Process/Data Collection
Content Area: Adult Health/Immune

Reference

Chernecky, C. & Berger, B. (2004). *Laboratory tests and diagnostic procedures* (4th ed). Philadelphia: Saunders, p. 745.

---

152. A nurse is preparing to assist a physician in performing a liver biopsy. The nurse assists the client to which position for this test to be performed?

1 Right lateral side-lying
2 Right Sims'
3 Prone with the hands crossed under the head
4 Supine with the right hand under the head

Answer: 4

Rationale: A supine position is assumed with the right hand placed under the head for a liver biopsy. The client also is asked to remain as still as possible during the test. Options 1, 2, and 3 are incorrect because the physician would not be able to access the liver.

Test-Taking Strategy: Think about the anatomical location of the liver. Recalling that the liver is located on the right side will direct you to option 4. Review this procedure and the various test-taking strategies if you had difficulty with this question.

Level of Cognitive Ability: Application
Client Needs: Physiological Integrity
Integrated Process: Nursing Process/Implementation
Content Area: Adult Health/Gastrointestinal

References

Chernecky, C. & Berger, B. (2004). *Laboratory tests and diagnostic procedures* (4th ed). Philadelphia: Saunders, p. 733.
Linton, A. & Maebius, N. (2003). *Introduction to medical-surgical nursing* (3rd ed). Philadelphia: Saunders, p. 720.

---

153. A nurse assists a male client with a diagnosis of obsessive-compulsive disorder prepare for bed. One hour later, the client calls the nurse and says he is feeling anxious and asks the nurse to sit and talk for a while. The nurse takes which appropriate initial action?

1 Asks the client if he would like an antianxiety medication
2 Tells the client that it is time for sleep and that they will talk tomorrow
3 Sits and talks with the client
4 Asks a male nursing assistant to sit with the client

Answer: 3

Rationale: The appropriate initial nursing action is to sit and talk if the client is expressing anxiety. Antianxiety medication may be necessary, but this is not the initial nursing action. A nursing assistant may not be able to alleviate the client's anxiety. Option 2 is an inappropriate action and places the client's feelings on hold.

Test-Taking Strategy: Note the key word "initial" and use therapeutic communication techniques. Recalling that it is best to address the client's feelings assists in directing you to option 3. Review care to the client with obsessive-compulsive disorder and the various test-taking strategies if you had difficulty with this question.

Level of Cognitive Ability: Application
Client Needs: Psychosocial Integrity
Integrated Process: Caring
Content Area: Mental Health

Reference

Morrison-Valfre, M. (2005). Foundations of mental health care (3rd ed). St. Louis: Mosby, pp. 72, 102-103.

154. A nurse reads in the client's record that the client suffered a severe emotional trauma 1 month ago and is now experiencing paralysis of the right arm. The nurse understands that the priority of care is to:

1 encourage the client to talk about his feelings.
2 check the client for organic causes of the paralysis.
3 refer the client to group therapy.
4 encourage the client to move and use the arm.

Answer: 2

Rationale: The priority of care is to assess for any physiological cause of the paralysis. Although a component of the plan of care is to encourage the client to discuss feelings, this is not the priority action. It is not appropriate to encourage the client to use the arm without ruling out a physiological cause of the paralysis. Although the client may be referred to group therapy, this also is not the priority action.

Test-Taking Strategy: Note the key word "priority." Use Maslow's Hierarchy of Needs theory and remember that physiological needs are the first priority. Option 2 is the only option that addresses a physiological need. Review care to the mental health client who experiences physiological disorders and the test-taking strategies for answering prioritizing questions if you had difficulty with this question.

Level of Cognitive Ability: Application
Client Needs: Physiological Integrity
Integrated Process: Nursing Process/Implementation
Content Area: Mental Health

Reference

Morrison-Valfre, M. (2005). *Foundations of mental health care* (3rd ed). St. Louis: Mosby, p. 225.

---

155. A nurse is assisting in developing a plan of care for a client admitted to the mental health unit with a diagnosis of obsessive-compulsive disorder who is experiencing severe anxiety. The nurse understands that a priority in the plan of care for this client is to:

1 monitor for repetitive behavior.
2 demand active participation in care.
3 educate the client about self-care demands.
4 establish a trusting nurse-client relationship.

Answer: 4

Rationale: The priority nursing action is to establish a trusting relationship with the client. Demanding anything from the client should never occur. The remaining options are appropriate components of the plan of care, but are not the priority. A trusting nurse-client relationship needs to be established first.

Test-Taking Strategy: Focus on the key word "priority" and note that the client is being admitted to the mental health unit. Recalling that a nurse-client relationship needs to be developed first assists in directing you to option 4. Review care to the client with obsessive-compulsive disorder and the test-taking strategies for answering prioritizing questions if you had difficulty with this question.

Level of Cognitive Ability: Application
Client Needs: Psychosocial Integrity
Integrated Process: Caring
Content Area: Mental Health

Reference

Morrison-Valfre, M. (2005). *Foundations of mental health care* (3rd ed). St. Louis: Mosby, p. 189.

156. A nurse plans to teach a client about breast cancer and the procedure for performing breast-self examination (BSE). Select all instructions that the nurse provides to the client.

___ If you are menstruating, the best time to do BSE is 2 or 3 days after your period ends.
___ If you notice discharge from the nipple, there is no need to be concerned because this is a common occurrence during menstruation.
___ Stand before a mirror to inspect both breasts.
___ Inspection should be done by pressing the hands firmly on the hips, bowing slightly toward the mirror as you pull your shoulders and elbows forward.
___ If you are premenopausal, you may feel lumps in the breast but these will be normal because of hormonal changes that occur.
___ Palpation can be done in the shower.
___ To palpate the breasts use three or four fingers, begin at the outer edge, press the flat part of your fingers in small circles, moving the circles slowly around the breast.
___ It is not necessary to palpate the armpit area or the area between the breast and the armpit.

Answer:
If you are menstruating, the best time to do BSE is 2 or 3 days after your period ends.

Stand before a mirror to inspect both breasts.

Inspection should be done by pressing the hands firmly on the hips, bowing slightly toward the mirror as you pull your shoulders and elbows forward.

Palpation can be done in the shower.

To palpate the breasts use three or four fingers, begin at the outer edge, press the flat part of your fingers in small circles, moving the circles slowly around the breast.

Rationale: If the client is menstruating, the best time to do BSE is 2 or 3 days after the period ends because the breasts are less likely to be tender or swollen. Any lumps or nipple discharge is a concern and is always reported to the health care provider for further evaluation. Inspection is done by standing before a mirror and by pressing the hands firmly on the hips, bowing slightly toward the mirror as the client pulls the shoulders and elbows forward. Palpation can be done in the shower and the client is taught to palpate the breasts using three or four fingers, beginning at the outer edge, pressing the flat part of the fingers in small circles, and moving the circles slowly around the breast. It is very important to palpate the armpit area or the area between the breast and the armpit and to report any masses or lumps noted in this area.

Test-Taking Strategy: The best strategy to use to answer the question is to visualize the procedure. Also recalling the anatomy of the breast and the characteristics of breast cancer will assist in answering this question. Review the procedure for breast self-examination and the various test-taking strategies if you had difficulty with this question.

Level of Cognitive Ability: Application
Client Needs: Health Promotion and Maintenance
Integrated Process: Teaching/Learning
Content Area: Adult Health/Oncology

Reference
Potter, P. & Perry, A. (2005) *Fundamentals of nursing* (6th ed). St. Louis: Mosby, p. 736.

---

157. A licensed practical nurse is supervising a nursing student who is performing a pulse oximetry measurement on a client with peripheral vascular disease. The nurse determines that the student is perform-

Answer: 4
Rationale: If the client has peripheral vascular disease, the pulse oximetry probe is placed on the earlobe or bridge of the nose because peripheral vasoconstriction or inadequate blood flow to the peripheral areas of the body interferes with the oxygen saturation measurement. For the

ing the procedure accurately if the student places the oximetry probe on which anatomical area?

1 Right index finger
2 Left thumb
3 One of the toes
4 Bridge of the nose

client with peripheral vascular disease, the pulse oximetry probe should be placed on the earlobe or bridge of the nose. Placing the probe on the anatomical areas noted in options 1, 2, and 3 will not provide an accurate measurement of the oxygen saturation measurement.

Test-Taking Strategy: Focus on the client's diagnosis, peripheral vascular disease, and recall the pathophysiology associated with the disease. Note that options 1, 2, and 3 are similar in that they indicate using a peripheral body area. Review the procedure for pulse oximetry measurement and the various test-taking strategies if you had difficulty with this question.

Level of Cognitive Ability: Comprehension
Client Needs: Physiological Integrity
Integrated Process: Teaching/Learning
Content Area: Leadership/Management

Reference

deWit, S. (2005). *Fundamental concepts and skills for nursing.* Philadelphia: Saunders, p. 496.

---

158. A nurse is reviewing the assessment data in the record of a client who she is assigned to care for and notes documentation that the client has pallor. The nurse determines that this skin color variation is most likely due to:

1 an increased amount of deposits of bilirubin in the tissues.
2 an increased amount of deoxygenated hemoglobin associated with hypoxia.
3 a reduced amount of oxyhemoglobin from decreased blood flow.
4 an increased amount of melanin in the tissues.

Answer: 3

Rationale: Pallor, a decrease in skin color, is due to a decreased amount of oxyhemoglobin resulting from decreased blood flow. Some causes of pallor include anemia or shock. Pallor can best be assessed in the face, conjunctivae, nailbeds, palms of the hands, or lips. A bluish discoloration (cyanosis) is due to increased amount of deoxygenated hemoglobin associated with hypoxia. A yellow-orange skin discoloration (jaundice) is due to increased amount of deposits of bilirubin in the tissues. A tan-brown skin color is due to increased amount of melanin in the tissues.

Test-Taking Strategy: Focus on the issue, pallor. Recalling that pallor refers to a pale skin color will direct you to option 3. Also noting the relationship of the word "pallor" to the description in option 3 will direct you to this option. Review skin assessment findings and the various test-taking strategies if you had difficulty with this question.

Level of Cognitive Ability: Comprehension
Client Needs: Physiological Integrity
Integrated Process: Nursing Process/Data Collection
Content Area: Adult Health/Integumentary

Reference

Potter, P. & Perry, A. (2005). *Fundamentals of nursing* (6th ed). St. Louis: Mosby, p. 689.

159. A nurse checks the client's skin for turgor. The nurse grasps a fold of the client's skin in which body area to best check for turgor?

1 Back of the hand
2 Sternal area
3 Top of the foot
4 Sacral area

Answer: 2

Rationale: Turgor refers to the skin's elasticity. To check the skin turgor, a fold of skin on the back of the forearm or sternal area is grasped with the fingertips and released. Normally the skin lifts easily and snaps back immediately into its normal resting position. The back of the hand is not the best area to assess turgor because the skin is normally loose and thin in this area. The sacral area and foot and ankle area are areas to assess for edema.

Test-Taking Strategy: Focus on the issue, checking skin turgor. Recalling that turgor refers to the skin's elasticity and visualizing each body area in the options will direct you to option 2. Review these data collection techniques and the various test-taking strategies if you had difficulty with this question.

Level of Cognitive Ability: Application
Client Needs: Health Promotion and Maintenance
Integrated Process: Nursing Process/Data Collection
Content Area: Adult Health/Integumentary

Reference

Potter, P. & Perry, A. (2005). *Fundamentals of nursing* (6th ed). St. Louis: Mosby, p. 691.

---

160. The nurse notes documentation that a client has cherry angiomas located on the abdomen. On inspection of the skin, the nurse expects to note which characteristic of this type of lesion?

1 Ruby red papules
2 Thickened skin areas
3 Pinpoint-sized red or purple spots
4 Areas of redness that are warm to touch

Answer: 1

Rationale: Cherry angiomas are noted as ruby red papules. Areas of skin thickening are noted as senile keratosis. Pinpoint-sized red or purple spots are known as petechiae. Areas of redness that are warm to touch are noted as erythema.

Test-Taking Strategy: Focus on the issue, cherry angiomas. Note the relationship between the word "cherry" and the words "ruby red" in option 1. Review the characteristics of various skin lesions and the various test-taking strategies if you had difficulty with this question.

Level of Cognitive Ability: Analysis
Client Needs: Health Promotion and Maintenance
Integrated Process: Nursing Process/Data Collection
Content Area: Adult Health/Integumentary

Reference

Potter, P. & Perry, A. (2005). *Fundamentals of nursing* (6th ed). St. Louis: Mosby, p. 691.

---

161. A hospitalized client with chronic renal failure has returned to the nursing unit after a hemodialysis treatment. The nurse checks pre- and postdialysis documentation of which parameters to determine the effectiveness of the procedure?

Answer: 2

Rationale: Following hemodialysis, the client's vital signs are monitored to determine whether the client is remaining hemodynamically stable and for comparison to predialysis measurements. The client's blood pressure and weight are expected to be reduced as a result of fluid removal. Laboratory studies are done as per protocol, but are neces-

1 Weight and blood urea nitrogen (BUN)
2 Blood pressure and weight
3 Potassium level and creatinine levels
4 BUN and creatinine levels

sarily done after the hemodialysis treatment has been ended.

Test-Taking Strategy: Focus on the issue, *determining the effectiveness of hemodialysis,* and note that this is an evaluation-type question. Also remember that when options contain two parts, both parts need to be correct in order for the option to be correct. Knowing that weight is an important variable allows you to eliminate options 3 and 4. From the remaining options, recalling that vital signs reflect hemodynamic stability will direct you to option 2. Review the parameters that will determine the effectiveness of hemodialysis and the various test-taking strategies if you had difficulty with this question.

Level of Cognitive Ability: Analysis
Client Needs: Physiological Integrity
Integrated Process: Nursing Process/Evaluation
Content Area: Adult Health/Renal

Reference
Christensen, B. & Kockrow, E. (2003). *Adult health nursing* (4th ed). St. Louis: Mosby, p. 444.

---

162. A nurse is caring for a client who is dying. The nurse assists to develop a plan of care understanding that which intervention is inappropriate in the care of the client?
1 Provide extremely thorough answers to each question asked by the client or family.
2 Suggest making referrals to other disciplines based on the client's stated needs.
3 Plan to balance the client's need for assistance with that for independence.
4 Offer to contact the clergy to support the client's spiritual needs.

Answer: 1
Rationale: In planning care for a dying client, the nurse provides information and answers questions to the extent most helpful to the client and family. The nurse suggests making referrals to other disciplines and clergy based on an identified need, and tries to balance the client's need for assistance with the need to maintain some measure of independence. Also, it is very helpful to spend time with the client.

Test-Taking Strategy: Note the key word "inappropriate." This indicates a false response question and that you need to select the option that is an incorrect intervention. Eliminate options 2 and 4 first because they are similar. From the remaining options, note the exaggerated detail of response implied in option 1, which makes it inappropriate. Review the psychosocial needs of the dying client and the various test-taking strategies if you had difficulty with this question.

Level of Cognitive Ability: Comprehension
Client Needs: Psychosocial Integrity
Integrated Process: Caring
Content Area: Fundamental Skills

Reference
Linton, A. & Maebius, N. (2003). *Introduction to medical-surgical nursing* (3rd ed). Philadelphia: Saunders, p. 312.

163. A nurse is planning to teach a client how to mix Regular and NPH insulin in the same syringe. Which of the following instructions is included in the teaching plan?

1 Take all of the air out of the bottle before mixing.
2 Draw up the Regular insulin first into the syringe.
3 Keep both bottles stored in the refrigerator for 1 month.
4 Shake the NPH insulin bottle in the hands before mixing.

Answer: 2

Rationale: Before mixing different types of insulin, the bottle should be rotated for at least 1 minute between both hands. This resuspends the insulin and helps warm the medication. The nurse should not shake the bottles. Shaking causes foaming and bubbles to form, which may trap particles of insulin and alter the dosage. Insulin may be maintained at room temperature. Additional bottles of insulin should be stored in the refrigerator for future use. Regular insulin is drawn up before NPH insulin. Air does not need to be removed from the insulin bottle.

Test-Taking Strategy: Visualize the procedure as you carefully read each option. When answering questions that relate to mixing insulin remember the letters "R.N."—draw the *R*egular insulin into the syringe before the *N*PH insulin. Review the procedures for administering insulin and the test-taking strategies for answering pharmacology questions if you had difficulty with this question.

Level of Cognitive Ability: Application
Client Needs: Physiological Integrity
Integrated Process: Nursing Process/Planning
Content Area: Pharmacology

Reference

Hodgson, B. & Kizior, R. (2005). *Saunders nursing drug handbook 2005.* Philadelphia: Saunders, p. 570.

---

164. A client has been taking lansoprazole (Prevacid). The nurse monitors the client for the relief of which of the following symptoms?

1 Constipation
2 Diarrhea
3 Flatulence
4 Heartburn

Answer: 4

Rationale: Lansoprazole is a gastric pump inhibitor (proton pump inhibitor). Its intended effect is relief of gastric irritation pain, often referred to as heartburn. The medication does not relieve constipation, diarrhea, or flatulence.

Test-Taking Strategy: Focus on the key words "relief of." Note the name of the medication and recall that most proton pump inhibitors medication names end with the letters "zole." This will direct you to option 4. Review this medication and the test-taking strategies for answering pharmacology questions if you had difficulty with this question.

Level of Cognitive Ability: Analysis
Client Needs: Physiological Integrity
Integrated Process: Nursing Process/Evaluation
Content Area: Pharmacology

Reference

Hodgson, B. & Kizior, R. (2005). *Saunders nursing drug handbook 2005.* Philadelphia: Saunders, p. 616.

165. A physician has written an order for ranitidine (Zantac) once daily. The nurse schedules administration of the medication:

1 at bedtime.
2 with supper.
3 just before lunch.
4 just before breakfast.

Answer: 1

Rationale: Ranitidine should be taken at bedtime when given as a single daily dose. This allows for its prolonged effect and the greatest protection of gastric mucosa around the clock. The other options are incorrect.

Test-Taking Strategy: Note the similarity in options 2, 3, and 4 in that these times indicate administration of the medication with food. Review this medication and the test-taking strategies for answering pharmacology questions if you had difficulty with this question.

Level of Cognitive Ability: Application
Client Needs: Physiological Integrity
Integrated Process: Nursing Process/Implementation
Content Area: Pharmacology

Reference

Hodgson, B. & Kizior, R. (2005). *Saunders nursing drug handbook 2005.* Philadelphia: Saunders, p. 926.

---

166. A client reports to the emergency department complaining that "his heart is skipping beats." After diagnostic studies, it is determined that the client is experiencing isolated premature ventricular contractions (PVCs) and has no underlying cardiac disease. The nurse provides dietary instructions to the client and tells him that which item is acceptable to consume?

1 Coffee
2 Tea
3 Cola
4 Apple juice

Answer: 4

Rationale: Clients experiencing a cardiac dysrhythmia such as PVCs should not consume caffeinated beverages because of the vasoconstriction effect associated with caffeine. Options 1, 2, and 3 are items that contain caffeine.

Test-Taking Strategy: Note the similarity between options 1, 2, and 3 in that they contain caffeine. Review the treatment for PVCs and the various test-taking strategies if you had difficulty with this question.

Level of Cognitive Ability: Application
Client Needs: Health Promotion and Maintenance
Integrated Process: Teaching/Learning
Content Area: Fundamental Skills

References

Black, J. & Hawks, J. (2005). *Medical-surgical nursing: clinical management for positive outcomes* (7th ed). Philadelphia: Saunders, p. 570.
Christensen, B. & Kockrow, E. (2003). *Adult health nursing* (4th ed). St. Louis: Mosby, p. 299.

---

167. A client is hospitalized with chest pain, and myocardial infarction is suspected. The client tells the nurse that the chest pain has returned, and the nurse administers one 0.4-mg nitroglycerin tablet sublingually as prescribed and notifies a registered nurse. What does the nurse do next before administering another sublingual nitroglycerin tablet if the pain is not relieved?

Answer: 2

Rationale: Nitroglycerin tablets are administered one every 5 minutes, not exceeding three tablets for chest pain as long as the client maintains a systolic blood pressure of 100 mm Hg or more. The nurse should check the client's blood pressure before administering a second nitroglycerin. The physician is notified if the chest pain is not relieved after administering the three tablets. If there is a sudden drop in blood pressure, the client is placed in the Trendelenburg (head-lowered) position and the physician is notified. Deep breathing will not relieve the chest pain that oc-

1 Ambulates the client to determine if activity worsens with exercise
2 Checks the client's blood pressure
3 Places the client in Trendelenburg position
4 Encourages the client to deep breathe

curs as a result of myocardial infarction. The client is immediately placed at rest if chest pain occurs; activity such as ambulation is contraindicated.

Test-Taking Strategy: Note the key word "next." Use the ABCs—airway, breathing, and circulation. This will direct you to option 2. Checking the blood pressure is a means of checking the client's circulatory status. Review care to the client experiencing chest pain and the test-taking strategies for answering pharmacology questions if you had difficulty with this question.

Level of Cognitive Ability: Application
Client Needs: Physiological Integrity
Integrated Process: Nursing Process/Implementation
Content Area: Adult Health/Cardiovascular

Reference
Christensen, B. & Kockrow, E. (2003). *Adult health nursing* (4th ed). St. Louis: Mosby, p. 313.

---

168. A licensed practical nurse is assisting a registered nurse in caring for a client with a suspected myocardial infarction who is experiencing chest pain unrelieved by nitroglycerin. A registered nurse administers morphine sulfate 5 mg intravenously as prescribed to treat the chest pain. After the administration of the morphine sulfate, the licensed practical nurse takes which priority action?
1 Places the call bell at the client's side and instructs the client to call the nurse if the chest pain is not relieved
2 Monitors the respirations and blood pressure
3 Monitors urinary output
4 Places the client in Trendelenburg position

Answer: 2
Rationale: Morphine sulfate is administered to control pain in cardiac clients. After administration, the nurse must monitor the client's heart rhythm and vital signs, especially the client's respirations. Signs of morphine sulfate toxicity include respiratory depression and hypotension. The client is placed in Trendelenburg position only if a sudden drop in blood pressure occurs; otherwise, a semi-Fowler's to high-Fowler's position is maintained. Urinary output is not directly related to the administration of this medication. The client with a suspected myocardial infarction should not be left alone.

Test-Taking Strategy: Note the key word "priority." Use the ABCs—airway, breathing, and circulation—to direct you to option 2. Review this medication and the test-taking strategies for answering prioritizing questions if you had difficulty with this question.

Level of Cognitive Ability: Application
Client Needs: Physiological Integrity
Integrated Process: Nursing Process/Implementation
Content Area: Adult Health/Cardiovascular

Reference
Hodgson, B. & Kizior, R. (2005). *Saunders nursing drug handbook 2005.* Philadelphia: Saunders, p. 734.

---

169. A mother brings her child to the emergency department and reports that her child states that dirt flew into his eye during softball practice. The nurse plans for which action first?

Answer: 1
Rationale: If a surface foreign body injury occurs to the eye, the nurse would first check visual acuity. The eye will then be checked for corneal abrasions followed by irrigating the eye with sterile normal saline to gently remove the particles. There is no reason to place ice on the eye. Plac-

1 Checks vision
2 Irrigates the eye with sterile saline
3 Removes the dirt
4 Places ice on the eye

ing ice on the eye would be done if the client sustained an eye contusion.

Test-Taking Strategy: Use the steps of the clinical problem-solving process (nursing process). Option 1 is the only option that relates to data collection. Options 2, 3, and 4 relate to implementation. Review content related to initial treatment of various eye injuries and the various test-taking strategies if you had difficulty with this question.

Level of Cognitive Ability: Application
Client Needs: Physiological Integrity
Integrated Process: Nursing Process/Implementation
Content Area: Child Health

Reference
Wong, D. & Hockenberry, M. (2003). *Nursing care of infants and children* (7th ed). St. Louis: Mosby, p. 1003.

---

170. A nurse is assisting residents involved in a hurricane and flood. Many of the older residents are emotionally despondent and refuse to evacuate their homes. With regard to rescue and relocation of the older residents the nurse plans to first:
1 attend to emotional needs.
2 attend to nutritional and basic needs.
3 contact families.
4 arrange for transportation to shelters.

Answer: 2
Rationale: Attending to people's basic needs of food, shelter, and clothing is the priority. Options 1, 3, and 4 may or may not be needed at a later date.

Test-Taking Strategy: Note the key word "first" and use Maslow's hierarchy of needs theory. Option 2 addresses basic physiological needs. Options 1, 3, and 4 address psychosocial needs and may be appropriate at a later date. Review the nurse's role in the event of a disaster and the test-taking strategies for answering prioritizing questions if you had difficulty with this question.

Level of Cognitive Ability: Application
Client Needs:Physiological Integrity
Integrated Process: Nursing Process/Planning
Content Area: Delegating/Prioritizing

Reference
Stuart, G. & Laraia, M. (2005). *Principles & practice of psychiatric nursing* (8th ed). St. Louis: Mosby, pp. 224, 234.

---

171. A nurse employed in an eye clinic notes documentation that a client's intraocular pressure in the right eye is 16 mm Hg and 18 mm Hg in the left eye. The nurse tells the client:
1 that the pressure is elevated in the left eye.
2 that the pressure is elevated in the right eye.
3 that the pressure is normal in both eyes.

Answer: 3
Rationale: Normal intraocular pressure ranges from 10 to 21 mm Hg. Therefore, the client's intraocular pressure is normal, and options 1, 2, and 4 are incorrect.

Test-Taking Strategy: Focus on the data presented in the question. Recalling that normal intraocular pressure ranges from 10 to 21 mm Hg will direct you to option 3. Review this normal finding and the various test-taking strategies if you had difficulty with this question.

4 that the pressure in both eyes is low, requiring treatment to increase it.

Level of Cognitive Ability: Application
Client Needs: Physiological Integrity
Integrated Process: Nursing Process/Implementation
Content Area: Adult Health/Eye

Reference

Linton, A. & Maebius, N. (2003). *Introduction to medical-surgical nursing* (3rd ed). Philadelphia: Saunders, p. 1051.

---

172. A stapedectomy is performed on a client with otosclerosis. The nurse prepares the client for discharge and provides the client with which home care instruction?

1 To lie on the operative ear with the head of the bed flat
2 That acute vertigo is expected to occur
3 That it is okay to sneeze or blow the nose as he usually does
4 That plans for air travel need to be delayed for at least 1 month

Answer: 4

Rationale: Following stapedectomy the client is instructed to lie on the nonoperative ear with the head of the bed elevated. The client should also avoid excessive exercise, straining, and activities that might lead to head trauma. If the client needs to blow the nose, it should be done gently, one nostril at a time and the client should sneeze with the mouth open. The acute onset of vertigo needs to be reported to the physician. No airplane travel is allowed for 1 month.

Test-Taking Strategy: Focus on the surgical procedure and its location to direct you to option 4. Also, eliminate option 1 because of the words "lie on the operative ear with the head of the bed flat," option 2 because of the words "acute vertigo," and option 3 because of the words "as he usually does." Review postoperative care following stapedectomy and the various test-taking strategies if you had difficulty with this question.

Level of Cognitive Ability: Application
Client Needs: Health Promotion and Maintenance
Integrated Process: Teaching/Learning
Content Area: Adult Health/Ear

References

Christensen, B. & Kockrow, E. (2003). *Adult health nursing* (4th ed). St. Louis: Mosby, p. 595.
Linton, A. & Maebius, N. (2003). *Introduction to medical-surgical nursing* (3rd ed). Philadelphia: Saunders, p. 1088.

---

173. A nurse reinforces instructions to a client about the measures to treat gout. The nurse determines that the client needs additional instructions if the client states that:

1 the intake of red meats need to be limited.
2 weight loss can help prevent an attack.
3 medication can help keep the uric acid level down.
4 fluid intake needs to be limited.

Answer: 4

Rationale: Medication therapy is a component of management for clients with gout, and the physician normally prescribes a medication that will promote uric acid excretion or to reduce its production for clients with chronic gout. Fluid intake is important to promote uric acid excretion. Weight loss can reduce the incidence of attacks and reduce uric acid levels. A decrease in the intake of red meats and organ meats will assist in controlling uric acid levels.

Test-Taking Strategy: Note the key words "needs additional instructions." These words indicate a false response question and direct you to look for the client statement that is incorrect. Recalling that in this disorder the client experiences an increased uric acid level and that measures need to be implemented to promote uric acid excretion will direct you to option 4. Review the management of gout and the test-taking strategies for answering false response questions if you had difficulty with this question.

Level of Cognitive Ability: Analysis
Client Needs: Health Promotion and Maintenance
Integrated Process: Nursing Process/Evaluation
Content Area: Adult Health/Musculoskeletal

Reference

Christensen, B. & Kockrow, E. (2003). *Adult health nursing* (4th ed). St. Louis: Mosby, p. 121.

---

174. Buck's extension traction will be applied to the right leg of a client who sustained a right hip fracture. The nurse develops a plan of care for the client and includes which intervention in the plan?

1 Apply lanolin to the skin before applying the traction.
2 Remove the traction weights once every 2 hours for 15 minutes.
3 Clean the pin sites with half-strength hydrogen peroxide once per shift.
4 Check the skin integrity of the right leg at least every 8 hours.

Answer: 4

Rationale: Buck's extension traction is a type of skin traction. It is important with skin traction to inspect the skin underneath at least once every 8 hours for irritation or inflammation. The nurse never releases the weights of traction unless specifically ordered by the physician. Applying lanolin to the skin could make the skin area slippery, making it difficult to maintain the belt or boot used for the skin traction. There are no pins to care for with skin traction.

Test-Taking Strategy: Focus on the issue, *Buck's extension traction.* Recalling that Buck's extension traction is a skin traction will assist in eliminating option 3. Eliminate option 2 next because the nurse never removes weights without a specific order to do so. From the remaining options, use the steps of the clinical problem-solving process (nursing process). Option 4 addresses data collection. Review care to the client in Buck's traction and the various test-taking strategies if you had difficulty with this question.

Level of Cognitive Ability: Application
Client Needs: Physiological Integrity
Integrated Process: Nursing Process/Planning
Content Area: Adult Health/Musculoskeletal

Reference

Christensen, B. & Kockrow, E. (2003). *Adult health nursing* (4th ed). St. Louis: Mosby, p. 153.

---

175. A client diagnosed with acquired immunodeficiency syndrome (AIDS) is hospitalized. The nurse reviews the plan of care and determines that which intervention is the priority?

1 Discussing the ways that the client contracted the AIDS virus
2 Identifying the ways that AIDS can be contracted by others

Answer: 3

Rationale: The client with AIDS has inadequate immune bodies and is at risk for infection. The priority nursing intervention would be to protect the client from infection. The nurse would also provide emotional support to the client but this is not the priority from the options provided. Discussing the ways that the client contracted the AIDS virus and the ways others can contract AIDS is not an appropriate priority intervention.

3 Instituting measures to prevent infection in the client
4 Providing emotional support to the client

Test-Taking Strategy: Note the key word "priority." Eliminate options 1 and 2 first because they are similar. Also use Maslow's hierarchy of needs theory. Remember that physiological needs are the priority. This will direct you to option 3. Review the priority needs of a client with AIDS and the test-taking strategies for answering prioritizing questions if you had difficulty with this question.

Level of Cognitive Ability: Comprehension
Client Needs: Physiological Integrity
Integrated Process: Nursing Process/Planning
Content Area: Adult Health/Immune

Reference
Christensen, B. & Kockrow, E. (2003). *Adult health nursing* (4th ed). St. Louis: Mosby, p. 694.

---

176. A client arrives to the emergency department with complaints of hives, itching, and difficulty swallowing, and states that "my throat feels as though it is closing off." The client states that he was visiting a relative who has two cats and two dogs and believes that he is allergic to cats. The nurse ensures that the client has a patent airway and then prepares the client for which initial intervention?
1 Administration of a subcutaneous injection of epinephrine (Adrenalin)
2 Administration of an intravenous glucocorticoid
3 Administration of normal saline solution
4 The application of ice to the throat

Answer: 1
Rationale: The initial action would be to maintain a patent airway. Once airway is established, the client would receive a subcutaneous injection of epinephrine. Intravenous corticosteroids and intravenous fluids may also be prescribed. The application of ice to the throat will not relieve the symptoms.

Test-Taking Strategy: Note the key word "initial." Use the ABCs—airway, breathing, and circulation—to direct you to option 1. Remember, once airway is established, the client will receive epinephrine. Review care to the client who experiences an allergic reaction and the various test-taking strategies if you had difficulty with this question.

Level of Cognitive Ability: Application
Client Needs: Physiological Integrity
Integrated Process: Nursing Process/Implementation
Content Area: Adult Health/Immune

References
Black, J. & Hawks, J. (2005). *Medical-surgical nursing: clinical management for positive outcomes* (7th ed). Philadelphia: Saunders, p. 2325.
Hodgson, B. & Kizior, R. (2005). *Saunders nursing drug handbook 2005.* Philadelphia: Saunders, p. 379.

---

177. A client with a spinal cord injury suddenly complains of a severe, pounding headache. The nurse quickly checks the client and notes that the client is diaphoretic, has an elevated blood pressure, and has a drop in the heart rate. The nurse suspects that the client is experiencing autonomic dysreflexia. The nurse elevates the head of the client's bed, and immediately:

Answer: 4
Rationale: Autonomic dysreflexia is an acute emergency that occurs as a result of exaggerated autonomic responses to stimuli that are innocuous in normal individuals. It occurs only after spinal shock has resolved. A number of stimuli may trigger this response, including a distended bladder (the most common cause); distension or contraction of the visceral organs, especially the bowel (from constipation, impaction); or stimulation of the skin. When autonomic hyperreflexia occurs, the client is immediately placed in a sitting position to lower the blood pressure. The nurse

1 Ensures the client that this is a normal response to injuries.
2 Checks to see if the client has an order for an antihypertensive.
3 Increases the rate of intravenous fluids.
4 Checks the client's bladder for distention.

then performs a rapid assessment to identify and alleviate the cause. The client's bladder is emptied immediately via a urinary catheter, the rectum is checked for the presence of a fecal mass, and the skin is examined for areas of pressure, irritation, or broken skin. A registered nurse is notified, the physician is contacted, and then the nurse documents the occurrence and the actions taken. Increasing the rate of intravenous fluids is an inappropriate action.

Test-Taking Strategy: Focus on the data in the question and note that the nurse has already elevated the head of the client's bed and checked the client's blood pressure. Next, recalling that autonomic dysreflexia occurs as a result of exaggerated autonomic responses to stimuli and that the stimuli need to be removed quickly will direct you to option 4. Review immediate interventions to treat autonomic dysreflexia and the various test-taking strategies if you had difficulty with this question.

Level of Cognitive Ability: Application
Client Needs: Physiological Integrity
Integrated Process: Nursing Process/Implementation
Content Area: Adult Health/Neurological

References
Christensen, B. & Kockrow, E. (2003). *Adult health nursing* (4th ed). St. Louis: Mosby, pp. 650-651.
Linton, A. & Maebius, N. (2003) *Introduction to medical-surgical nursing* (3rd ed). Philadelphia: Saunders, p. 446.

---

178. A client who is recovering from a cerebrovascular accident (CVA) has residual dysphagia. To check the client's swallowing ability the nurse should do which of the following?
1 Ask the client to swallow some water
2 Ask the client to swallow a teaspoon of applesauce
3 Ask the client to produce an audible cough
4 Ask the client to suck on a piece of hard candy

Answer: 3
Rationale: To assess the client's readiness and ability to swallow the nurse should check the client's level of consciousness (client needs to be alert), check for a gag reflex (gag reflex must be present), have the client produce an audible cough (client must be able to produce an audible cough), and ask the client to produce a voluntary swallow (client must be able to do this). The nurse should not give the client a liquid or food item and should not ask the client to suck on a piece of hard candy or any other item because of the risk of aspiration.

Test-Taking Strategy: Eliminate options 1, 2, and 4 first because they are similar and would place the client at risk for aspiration. Also, use the ABCs—airway, breathing, and circulation—to direct you to option 3. Review care of the client with residual dysphagia and the various test-taking strategies if you had difficulty with this question.

Level of Cognitive Ability: Application
Client Needs: Safe, Effective Care Environment
Integrated Process: Nursing Process/Implementation
Content Area: Adult Health/Neurological

Reference
Christensen, B. & Kockrow, E. (2003). *Adult health nursing* (4th ed). St. Louis: Mosby, p. 620.

179. A nurse is assisting in developing a plan of care for a client who is experiencing homonymous hemianopia following a cerebrovascular accident (CVA). The nurse suggests interventions that will promote a safe environment, knowing that in this disorder:

1 the client is unable to carry out a skilled act such as dressing in the absence of paralysis.
2 the client has lost the ability to recognize familiar objects through the senses.
3 the client has paralysis of the sympathetic nerves of the eye, causing sinking of the eyeball.
4 the client has a visual loss in the same half of the visual field of each eye.

Answer: 4
Rationale: Homonymous hemianopia is a visual loss in the same half of the visual field of each eye so the client has only half of normal vision. Option 1 describes apraxia. Option 2 describes agnosia. Option 3 describes Horner's syndrome.

Test-Taking Strategy: Focus on the issue, homonymous hemianopia. Use medical terminology noting that *hemi* means half and *op* refers to the eye. This will direct you to option 4. Review care for the client with homonymous hemianopia and the various test-taking strategies if you had difficulty with this question.

Level of Cognitive Ability: Application
Client Needs: Safe, Effective Care Environment
Integrated Process: Nursing Process/Planning
Content Area: Adult Health/Neurological

Reference
Linton, A. & Maebius, N. (2003). *Introduction to medical-surgical nursing* (3rd ed). Philadelphia: Saunders, pp. 416, 426.

---

180. A nurse reinforces home care instructions with a client with Parkinson's disease about measures to control a right-sided hand tremor. The nurse tells the client to:

1 use the right hand only to perform tasks.
2 squeeze a rubber ball with the right hand.
3 use the left hand only to perform tasks.
4 sleep on the unaffected side.

Answer: 2
Rationale: If the client has a tremor, the client is instructed to use both hands to accomplish a task. The client is also instructed to hold change in a pocket or to squeeze a rubber ball with the affected hand. The client should sleep on the side that has the tremor to control it.

Test-Taking Strategy: Eliminate options 1 and 3 first because of the absolute word "only." From the remaining options, visualize each and think about each effect in terms of controlling the tremor. This will direct you to option 2. Review client teaching points for Parkinson's disease and the various test-taking strategies if you had difficulty with this question.

Level of Cognitive Ability: Application
Client Needs: Health Promotion and Maintenance
Integrated Process: Teaching/Learning
Content Area: Adult Health/Neurological

References
Black, J. & Hawks, J. (2005). *Medical-surgical nursing: clinical management for positive outcomes* (7th ed). Philadelphia: Saunders, p. 2174.
Linton, A. & Maebius, N. (2003). *Introduction to medical-surgical nursing* (3rd ed). Philadelphia: Saunders, pp. 397-398.

---

181. A nurse answers the call bell of a client who has an internal cervical radiation implant. The client states that she thinks that the implant fell out. The nurse checks the client and sees the implant lying in the bed. The nurse immediately uses a long-handled forceps to pick up the im-

Answer: 1
Rationale: A lead container (called a pig) and a pair of long-handled forceps should be kept in the client's room at all times during internal radiation therapy. If the implant becomes dislodged, the nurse should pick up the implant with long-handled forceps and place it in the pig. A registered nurse is informed. The radiation therapist and radiation safety officer are also notified immediately of the situ-

plant and places the implant into the lead container (pig) that is in the client's room. Which action should the nurse take next?

1 Notify a registered nurse
2 Call a security officer and ask the officer to send someone to guard the client's room until the situation is resolved
3 Call for transport personnel to deliver the lead container (pig) to the radiation department
4 Ask another nurse to assist in reinserting the implant

ation so that they can retrieve and secure the radiation source. The physician is also called after taking action to maintain the safety of the client and others. The nurse does not reinsert a radiation implant device. Options 2 and 3 are incorrect and can expose individuals to the radiation.

Test Taking Strategy: Note the key word "next." Option 4 can be eliminated first because inserting a radiation device is not a nursing activity. Recalling that the nurse needs to protect him- or herself and others from exposure to the radiation will assist in eliminating options 2 and 3. Additionally these options are similar. Review the measures related to a dislodged implant and the various test-taking strategies if you had difficulty with this question.

Level of Cognitive Ability: Application
Client Needs: Safe, Effective Care Environment
Integrated Process: Nursing Process/Implementation
Content Area: Adult Health/Oncology

Reference
Black, J. & Hawks, J. (2005). *Medical-surgical nursing: clinical management for positive outcomes* (7th ed). Philadelphia: Saunders, p. 363.

---

182. A nurse is teaching a nursing assistant how to measure a carotid pulse. The nurse tells the nursing assistant to measure the pulse on only one side of the client's neck primarily:

1 so that the client will not feel a sense of choking.
2 because it will provide a more accurate determination of the quality of the pulse.
3 because the pulse rate will be easier to count.
4 to prevent dizziness and a drop in the heart rate.

Answer: 4
Rationale: Applying pressure to both carotid arteries at the same time is contraindicated. Excess pressure to the baroreceptors in the carotid vessels could cause the heart rate and blood pressure to reflexively drop and cause syncope. In addition, the manual pressure could interfere with the flow of blood to the brain.

Test-Taking Strategy: Note the key word "primarily." Note also that option 4 describes the greatest danger to the client. Review the function and location of baroreceptors in the carotid vessels and the various test-taking strategies if you had difficulty with this question.

Level of Cognitive Ability: Application
Client Needs: Physiological Integrity
Integrated Process: Teaching/Learning
Content Area: Leadership/Management

Reference
Black, J. & Hawks, J. (2005). *Medical-surgical nursing: clinical management for positive outcomes* (7th ed). Philadelphia: Saunders, p. 1482.

---

183. Ondansetron (Zofran) is administered to a client receiving chemotherapy. The nurse determines that the medication is effective if the client states that:

1 pain is minimal.
2 she is not experiencing any nausea.

Answer: 2
Rationale: Ondansetron is an antiemetic that is used in the treatment of nausea and vomiting associated with chemotherapy, as well as postoperative nausea and vomiting. Options 1, 3, and 4 are unrelated to the intended effects of this medication.

3 the intravenous site is not burning.
4 she feels sleepy.

Test-Taking Strategy: Note the key words "medication is effective." Focus on the data in the question and note that the client is receiving the medication during chemotherapy. Recalling that chemotherapy can cause nausea and vomiting will direct you to the correct option. Review the action of this medication and the test-taking strategies for answering pharmacology questions if you had difficulty with this question.

Level of Cognitive Ability: Analysis
Client Needs: Physiological Integrity
Integrated Process: Nursing Process/Evaluation
Content Area: Pharmacology

Reference
Hodgson, B. & Kizior, R. (2005). *Saunders nursing drug handbook 2005.* Philadelphia: Saunders, p. 802.

---

184. A nurse is preparing to perform oropharyngeal suctioning on a client who has coughed, resulting in secretions in the mouth and is unable to expectorate the secretions adequately. The nurse determines that there is a physician's order for the procedure and explains the procedure to the client. Number in order of priority the actions that the nurse should take to perform this procedure safely. Number 1 is the first action and Number 7 is the last action.

___ Remove the client's oxygen mask.
___ Wash hands.
___ Attach the suction catheter to the connecting tubing.
___ Apply a clean disposable glove to the dominant hand.
___ Encourage the client to cough and repeat the suctioning if necessary.
___ Insert the catheter into the client's mouth and move the catheter around the mouth, pharynx, and gum line until secretions are cleared.
___ Place the oxygen mask on the client.

Answer: 4132657

Rationale: The nurse always washes the hands before performing any procedure, then dons a clean glove. A clean rather than a sterile glove can be used in this procedure because the oral cavity is not sterile. The nurse may also consider applying a mask or face shield because suctioning may cause splashing of body fluids. The nurse then completes preparation by attaching the suction catheter to the connecting suction tubing. The nurse removes the oxygen mask just before implementing the procedure so that the client is oxygenated as much as possible (remember, suctioning can deplete oxygen). The catheter is then inserted into the client's mouth until secretions are cleared. If the client is not tolerating the procedure, the catheter is removed and the oxygen mask is reapplied. The nurse then encourages the client to cough because coughing moves secretions from the lower to upper airways into the mouth. At this point, suctioning is repeated if necessary. The oxygen mask is then reapplied.

Test-Taking Strategy: The best strategy to use to answer this question is to first focus on the data in the question and then to visualize the procedure. Remember that hands are always washed first. Next remember that any preparation activities are done before removing the client's oxygen mask and that the client's oxygen is reapplied after completion of the procedure. Review the procedure for oropharyngeal suctioning and the test-taking strategies for answering prioritizing questions if you had difficulty with this question.

Level of Cognitive Ability: Application
Client Needs: Safe, Effective Care Environment
Integrated Process: Nursing Process/Implementation
Content Area: Delegating/Prioritizing

Reference
Potter, P. & Perry, A. (2005). *Fundamentals of nursing* (6th ed). St. Louis: Mosby, p. 1103.

185. A nurse is checking a 1-hour post-operative client following a right pulmonary wedge resection. The nurse notes the presence of 200 mL of bloody drainage in the client's collection chamber of the chest tube drainage system. Which action by the nurse is appropriate at this time?

1. Irrigate the chest tube.
2. Lower the amount of suction being applied.
3. Document the findings.
4. Notify a registered nurse immediately.

Answer: 3

Rationale: Between 100 and 300 mL of fluid may drain from the pleural chest tube in an adult during the first 3 hours after insertion. This rate will decrease after 2 hours (500 to 1000 mL can be expected in the first 24 hours). Drainage is grossly bloody in the first several hours after surgery and then changes to serous. Therefore, in this situation the nurse would document the findings. Lowering the amount of suctioning being applied is inappropriate and is NOT done without a physician's order. Chest tubes are never irrigated by the nurse. If there are excessive amounts and/or the continued presence of frank bloody drainage after the first several hours of surgery, it should be reported immediately to a registered nurse, who then contacts the physician.

Test-Taking Strategy: Focus on the data in the question and note the key words "1-hour postoperative" and "200 mL of bloody drainage." Option 1 can be easily eliminated because the nurse would never irrigate a chest tube. Option 2 can be eliminated next because the amount of suction would not be lowered without a physician's order. From the remaining, focusing on the key words will direct you to option 3 by recalling that these findings are expected at this postoperative time. Review care to the client following right pulmonary wedge resection and the various test-taking strategies if you had difficulty with this question.

Level of Cognitive Ability: Application
Client Needs: Physiological Integrity
Integrated Process: Nursing Process/Implementation
Content Area: Adult Health/Respiratory

Reference

Potter, P. & Perry, A. (2005). *Fundamentals of nursing* (6th ed). St. Louis: Mosby, p. 1120.

---

186. A nurse has provided instructions to a client with chronic obstructive pulmonary disease about the procedure for performing pursed-lip breathing. The nurse observes the client perform the procedure and determines that the client is performing it correctly if the client:

1. takes a deep breath and exhales quickly.
2. monitors inhalation time and ensures that exhalation time is less than inhalation time.
3. lies on the side in a supine position to perform the procedure.
4. sits in an upright position, takes a deep breath, and exhales slowly.

Answer: 4

Rationale: Pursed-lip breathing involves deep inspiration and prolonged expiration through pursed lips to prevent alveolar collapse. While sitting up, the client is instructed to take a deep breath and to exhale slowly through pursed lips. Therefore, options 1, 2, and 3 are incorrect.

Test-Taking Strategy: Eliminate options 1 and 2 first because they are similar. From the remaining options note the client's diagnosis and recall that clients with respiratory conditions are not positioned supine because this position affects respiratory status and will increase the work of breathing, resulting in dyspnea. Review the procedure for pursed-lip breathing and the various test-taking strategies if you had difficulty with this question.

Level of Cognitive Ability: Analysis
Client Needs: Health Promotion and Maintenance

Integrated Process: Nursing Process/Evaluation
Content Area: Adult Health/Respiratory

Reference

Potter, P. & Perry, A. (2005). *Fundamentals of nursing* (6th ed). St. Louis: Mosby, p. 1130.

---

187. Artificial rupture of the membranes is done to induce labor on a client. Following this procedure the nurse immediately:

1 cleans the client's perineal area.
2 places the client in a comfortable position.
3 informs the client that a wet feeling in the perineal area is normal and expected.
4 checks the fetal heart rate.

Answer: 4
Rationale: Artificial rupture of the membranes may be done to augment or induce labor or to facilitate placement of internal monitors when fetal status indicates the need for some form of direct assessment. Because the umbilical cord can prolapse when the membranes rupture, the fetal heart rate and fetal pattern should be monitored immediately and for several minutes following the procedure to ascertain fetal well-being. Although options 1, 2, and 3 are appropriate, they are not the priority concern, Additionally, in the preprocedure period, the client should be told that a wet feeling in the perineal area is normal and expected.

Test-Taking Strategy: Use the ABCs—airway, breathing, and circulation—to direct you to option 4. Also, use the steps of the clinical problem-solving process (nursing process) to direct you to option 4 because it is the only option that addresses data collection. Review care to the client following artificial rupture of the membranes and the test-taking strategies for answering prioritizing questions if you had difficulty with this question.

Level of Cognitive Ability: Application
Client Needs: Physiological Integrity
Integrated Process: Nursing Process/Implementation
Content Area: Maternity/Intrapartum

Reference

Leifer, G. (2003). *Introduction to maternity & pediatric nursing* (4th ed). Philadelphia: Saunders, p. 176.

---

188. A client in labor has been repositioned from side to side every 30 minutes. The client tells the nurse that she is tired of having to lie on her side and would like to lie on her back for a while. The nurse should:

1 tell the client that the supine position is contraindicated during labor.
2 position the client supine and place a pillow under one hip to act as a wedge.
3 tell the client that the obstetrician will need to be called to obtain an order for lying in the supine position.

Answer: 2
Rationale: The client in labor should be assisted to change positions every 30 to 60 minutes. The side-lying (lateral) position is the preferred position because it promotes optimal uteroplacental blood flow and increases fetal oxygenation. If the client wants to lie supine, the nurse may place a pillow under one hip as a wedge to prevent the uterus from compressing the aorta and vena cava. A physician's order is not needed to reposition this client.

Test-Taking Strategy: Eliminate options 1 and 4 first because they are similar. Next eliminate option 3, recalling that a physician's order is not required to reposition this client. Review care to the client in labor and the various test-taking strategies if you had difficulty with this question.

4 tell the client that bed rest lying on one side or the other is necessary.

Level of Cognitive Ability: Application
Client Needs: Physiological Integrity
Integrated Process: Nursing Process/Implementation
Content Area: Maternity/Intrapartum

Reference
Leifer, G. (2005). *Maternity nursing* (9th ed). Philadelphia: Saunders, p. 104.

---

189. A client in labor tells the nurse that she suddenly has a wet feeling in the vaginal area. The nurse quickly checks the client and notes the presence of a large amount of bright red blood. The nurse should immediately:

1 notify a registered nurse.
2 prepare the client for an emergency cesarean birth.
3 prepare to perform a vaginal examination.
4 prepare for the insertion of an intravenous catheter.

Answer: 1
Rationale: Vaginal bleeding (bright red, dark red, or in an amount in excess of that expected during normal cervical dilation) requires immediate notification of a registered nurse, who then contacts the obstetrician. This finding indicates an emergency situation and could have occurred as a result of placenta previa or placental separation. Although the nurse will prepare the client for an emergency cesarean section and prepares for the insertion of an intravenous catheter, these are not the immediate actions. A vaginal examination is not performed on a pregnant client who is bleeding vaginally.

Test-Taking Strategy: Note the key word "immediately" and focus on the data in the question. Noting the words "large amount of bright red blood" will direct you to option 1. Remember when an emergency situation is presented in the question, it is likely that the correct option will be to notify a registered nurse. Review care to the client in labor, the test-taking strategies for answering prioritizing questions, and those related to contacting a registered nurse if you had difficulty with this question.

Level of Cognitive Ability: Application
Client Needs: Physiological Integrity
Integrated Process: Nursing Process/Implementation
Content Area: Maternity/Intrapartum

Reference
Leifer, G. (2005). *Maternity nursing* (9th ed). Philadelphia: Saunders, p. 216.

---

190. A client with a diagnosis of suspected food poisoning is admitted to the hospital because of dehydration. The nurse expects to note which finding on data collection of this client?

1 Dry mucous membranes
2 Decreased pulse
3 Decreased respiratory rate
4 Increased urine output

Answer: 1
Rationale: A client with dehydration will have dry mucous membranes because of deficient fluid volume. The client will also have an increased depth and rate of respirations and an increased pulse rate. The deficient fluid volume is perceived by the body as decreased oxygen levels (hypoxia), and increased respirations and an increased pulse rate is an attempt to maintain oxygen delivery. Other findings of deficient fluid volume are weight loss, poor skin turgor, decreased urine volume, concentrated urine with increased specific gravity, increased hematocrit, and altered level of consciousness.

Test-Taking Strategy: Focus on the issue, *dehydration (deficient fluid volume)*. Note the relationship between the issue and the finding in option 1. Review the signs of dehydration and the various test-taking strategies if you had difficulty with this question.

Level of Cognitive Ability: Analysis
Client Needs: Physiological Integrity
Integrated Process: Nursing Process/Data Collection
Content Area: Adult Health/Gastrointestinal

Reference

Linton, A. & Maebius, N. (2003). *Introduction to medical-surgical nursing* (3rd ed). Philadelphia: Saunders, p. 159.

---

191. A nurse notes that a client's serum potassium level is 5.8 mEq/L. The nurse interprets that this is an expected finding in the client with which problem?

1 Diarrhea
2 Diabetes insipidus
3 Burn injury
4 Pulmonary edema being treated with loop diuretics

Answer: 3

Rationale: A serum potassium level greater than 5.1 mEq/L indicates hyperkalemia and requires physician notification. Burn injuries is a cause of hyperkalemia. Other common causes of hyperkalemia include adrenal insufficiency (Addison's disease), renal failure, and the use of potassium-sparing diuretics. The client with diarrhea or diabetes insipidus, or the client being treated with loop diuretics is at risk for hypokalemia.

Test-Taking Strategy: Eliminate options 1, 2, and 4 because they are similar and all indicate that the client is experiencing body fluid losses, thus a loss of potassium. Review the causes of hyperkalemia and the various test-taking strategies if you had difficulty with this question.

Level of Cognitive Ability: Analysis
Client Needs: Physiological Integrity
Integrated Process: Nursing Process/Data Collection
Content Area: Adult Health/Integumentary

Reference

Linton, A. & Maebius, N. (2003). *Introduction to medical-surgical nursing* (3rd ed). Philadelphia: Saunders, p. 783.

---

192. A nurse is monitoring a client with hyperparathyroidism for signs of hypercalcemia. The nurse expects to note which finding if hypercalcemia is present?

1 Hyperactive deep tendon reflexes
2 Positive Chvostek's sign
3 Diminished bowel sounds
4 Paresthesias

Answer: 3

Rationale: Signs of hypercalcemia include decreased gastrointestinal motility, muscle weakness, diminished or absent deep tendon reflexes, increased urine output, and an increased heart rate and blood pressure. Options 1, 2, and 4 are signs of hypocalcemia.

Test-Taking Strategy: Eliminate options 1, 2, and 4 because they are similar and reflect a hyperactivity of the neuromuscular system. Review the signs of hypercalcemia and the various test-taking strategies if you had difficulty with this question.

Level of Cognitive Ability: Analysis
Client Needs: Physiological Integrity
Integrated Process: Nursing Process/Data Collection
Content Area: Adult Health/Endocrine

References

Christensen, B. & Kockrow, E. (2003). *Adult health nursing* (4th ed). St. Louis: Mosby, p. 469.
Linton, A. & Maebius, N. (2003). *Introduction to medical-surgical nursing* (3rd ed). Philadelphia: Saunders, p. 783.

---

193. A nurse is reviewing the assessment findings and laboratory results of a child diagnosed with new-onset glomerulonephritis. Which of the following findings does the nurse most likely expect to note?

1 Elevated creatinine levels
2 Hypotension
3 Low serum potassium
4 Tea-colored urine

Answer: 4

Rationale: Gross hematuria resulting in dark brown or tea-colored urine is a classic symptom of glomerulonephritis. Hypertension is also a common finding in glomerulonephritis. Blood urea nitrogen levels and creatinine levels are elevated only when there is an 80% decrease in glomerular filtration rate and renal insufficiency is severe. A high potassium level results from inadequate glomerular filtration.

Test-Taking Strategy: Note that the child is experiencing a renal disorder and note the key words "new-onset" and "most likely." Recalling that the creatinine level elevates only when there is an 80% decrease in glomerular filtration rate will assist in eliminating option 1. Next eliminate options 2 and 3, knowing that hypertension rather than hypotension and hyperkalemia rather than hypokalemia will occur in this renal disorder. Review the clinical manifestations associated with glomerulonephritis and the various test-taking strategies if you had difficulty with this question.

Level of Cognitive Ability: Analysis
Client Needs: Physiological Integrity
Integrated Process: Nursing Process/Data Collection
Content Area: Child Health

Reference

Price, D. & Gwin, J. (2005). *Thompson's pediatric nursing* (9th ed). Philadelphia: Saunders, p. 245.

---

194. A child newly diagnosed with type 1 diabetes mellitus who is receiving insulin suddenly experiences signs of a hypoglycemic reaction. The nurse should immediately give the child:

1 a teaspoon of honey.
2 a teaspoon of sugar.
3 ½ cup of diet cola.
4 8 ounces of skim milk.

Answer: 4

Rationale: Hypoglycemia is immediately treated with 15 g of carbohydrate. Glucose tablets or glucose gel may be administered. Other items used to treat hypoglycemia include ½ cup of fruit juice, ½ cup of regular (nondiet) soft drink, 8 ounces of skim milk, 6 to 10 hard candies, 4 cubes of sugar or 4 teaspoons of sugar, 6 saltines, 3 graham crackers, or 1 tablespoon of honey or syrup. The items in options 1, 2, and 3 do not adequately treat hypoglycemia.

Test-Taking Strategy: Eliminate options 1 and 2 first because they are similar. From the remaining options, select option 4 because a diet cola does not contain the adequate amount of carbohydrate needed to treat hypoglycemia. Review the treatment measures for hypoglycemia and the various test-taking strategies if you had difficulty with this question.

Level of Cognitive Ability: Application
Client Needs: Physiological Integrity
Integrated Process: Nursing Process/Implementation
Content Area: Child Health

Reference

Price, D. & Gwin, J. (2005). *Thompson's pediatric nursing* (9th ed). Philadelphia: Saunders, p. 285.

---

195. A child with a diagnosis of pertussis (whooping cough) is being admitted to the pediatric unit. As soon as the child arrives to the unit, the nurse should first:

1 place the child on a pulse oximeter.
2 weigh the child.
3 take the child's temperature.
4 prepare for the administration of the prescribed antibiotic.

Answer: 1

Rationale: To adequately determine if the child is getting enough oxygen, the child is placed on a pulse oximeter. The pulse oximeter provides ongoing information on the child's oxygen level. The child is also immediately placed on a cardiorespiratory monitor to provide early identification of periods of apnea and bradycardia. The nurse then checks the child's temperature and weight and ask the parents about the child. An antibiotic may be prescribed, but the child's airway status needs to be assessed first.

Test-Taking Strategy: Note the key word "first." Focus on the child's diagnosis and use the ABCs—airway, breathing, and circulation. This will direct you to option 1. Review care to the child with pertussis and the test-taking strategies for answering prioritizing questions if you had difficulty with this question.

Level of Cognitive Ability: Application
Client Needs: Physiological Integrity
Integrated Process: Nursing Process/Implementation
Content Area: Delegating/Prioritizing

References

Leifer, G. (2003). *Introduction to maternity & pediatric nursing* (4th ed). Philadelphia: Saunders, p. 744.
Price, D. & Gwin, J. (2005). *Thompson's pediatric nursing* (9th ed). Philadelphia: Saunders, p. 255.

---

196. A nurse is collecting data on a child with increased intracranial pressure who has been exhibiting decorticate posturing. The nurse notes extension of the upper and lower extremities with internal rotation of the upper arms and wrists and knees and feet. The nurse determines that the child's condition:

1 has improved.
2 indicates decreased intracranial pressure.

Answer: 3

Rationale: In decorticate posturing, the nurse will note flexion of the upper extremities and extension of the lower extremities. In decerebrate posturing, the nurse notes extension of the upper and lower extremities with internal rotation of the upper arms and wrists and the knees and feet. The progression from decorticate to decerebrate posturing usually indicates deteriorating neurological function. This needs to be reported to a registered nurse immediately and warrants physician notification. Options 1, 2, and 4 are inaccurate interpretations.

3 indicates a deterioration in neurological function.
4 is unchanged.

Test-Taking Strategy: Eliminate options 1 and 2 first because they are similar. From the remaining options, recalling the significance of decerebrate posturing will direct you to option 3. Review the significance of posturing and the various test-taking strategies if you had difficulty with this question.

Level of Cognitive Ability: Analysis
Client Needs: Physiological Integrity
Integrated Process: Nursing Process/Data Collection
Content Area: Child Health

Reference

Price, D. & Gwin, J. (2005). *Thompson's pediatric nursing* (9th ed). Philadelphia: Saunders, p. 203.

---

197. A nurse in the newborn nursery is monitoring a neonate born to a mother with diabetes mellitus. The nurse determines that the neonate is at risk for which disorder?
1 Hypercalcemia
2 Hypobilirubinemia
3 Hyperglycemia
4 Hypomagnesemia

Answer: 4
Rationale: The major neonatal complications of preexisting diabetes mellitus in the mother are hypoglycemia, hypocalcemia, hypomagnesemia, hyperbilirubinemia, and polycythemia. Congenital anomalies, macrosomia, birth trauma, perinatal asphyxia, respiratory distress syndrome, and cardiomyopathy are also problems seen in newborns of diabetic mothers.

Test-Taking Strategy: Focusing on the mother's diagnosis will assist in eliminating option 3. From the remaining options it is necessary to know the complications of the neonate of a mother with diabetes mellitus. Review the complications associated with the neonate born to the mother with diabetes mellitus and the various test-taking strategies if you had difficulty with this question.

Level of Cognitive Ability: Analysis
Client Needs: Physiological Integrity
Integrated Process: Nursing Process/Data Collection
Content Area: Maternity/Postpartum

Reference

Lowdermilk, D. & Perry, A. (2004). *Maternity & women's health care* (8th ed). St. Louis: Mosby, p. 1057.

---

198. A nurse is collecting data on a client in the fourth stage of labor and notes that the uterine fundus is firmly contracted and is midline at the level of the umbilicus. Based on this finding, the nurse should:
1 massage the fundus.
2 notify a registered nurse.
3 assist the mother to void.
4 record the findings.

Answer: 4
Rationale: In the postpartum period, the nurse checks for uterine atony and checks the consistency and location of the uterine fundus. The uterine fundus should be firmly contracted, at or near the level of the umbilicus, and midline. Therefore the nurse would record the findings. Because the finding is normal, options 1, 2, and 3 are not necessary. The nurse should massage the uterine fundus if it is soft and boggy. The registered nurse is notified if the client experiences excessive bleeding (the registered nurse then contacts the physician). A full bladder may cause a displaced fundus and one that is above the level of the umbilicus.

Test-Taking Strategy: Use the process of elimination and focus on the data in the question. Recalling the normal location and consistency of the fundus will direct you to option 4. Review the expected postpartum findings if you had difficulty with this question.

Level of Cognitive Ability: Application
Client Needs: Physiological Integrity
Integrated Process: Nursing Process/Implementation
Content Area: Maternity/Postpartum

Reference
Murray, S., McKinney, E., & Gorrie, T. (2002). *Foundations of maternal-newborn nursing* (3rd ed). Philadelphia: Saunders, p. 779.

---

199. A client in the second trimester of pregnancy is admitted to the maternity unit with a diagnosis of abruptio placentae. The nurse expects to note which clinical manifestation associated with this disorder?

1 Painless vaginal bleeding
2 Soft relaxed uterus with normal tone
3 Uterine hypertonicity
4 Nontender uterus

Answer: 3
Rationale: In abruptio placentae, abdominal pain, uterine tenderness, and uterine hypertonicity are present. Uterine tenderness accompanies placental abruption, especially with a central abruption in which blood becomes trapped behind the placenta. The abdomen will feel hard and boardlike upon palpation as the blood penetrates the myometrium and causes uterine irritability. Excessive uterine activity with poor relaxation between contractions is present. Painless bright red vaginal bleeding, a soft relaxed uterus with normal tone, and a nontender uterus are signs of placenta previa.

Test-Taking Strategy: Eliminate options 1 and 4 first because they are similar. From the remaining options note that option 3 indicates a sign opposite to the sign in option 2. This provides a clue that one of these options is the correct one. Recalling the signs of abruptio placentae will direct you to option 3. Review these signs and the various test-taking strategies if you had difficulty with this question.

Level of Cognitive Ability: Analysis
Client Needs: Physiological Integrity
Integrated Process: Nursing Process/Data Collection
Content Area: Maternity/Antepartum

Reference
Leifer, G. (2005). *Maternity nursing* (9th ed). Philadelphia: Saunders, p. 218.

---

200. A nurse is collecting data on a client with severe preeclampsia. Which sign indicates an improvement in the client's condition?

1 Protein in the urine is trace
2 Blood urea nitrogen is 40 mg/dL
3 Blood pressure is 148/102 mm Hg

Answer: 1
Rationale: Preeclampsia is considered mild when the diastolic blood pressure does not exceed 100 mm Hg; proteinuria is no more than 500 mg/day (trace to 1+), and symptoms such as headache, visual disturbances, or abdominal pain are absent. In addition, signs of kidney or liver involvement are absent. An elevated blood urea nitrogen level indicates the presence of kidney damage as a result of the preeclampsia.

4 Client complains of abdominal pain

Test-Taking Strategy: Use the process of elimination, noting the key words "severe preeclampsia" and "improvement in the client's condition." Note the key word "trace" in option 1. This is the only option that is not indicative of severe preeclampsia. Review the signs of mild and severe preeclampsia, the signs that indicate improvement, and the various test-taking strategies if you had difficulty with this question.

Level of Cognitive Ability: Analysis
Client Needs: Physiological Integrity
Integrated Process: Nursing Process/Evaluation
Content Area: Maternity/Antepartum

Reference

Lowdermilk, D. & Perry, A. (2004). *Maternity & women's health care* (8th ed). St. Louis: Mosby, p. 839.

---

201. A nurse assists in developing a plan of care for a client with a new diagnosis of Graves' disease. The nurse suggests including which of the following in the plan?

1 Provide a diet low in calories and protein.
2 Keep the room temperature cool.
3 Encourage frequent ambulation and other physical activities.
4 Place extra blankets on the client's bed.

Answer: 2

Rationale: Graves' disease is a form of hyperthyroidism and is characterized by a hypermetabolic state. The client benefits most from an environment that is restful both physically and mentally; therefore, the client is encouraged to rest. To compensate for the hypermetabolic state, the client needs a diet that is high in calories and high in protein. These clients experience heat intolerance and diaphoresis and require a cool environment.

Test-Taking Strategy: Focus on the client's diagnosis. Recalling that Graves' disease is characterized by a hypermetabolic state will direct you to option 2. Review care to the client with Graves' disease and the various test-taking strategies if you had difficulty with this question.

Level of Cognitive Ability: Application
Client Needs: Physiological Integrity
Integrated Process: Nursing Process/Planning
Content Area: Adult Health/Endocrine

References

Black, J. & Hawks, J. (2005). *Medical-surgical nursing: clinical management for positive outcomes* (7th ed). Philadelphia: Saunders, p.1199.
Christensen, B. & Kockrow, E. (2003). *Adult health nursing* (4th ed). St. Louis: Mosby, p. 463.

---

202. A nurse is caring for a hospitalized client with a diagnosis of acute pancreatitis. The nurse assists the client to which position that will decrease the abdominal pain?

1 Prone
2 Supine with the legs straight

Answer: 4

Rationale: Correct positioning will assist in providing comfort to the client with acute pancreatitis. These positions include a side-lying position with the knees curled up to the chest and a pillow pressed against the abdomen or upright in a sitting position with the trunk flexed. Options 1, 2, and 3 are incorrect.

3 Side-lying with the head of the bed flat
4 Upright in a sitting position with the trunk flexed

Test-Taking Strategy: Focus on the client's diagnosis and evaluate each of the options in terms of the amount of stretching or flexing of the abdominal wall that the action will cause. Also note that options 1, 2, and 3 are similar in that they are flat positions. Review the positions that will reduce pain in the client with acute pancreatitis and the various test-taking strategies if you had difficulty with this question.

Level of Cognitive Ability: Application
Client Needs: Physiological Integrity
Integrated Process: Nursing Process/Implementation
Content Area: Adult Health/Gastrointestinal

Reference

Christensen, B. & Kockrow, E. (2003). *Adult health nursing* (4th ed). St. Louis: Mosby, p. 243.

---

203. A client is diagnosed with viral hepatitis and the nurse reinforces home care instructions to the client. The nurse determines that the client understands the instructions if the client makes which statement?
1 "I need to remain in bed for the next 6 weeks."
2 "I can take acetaminophen (Tylenol) for any discomfort."
3 "I need to eat small frequent meals that are low in fat and protein."
4 "I need to limit my intake of alcohol."

Answer: 3
Rationale: Fatigue is a normal response to hepatic cellular damage. During the acute stage, rest is an essential intervention to reduce the liver's metabolic demands and increase its blood supply, but bed rest for 6 weeks is unnecessary. The client should avoid taking medications, including acetaminophen (which is hepatotoxic), unless prescribed by the physician. The client needs to avoid all alcohol consumption. The client should consume small frequent meals that are low in fat and protein to reduce the workload of the liver.

Test-Taking Strategy: Eliminate option 4 first, recalling that the client needs to avoid (not limit) alcohol intake. Next eliminate option 1 because of the words "next 6 weeks." From the remaining options, recalling that acetaminophen is hepatotoxic will assist in eliminating option 2. Review instructions for the client with viral hepatitis and the various test-taking strategies if you had difficulty with this question.

Level of Cognitive Ability: Application
Client Needs: Physiological Integrity
Integrated Process: Teaching/Learning
Content Area: Adult Health/Gastrointestinal

Reference

Christensen, B. & Kockrow, E. (2003). *Adult health nursing* (4th ed). St. Louis: Mosby, p. 231.

---

204. The nurse teaches a client with gastroesophageal reflux disease (GERD) about the measures to prevent reflux while sleeping. The nurse determines that the client needs additional instructions if the client states:

Answer: 3
Rationale: Elevation of the head of the bed 6 to 8 inches will prevent nocturnal reflux. The client is instructed to avoid eating within 3 hours from bedtime to prevent nocturnal reflux. Antacids and histamine receptor antagonists may be prescribed for the client and are frequently prescribed at bedtime. Losing weight (if overweight) will decrease the gastroesophageal pressure gradient.

1 "I shouldn't eat anything at bedtime."
2 "I should take an antacid at bedtime."
3 "I should sleep flat on my back."
4 "Losing weight will decrease some of the stomach pressure."

Test-Taking Strategy: Note the key words "needs additional instructions." These words indicate a false response question and tell you that you are looking for the option that is an incorrect client statement. Recalling that a backward flow of gastric contents occurs in this disorder will direct you to option 3. Review these client teaching points and the test-taking strategies for answering false response questions if you had difficulty with this question.

Level of Cognitive Ability: Analysis
Client Needs: Health Promotion and Maintenance
Integrated Process: Teaching/Learning
Content Area: Adult Health/Gastrointestinal

Reference
Black, J. & Hawks, J. (2005). *Medical-surgical nursing: clinical management for positive outcomes* (7th ed). Philadelphia: Saunders, pp. 732-733.

---

205. Digoxin (Lanoxin) is prescribed for a client with heart failure. The nurse checks which most important item before administering the medication?
1 Temperature
2 Pulse oximetry
3 Blood pressure
4 Apical heart rate

Answer: 4
Rationale: Digoxin is a cardiac glycoside used in the treatment of heart failure. The nurse would check the apical heart rate for 1 minute. In the adult, if the heart rate is below 60 beats per minute, the medication is withheld and the physician is notified. Although the nurse may check the client's temperature, pulse oximetry, and blood pressure, these are not specifically associated with this medication.

Test-Taking Strategy: Focus on the data in the question. Note the relationship between the client's diagnosis and option 4. Review this medication and the test-taking strategies for answering pharmacology questions if you have difficulty with the question.

Level of Cognitive Ability: Application
Client Needs: Physiological Integrity
Integrated Process: Nursing Process/Implementation
Content Area: Pharmacology

Reference
Lehne, R. (2004). *Pharmacology for nursing care* (5th ed). Phildadelphia: Saunders, p. 481.

Index